Zoonoses

Second edition

Zoonoses

SECOND EDITION

Martin Shakespeare
RD, BPharm, MRPharmS, DipAgVet, DipCP(DES), RNR
Pharmacist, UK

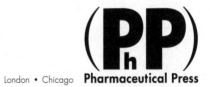

London • Chicago **Pharmaceutical Press**

Published by the Pharmaceutical Press
An imprint of RPS Publishing

1 Lambeth High Street, London SE1 7JN, UK
100 South Atkinson Road, Suite 200, Grayslake, IL 60030–7820, USA

© Pharmaceutical Press 2009

(**PP**) is a trade mark of RPS Publishing
RPS Publishing is the publishing organisation of the Royal Pharmaceutical Society
of Great Britain

First edition published in 2002
Second edition published in 2009

Typeset by J&L Composition, Scarborough, North Yorkshire
Printed in Great Britain by TJ International, Padstow, Cornwall

ISBN 978 0 85369 753 4

Contents

Preface

Like the first edition of *Zoonoses*, the second edition is aimed at trained and trainee healthcare professionals. It seeks to provide, in a compact format, an introduction and easily accessible reference for the more commonly encountered zoonotic diseases and some discussion of the issues surrounding zoonoses, and their societal and economic impact. This volume discusses zoonoses not only within the context of domestic disease, but also in the wider world. Healthcare and healthcare problems become more international every day, with the massive increase in numbers of people travelling from place to place for business or pleasure. This makes it increasingly necessary for us, as healthcare professionals, to widen our horizons, so that we can respond appropriately to patient needs.

Zoonoses pose a constant challenge to healthcare and our society, and I hope that even dipping into the volume will give readers some awareness of the ways in which these conditions are so important in our history, infrastructure and lives.

There is an emphasis on those zoonoses that are considered to be significant, established or emerging in the UK or the USA, and that are likely to present in domestic healthcare settings in the sections on companion and domestic animals. However, for some sections of the volume, conditions or disease states have been included that have a worldwide significance, not only for completeness, but also for information and educational purposes.

Since the first edition, several changes in disease patterns around the world have occurred in the world. The section on bird flu has been revised and expanded, and some other sections have been reduced to reflect diminishing interest. This volume still includes a chapter, designated Pandora's box (Chapter 6), that aims to dispel some of the mythology surrounding the more emotive and dramatic zoonoses found elsewhere in the world, especially those where media reporting may be too dramatic for more scientific tastes. This also now includes a section on bioterrorism, including the Amerithrax incident in September 2001.

I hope that readers will find this second edition as rewarding to read as I found it challenging and interesting to write.

Martin Shakespeare
January 2009

Acknowledgements

I would like to dedicate this edition to my mother and father, both of whom have died since the first edition was published. My thanks go to my wife, Josephine Sheppard, who has supported and encouraged me to continue to pursue my interest in this area of study. Without her, none of this would have happened. My thanks also go to the members and Committee of the Veterinary Group of the Royal Pharmaceutical Society of Great Britain and the staff of the Pharmaceutical Press.

About the author

Martin Shakespeare graduated in 1980 with a Bachelor of Pharmacy degree from the London School of Pharmacy, University of London, and went on to undertake his preregistration year at St Bartholomew's Hospital, London. After registration, he continued his studies by undertaking the Diploma in Crop Protection at Harper Adams Agricultural College, Shropshire.

While working in community pharmacy, he completed the Diploma in Agricultural and Veterinary Pharmacy in 1986. His subsequent career has been varied. A long-standing interest in zoonoses led to Martin being invited to make a presentation at the British Pharmaceutical Conference in 1999. The writing of an education package for the Scottish Centre for Post Qualification Pharmaceutical Education on zoonoses for pharmacists followed in early 2000, with the material being developed and expanded to produce the first edition of *Zoonoses*. Martin currently works for the Royal Navy.

1

Introduction to zoonoses

A basic definition

In the study of any scientific subject it is important that the terms used are understood from the outset. So, what is a zoonosis? The best scientifically agreed definition is that developed and used by the World Health Organization (WHO), which defines a zoonosis as:

Those diseases and infections which are naturally transmitted between vertebrate animals and man.

As with many definitions, some of the conditions that are generally classified as zoonoses may lie outside the strict definition, e.g. ciguatera and the related complex of shellfish poisonings are the result of ingested toxins, not an infective agent, and shellfish are invertebrates; however, as this condition is not easily placed into any other disease classification, and can be caused by eating fish, it is generally accepted as being zoonotic.

Other afflictions, such as malaria, that most people assume to be zoonoses are not. The malarial mosquitoes are only a vector for the disease, with the reservoir of infection being infected humans, rather than animals. In this particular case, the confusion arises because some animals can be a temporary alternative food supply for the mature mosquito, but do not show clinical signs of suffering from the disease in significant numbers. A comparison of malaria with other mosquito-borne infections, such as West Nile virus (WNV), where the infective reservoir may be one of many animal species, and particularly birds, highlights the difference.

Causative pathogens

The causative organisms responsible for zoonoses are very diverse and representative of a wide range of pathogens, or parasites (Table 1.1).

Table 1.1 Types of causative agent	
Types of causative agent	**Examples**
Arthropods	Scabies (also as vectors)
Bacteria	Brucellosis, tuberculosis
Fungi	*Cryptococcus*, ringworm
Helminths	Ascariasis, *Toxocara*
Prions	BSE/vCJD
Protozoa	Toxoplasmosis, cryptosporidia
Rickettsia	Q fever
Viruses	Ebola, rabies

BSE, bovine spongiform encephalopathy; vCJD, variant Creutzfeldt–Jakob disease.

The range of symptoms and effects that this extensive range of causative organisms produce in both their animal hosts and humans is just as diverse, from the asymptomatic, through the slightly inconvenient, to some associated cases with fatalities in excess of 50% of infected individuals. This can reach more than 90% in an outbreak of Ebola virus. An outbreak of Ebola in the Republic of The Democratic Republic of the Congo in May 2005 killed 9 of the 11 confirmed human cases; previous outbreaks in the Sudan, in 2004, killed 7 of 17 confirmed cases, and in a major outbreak in Gulu district, northern Uganda, during the autumn of 2000, over 150 died, including many healthcare workers. Fortunately it is not native to Europe or the Americas, and rare in its normal range of sub-Saharan Africa.[1]

It can be seen that the causative pathogen of a zoonosis usually comes from a class of organism already capable of causing disease in single-species groups. The important difference between those pathogens responsible for zoonotic disease and other members of the same group or family of pathogens lies in their ability to cause disease across at least two groups of species, of which human beings, implicitly by the definition of a zoonosis, must be one. The process of the spread of the disease or pathogen into another species is known as 'crossing or jumping the species gap'.

This ability is the one common factor in all pathogens responsible for zoonotic infections. Regardless of type, they must have the ability to cross between an animal and a human host under suitable circumstances or conditions. Any disease that can cross the species gap is described as having a zoonotic potential. Although this is essential, the importance of the pathogen in epidemiological or healthcare terms rests on the ease with which it makes this transfer. A highly virulent pathogen that requires extreme circumstances for cross-species transfer poses little or no general threat, although significant for the individual infected. An organism capable of transferring easily from the animal source with occasional serious sequelae in infected human patients will in practice be more significant.

Foot-and-mouth disease, although of undoubted virulence in cattle, is so difficult for a human to contract, and the necessary circumstances so extreme for transfer to occur, that the disease is almost not classed as zoonotic, with only 40 confirmed cases being reported to the WHO in the last century. On the other side of the coin, if an extensive survey of blood donations is accurate, more than 40% of the residents of the UK have at one time or another been infected with *Toxoplasma gondii*. In the USA, it is estimated that 60 million people (22% of the population) are infected, although few have symptoms.[2]

It is essential to recognise that only *some* animal diseases have a zoonotic potential, but all zoonoses have to, by definition, have an animal host. Some other diseases, although classed or viewed as zoonoses, are actually environmental pathogens, capable of affecting both animals and humans. The reasoning behind classifying these pathogens as zoonotic lies in the animal forming an additional and perhaps more efficient transmitter of the disease to humans than solely environmental exposure. In these and other zoonoses, the animal host not only can act just as a reservoir of infection, but is also often capable of amplifying the infection by allowing the organism to multiply, sometimes with the host remaining asymptomatic.

Some organisms with a zoonotic potential do not cause currently recognised disease states; however, the more investigations undertaken, the greater our knowledge and the more complex our outfit of investigative tools, the more zoonoses are identified. Changes in farming practice, dietary preference or other factors, may also allow previously unknown organisms to move into a position where they can begin to pose a threat to human health.

An example of a zoonotic pathogen under intensive investigation is *Mycobacterium avium* var. *paratuberculosis*, the causative organism of Johne's disease in cattle worldwide. Infection in humans with this bacterium, and the subsequent development of Crohn's disease, has been anecdotally linked for many years. Transmission of the pathogen from cattle to humans by ingestion of infected dairy products has been demonstrated. Arguments between experts in the field continue over the evidence relating to the clinical role of the bacterium, with no firm conclusion as to a causal linkage. The organism is difficult to culture in the laboratory because, as with many species of *mycobacteria*, it is notoriously slow growing and requires specific and optimal conditions. This may partly explain why it has been isolated from only some samples obtained from Crohn's disease sufferers, and not all. Much research is being undertaken to determine or disprove any linkage between the affliction and the organism.[3]

Linking cause and effect can be difficult because of the long incubation or pre-patent period associated with some zoonotic diseases. Infection with Lyme disease, a tick-borne zoonosis of deer, may become evident in humans only when the serious sequelae of cardiac damage, neuropathies or arthritis appear many years afterwards.

Many cases of zoonoses go undetected or resolve spontaneously, often as a result of antibiotic use for another condition destroying the zoonotic pathogen before either the end of the pre-patent period or the appearance of clinical signs. With blind usage of broad-spectrum antibiotics becoming less common as part of antimicrobial resistance strategies, the use of specific agents against cultures of sensitive organisms may well emerge as the norm. It is possible that this will lead to more cases of long pre-patent zoonotic disease and an increase in clinical significance, because there will be a failure to eradicate the pathogen before it can pose a risk to susceptible infected individuals.[4]

There is a need, which has been addressed in some cases, for the significance and scale of infection with some zoonotic pathogens to be evaluated. Until screening for *Chlamydia* spp. and *Toxoplasma* spp. was developed it was impossible to determine the incidence of these infections in pregnant women. Many cases of spontaneous abortion attributable to these pathogens had been blamed on a wide range of other causes. It was only with retrospective investigations of serological markers that the true incidence of infection and causal attribution could be made. These investigations have allowed the development of harm-reduction and prevention strategies which, coupled with health information campaigns, have reduced the significance of these diseases for human morbidity and mortality.[2]

Emerging zoonoses

Healthcare is constantly changing, with new products and techniques affecting practice. There is a continual challenge from newly identified pathogens and diseases often identified and differentially diagnosed only by the improvement in or development of testing technologies.

About 80% of these new diseases and pathogens are zoonotic. The emergence of a new zoonosis may not be linked just to the ability of the causative agent to cross the species barrier, although this is a significant factor. The pathogen must have the opportunity to cross that barrier, always including interspecies contact, which is often related to a variety of other external factors. A change in the ecosystem, the meteorological pattern, global warming, farming practice or food handling can significantly alter the potential that a known or unknown pathogen has to cause disease in humans, with humans coming into closer or more prolonged contact with carrier species. After this contact there needs to be pathogen transmission, either directly or via a vector, such as a biting insect, and this transmission must be sustainable, with the pathogen in some cases colonising the vector if there is one. Once these condition have been met, the pathogen may also adapt to human physiology and immunology.[5]

The disease states discussed in this volume to date are mostly well known, recognised, detectable and classifiable. Their clinical course, the likely infective pathway and any treatment are well documented. For emerging diseases, some or all of these parameters are either less well known or remain subjects for speculation. The conclusion that the disease identified is zoonotic may be made from detecting, culturing and typing the causative organism in affected humans and animals; however, the linkage between the two, i.e. the transmission pathway and infective route, is sometimes neither well defined nor practically demonstrable. Treatment regimens may not be defined due to a lack of success with empirical treatment or the inability to identify a useful drug or treatment regimen before either death or recovery intervenes.

Another factor that often characterises an emergent pathogen is its ability to undergo gradual genetic modification, in a manner reminiscent of Darwin's finches, so that it reinvents itself as better adapted to exist in a particular population. This change can enable an organism, which is benign in other species, to become an efficient pathogen in humans or animals. Another factor is exposure: in many parts of the world forest clearance or the pressure on other habitats brings humans and animals into close proximity. Sometimes these will be species or populations that have previously remained apart. As we know from the introduction of smallpox into the Americas by the Spanish, the result of the exposure of previously unexposed groups to a novel pathogen can produce devastating effects.

It is not only pathogens that can migrate: the trade in used tyres has successfully spread malarial mosquitoes from one country to another in the stagnant water held in these unusual receptacles. Non-degradable plastic containers, abandoned in large numbers across the world, are capable of trapping rainwater and make viable alternatives to traditional wetland habitats for mosquitoes to maintain breeding populations. A rise in the density of a vector population can allow a previously species-discrete pathogen with a zoonotic potential to break out of its normal niche.[6]

In the UK, most of the landscape and its fauna have been shaped by humans, so that all major predator species have been eradicated and other wild species have become extinct. Thus the opportunity to encounter an isolated population of another species with an associated reservoir of a major zoonotic pathogen is minimal, although the arrival of migratory birds and the existence of vector populations, such as mosquitoes capable of spreading a disease organism, continue to be a cause for concern.

This is not the only route for emergence; the unexpected can still happen when the safeguards of good practice or common sense are ignored. In terms of common sense, feeding dead sheep to cattle defies belief, and has led to unforeseen but nevertheless dramatic consequences.

The USA has seen a number of emerging pathogens, of which West Nile virus (WNV) has in recent years been the most spectacular. Changes in migratory bird patterns and the increase in suitable mosquito vector populations within the areas now under the birds' flight paths have led to the infection spreading first into the eastern seaboard, and now across virtually all of mainland USA. It is of note that this particular disease requires both of these factors to be present in the same geographical location for it to become a threat. The presence of infected birds or suitable mosquitoes alone is not enough to precipitate an outbreak, thus providing an opportunity to control the disease.

Many emerging pathogens are seen in tropical and subtropical areas, because either the relationship of humans with animals is closer or environmental factors such as extreme heat encourage workers to be less careful with their use of protective clothing. High levels of ambient environmental heat and humidity allow pathogens to survive in the environment for longer and multiply faster on a susceptible host. The presence of humans in previously undisturbed rain forest or other ecosystems can lead to circumstances in which exposure to novel pathogens occurs.

The careful study of the associated epidemiology of emerging diseases, and their routes of infection and natural reservoirs, is the only way to gain the insights necessary to put in place the measures needed to prevent epidemic zoonose outbreaks. This is true for several of the zoonoses mentioned in this chapter; scientists and health professionals involved in the control of the outbreaks had to make informed assumptions from the case profiles or epidemiological pattern. It is only on subsequent investigation that their assumptions can be proved. Wherever the assumptions or deductions made are of importance they are included in the text, as examples of the processes essential to disease management.

A factor that needs to be considered in relation to all the diseases explored in this section is that emerging infections or diseases may actually be re-emerging. Systems break down, and the reasons for public or personal health measures may become forgotten or lost in the mists of time. Several pathogens that were scourges of past ages are showing a resurgence, with outbreaks highlighting ageing or decaying infrastructure systems, such as sewage or water treatment, and the failure of consumers to know, understand or heed common-sense warnings related to animal handling or food preparation.[7]

It also worthy of note that the knowledge base of most healthcare practitioners does not extend beyond their years; we are all children of our times. Symptoms and signs that would historically have sent alarm messages are ignored, or pass unseen. The lesson from the current outbreaks of human tuberculosis in the UK is that pathogens can only rarely be designated as eradicated; they are more likely to be in a state of abeyance, awaiting the chance to go on a rampage of infection.

The price of our continued safety in western Europe and the USA, behind the ramparts of our healthcare and social systems, is constant vigilance. Worldwide this role is borne by public organisations charged with the monitoring of public, human and animal health. In addition, the WHO and other organisations, such as the Institut Pasteur, have networks of laboratories worldwide that undertake surveillance on a spectrum of diseases, some of zoonotic origin.

Detection and identification are assisted by continual testing of indicator populations for susceptible species. In the USA the presence of WNV is monitored by just such a programme, using regularly inspected captive domesticated birds to determine ambient levels of the causative organism. Similar to the canary in a cage in a submarine or mine, these precautions are designed to alert the experts and the populations for which they are responsible to the likelihood of an outbreak.

In the event of an outbreak of a zoonotic disease, there is a requirement for the lead organisation to be identified quickly and for it to take charge of all aspects of the outbreak. On occasions this is a difficult process, because rivalry and maintenance of jurisdiction often become more of an issue than the disease itself. It behoves anybody involved with an outbreak to remember that all other issues are peripheral to controlling the disease and preventing human casualties and fatalities.

Routes of transmission

A potential zoonosis may not necessarily cause detectable symptomatic disease in the animal host, nor is transmission to humans certain from every exposure to the pathogen. As with any other infection, the size of inoculum necessary to initiate progress to clinical disease varies from causative organism to causative organism, and also depends on the route of transmission. The level of inoculum necessary in an infection of a human by *Yersinia pestis* (the causative pathogen of the plague) is believed to be a single bacterium delivered by a bite from an infected flea. *Bacillus anthracis* (anthrax) is also claimed to be capable of causing the cutaneous form of the disease from the infection of an existing skin abrasion by a single viable spore.

These two cases are exceptional and stem from infection occurring by direct injection of the organisms into the bloodstream, or infection of an existing wound or laceration; they are also coupled to the aggressiveness and pathogenicity of the organism concerned. Moderate-sized inocula or repeated infection with small cumulative amounts of pathogen are considered to be more the norm.

An exceptionally large inoculum may be necessary, e.g. in certain types of food poisoning. Necrotic enteritis or pigbel is caused by the ingestion of large quantities of the exotoxin from *Clostridium perfringens*, with or without the living organism being present. In most recorded cases the infective dose of the toxin is estimated to be produced by $> 10^8$ cells of the pathogen. The ensuing intestinal damage caused by the toxin, with overwhelming colonisation of the gut by either the associated pathogen or other opportunistic bacteria, leads to septicaemia which may be rapidly overwhelming, with fatal outcome.[8]

The mode of transmission varies from zoonosis to zoonosis, and can also vary for the same causative organism from host species to host species (Table 1.2). Transmission from animal to human can be not only by direct, but also by indirect contact. Indirect spread by physical contact with a previously infected object or surface is known as fomite spread.

Direct transmission may be by contact with infected body fluids such as fresh blood, saliva, urine or faeces, especially into open wounds, inhalation of infected aerosols or accidental ingestion of infected material.

Indirect spread may also involve animal-associated organic residues, such as urine, faecal matter or tears, and nasal secretions. *Chlamydophila psittaci* can be spread by inhalation of dried bird faeces and causes psittacosis (also known as ornithosis) in humans – the parrot's disease of comedy. A serious clinical case is no laughing matter for a human victim, because it can lead to serious sequelae including death in rare cases. The same pathogen is also endemic in sheep, but the route of transmission is very different as the organism is transferred to humans by contact with contaminated fluids or tissues.

The disease presentation and the clinical course associated with a particular pathogen may also vary depending on the route and mode of infection.

Table 1.2 Mode of transmission
Aerosol inhalation
Blood, saliva
Faeces, urine
Fomite contact
Food and water
Oral or physical contact
Parasitic vectors (fleas, mosquitoes, lice, ticks)
Scratches, bites or wounds
Skin, hair or wool

C. psittaci also affords an excellent, and dramatic example of how dissimilar the pattern of disease can be depending on the route of infection. The form of the illness associated with infection acquired from avian sources usually presents as a flu-like illness with fever and chills, followed by pneumonia and associated dry cough. It seldom causes systemic disease; however, in rare cases it can progress to a septic form with hepatitis, endocarditis and ultimately death.

By contrast, infections of sheep origin can demonstrate rapid progression to systemic disease with serious consequences, especially in pregnant women. Colonisation of the placenta occurs and can be fatal for both mother and baby, with late term abortion and neonate death. This particular pathogen is virulent enough for even the most indirect contact to be sufficient to spread the disease. Following investigations of reported cases, pregnant women whose partners work in close contact with sheep are advised not even to handle unwashed overalls which may be contaminated with blood or secretions from ewes or lambs, and wherever possible to avoid contact with pre-, peri- or postpartum ewes or young lambs.

In most diseases infection is by more obvious routes. The transfer of whole blood or exuding plasma from an infected individual forms a very effective and direct transmission route for many pathogens. Farcy or glanders caused by *Burkholderia mallei* is seen in humans after contamination of cuts and grazes by exudate from wounds on horses and other equids. Jockeys or stable hands in countries where the disease is endemic are especially at risk. Although the last case was seen in the UK in 1928, and in the USA in 1945, the disease is still seen in many other countries. Horse racing and other equine pursuits are international, and horses transferred into and out of the UK to other race venues are carefully monitored for this and other diseases; however this only protects the equids, not the rider. There is a potential risk to the growing number of leisure horse owners and riders who may not be aware of the significance or risk that this infection may pose, and may choose to ride while abroad, where the disease may be endemic.

Ingestion

Ingestion of contaminated foodstuffs or water also offers an effective route for a zoonotic pathogen to cross the species barrier. Unpasteurised milk has historically been recognised as a source of several important zoonoses, and is becoming increasingly important in the USA because raw milk consumption has increased in the last decade. Classic tuberculosis (TB) (*Mycobacterium bovis*) of animal origin was spread widely in the past by infected dairy produce. The introduction and refinement of a system of milking, storage, treatment and distribution with strict temperature and bacterial monitoring, coupled with establishment of a comprehensive herd-screening programme, have virtually eliminated the bovine-derived infection from the human population. In the 1830s, when the first Euston station in London was built on a site previously occupied by a particularly infected and disreputable urban dairy, several medical authorities of the day claimed the demolition of the dairy to be one of the most significant factors in an observed reduction of infections linked to the consumption of milk by young children in the city. It was not until 1882 that Koch identified the causative organism in milk and that any major advances were made in prevention strategies. Most cases of TB in the UK are now considered to be of human origin and are caused by *Mycobacterium tuberculosis hominis* which is non-zoonotic.[9]

TB is not the only disease that can spread by ingestion of dairy produce. Milk can also carry the causative organism of Q fever (*Coxiella burnetii*), which usually causes a mild illness similar to flu, but in rare cases can cause pneumonia, hepatic and cardiac damage, and death. The use of effective pasteurisation is still tremendously important in preventing this and other diseases spreading from this source, and has been refined and improved over time as research has identified the optimal temperature and time necessary to produce effective disinfection. That said, on occasions systems fail and this can allow pathogens to survive and cause infection.

Contamination of water or food by faecal matter or urine causes many infections. Direct ingestion of faecal matter, especially by children, can also occur. This process, known as pica, is especially significant in infection with *Toxocara* spp. and *Toxoplasma gondii*. Weil's disease, caused by *Leptospira* spp., follows consumption of water contaminated with infected bovine, equine or rodent urine. Such consumption may be unwitting or accidental, and is most common among devotees of water sports and other outdoor pursuits. Many cases of Q fever are related to the occupational exposure of stock workers to the infected urine of cattle in their charge, rather than to ingestion of contaminated dairy produce.

Meat, especially poorly cooked or incorrectly stored comminuted meat products such as beef burgers or sausages, can carry a wide variety of organisms, some responsible for potentially harmful zoonotic infections. The pathogens usually cause self-limiting diarrhoea and other gastrointestinal disturbances in otherwise healthy individuals, but can be fatal for already debilitated individuals. There is believed to be dramatic under-reporting of food poisoning, with an estimated 10 cases for every one of the approximately 71 000 reported to the Health Protection Agency (HPA) in England and Wales in 2006.[10]

From the early 1990s, in the UK, the zoonotic disease that exercised the imagination of the British public and healthcare professionals was the dietary and societal impact of bovine spongiform encephalopathy/variant Creutzfeldt–Jakob disease (BSE/vCJD) linked to the consumption of beef derived from infected cattle. The theory that this disease is caused by a prion is now fairly widely accepted as the most likely explanation for the pattern of infection and disease. A prion is defined as a polypeptide entity with no nucleic acid, consisting solely of a sequence of amino acids. Once inside the body of the host it is capable of replicating intracellularly, especially in nervous tissue. After migration of the prion, it leads to the development of a spongiform encephalopathy, where the brain and central nervous system are affected.

At postmortem examination, the appearance of areas of the brain is similar to a sponge. Proteinaceous sheets are found in the remaining cell structure, and large vacuoles or spaces in between the sheets give confirmation of the diagnosis. The emergence of this disease has had a profound effect on the meat and livestock trade, from farmer to retailer. The final death toll is hard to predict; however, the rate of infection/fatality has reduced dramatically since the outbreak was identified, and both husbandry and slaughter techniques have been modified to reduce infectious risk over the period since the first identification and characterisation of the infection.[11]

Other organisms associated with the ingestion of infected meat and meat products have also hit the headlines. Salmonella infection originating from a chain of Chinese takeaways in Lanarkshire was a 9-day wonder and caused several people to receive hospital treatment. The most significant and deadly outbreak of *Escherichia coli* (enterohaemorrhagic *E. coli* or EHEC) O157 in the UK remains the one linked to J Barr, butchers and bakers, of Wishaw, Scotland in 1996. The total fatalities associated with the outbreak reached 21 following the consumption of contaminated meat products. A recent outbreak in Leeds during July 2006 was also associated with a butcher with multiple outlets across the city.

This outbreak and others demonstrate the continuing lack of knowledge displayed by the general public relating to the safe storage and preparation of food. Following the establishment of the Food Standards Agency (FSA) in the wake of the Wishaw outbreak, it has been given the role of watchdog and educator. It is also responsible for making policy and enforcing standards across the food industry in production, distribution and retailing.[12]

Under government sponsorship, lessons on food safety have now been introduced into the curriculum in secondary schools in an attempt to address the lack of understanding and knowledge. Until the level of education of the public at large relating to the handling, storage and cooking of food improves, it is likely that further high-profile cases of infection related to food-borne zoonoses will occur.

Direct contact

Physical damage of the skin or body tissue can lead to open wounds capable of acting as a window for opportunistic pathogen transfer. The obvious individuals likely to fall victim to infections from this route of infection are people who handle animals in the course of their work, be they agricultural workers, abbatoir workers, veterinary surgeons or animal rescue workers. A less obvious group at risk from this mode of transmission is any pet owner, especially those foolish enough to allow their animal to kiss or lick them. Anybody who is bitten or scratched by an animal is placed at an increased risk of contracting zoonotic diseases.

Rabies, fortunately currently not present in the UK but widely distributed in continental Europe, the Americas and most of the rest of the world, can be transferred by the bite of an infected animal. Scratches inflicted by an infected cat can transfer *Bartonella henselae*, the causative organism of Cat Scratch Disease, to humans; however, there have also been reported cases where owners have been infected after being foolish enough to allow cats to lick their open wounds.[13]

Physical contact does not pose a risk just from the living animal. Animal skins, hair or wool can act as a physical reservoir, particularly in anthrax. Once known in its pulmonary form as Woolsorter's Disease, infection can occur following inhalation of spores from infected fleeces or hides during processing. An isolated case in August 2000 in Bradford in a textile worker is a striking example of re-emergence of a supposedly eradicated condition. In 2006, two drummers, in unrelated incidents – one in the USA and one in Scotland – both contracted inhalational anthrax, with a further case occurring in a drum maker in the USA in October 2008. In the past, customs officials in the USA and the UK impounded goatskin bags brought from Haiti by tourists because these were found to be heavily contaminated with anthrax spores.

Fomite spread

Touching an object or surface that has been in physical contact with an infected animal can also lead to infection. This is known as fomite spread, and is significant in ringworm and anthrax in its cutaneous form. The inoculum on the fomites may consist of active organism, spores or encysted forms. After infection, surface colonisation may occur or disease progression may occur after the introduction of the initial inoculum into wounds, inhalation or ingestion.

Vectors

Transmission of zoonotic pathogens may also be caused by the involvement of vector species, particularly fleas, mosquitoes, lice and ticks. Physical contact with animals can lead to transfer of arthropod vectors; however, these vectors can also be encountered in the wider environment. Once infected, arthropods may act not only as an infective vector, but also as a persistent or temporary reservoir of infection with vertical transmission from generation to generation via an infected mother to her eggs (trans-ovarian transfer). Interestingly, controlling the arthropod vector is usually the mainstay of prevention in many of these infections, because, without the vector, humans and infected animals may occupy the same geographical area without disease transfer taking place. The absence or control of the vector may not arrest the disease in the animal host; however, it can prevent or reduce the spread into the human population.

The spread of Lyme disease from deer to humans occurs mainly through being bitten by a tick such as *Ixodes dammini*. In areas where it is endemic, clearance of low vegetation in woods and around footpaths where the tick loiters awaiting its next host reduces infection rates.[4]

Flea control by the use of insecticides or development-arresting agents, in both domestic and commercial settings, is not only effective at preventing the irritation associated with the mental and physical effects of the bite, but also important in the control of possible zoonoses. Fleas are usually host specific, especially as adults, when the female will try to obtain a blood meal only from a preferred host; if the preferred host is not available, it will prey on any warm-blooded host. It is therefore not sufficient to control fleas but also the normally associated host must be controlled. This is particularly important in arresting the spread of *Yersinia pestis*, the causative organism of plague, where both rats and their fleas require control and eradication.

Mosquitoes can also be vectors in the spread of specific zoonoses. The first outbreak of WNV in New York in 2000 was initially believed to be St Louis Encephalitis. Carried by migratory birds, transmission to humans follows the bite of infected culicoides mosquitoes, which have previously obtained a blood meal from a diseased bird. An increase in the number of mosquitoes in the urban New York area had followed discontinuation of pesticide spraying on areas of standing fresh water, including Central Park, where mosquito larvae develop. Coupled to a change in weather conditions, which altered patterns of migration for infected birds, host, pathogen and suitable vector were all co-located, leading to the outbreak. The disease has subsequently spread widely across the USA and Canada.[14]

Humans preyed on by a vector are infected only if the vector has previously bitten an infected host. In most cases the vector is essential for the pathogen to cross the species barrier. Controlling the vector can therefore stop or slow transmission and spread of the pathogen, and its associated disease. Once across the species barrier, infection spreads within the human population, following similar pathways to any other diseases if the pathogen has the potential for human-to-human transmission. These can include physical and sexual contact, inhalation and ingestion.

Importance of zoonoses

The importance of zoonoses in terms of human health and well-being cannot be underestimated. They affect how we live our lives, not only in a narrow health-related sense but also in a much wider cultural context. The threat that zoonotic diseases pose has shaped human history and many aspects of the infrastructure of our physical and social environment, including animal welfare – both domesticated and wild – food safety, and public health and hygiene.

The emphasis on the importance placed on zoonoses is reflected in the UK by the establishment of the joint Human Animal Infections and Risk Surveillance (HAIRS) group. This is a multi-agency, cross-disciplinary group with members from the HPA, the Department for Environment, Food and Rural Affairs (DEFRA), the Veterinary Laboratories Agency (VLA) and the Department of Health (DH); it is chaired by the HPA's Department of Emerging Infections and Zoonoses (EIZ) at the Centre for Infections (CFI). The group meets monthly to identify and discuss infections with potential for interspecies transfer (particularly zoonotic infections) which may pose a threat to public health in the UK.

The HAIRS group undertakes systematic examination of formal and informal reports on infectious incidents in animal and human populations globally. A wide range of sources of information is scanned, including informal news reports and bulletins, early warning communications, surveillance data and peer-reviewed scientific literature. The multidisciplinary nature of the HAIRS group enables it to assess these reports in an objective and scientific manner.

If infections are thought to be of potential significance, they are included in the *Infectious Disease Surveillance and Monitoring System for Animal and Human Health: Summary of notable events/incidents of public health significance* which is produced monthly and circulated to a wide audience within health (both human and animal) bodies and government.

The Centers for Disease Control and Prevention (CDC) undertakes a similar role in the USA, monitoring emerging diseases, and advising federally on countermeasures, treatment and epidemiology.

The earliest encounters of humans and zoonosis will have occurred before the start of written history. Handing on to the next generation the knowledge necessary to avoid illness or death from such diseases, in association with measures necessary to control other illnesses, has become part of certain religious conventions and proscriptions. This is particularly true when we consider food-borne zoonoses. The rules relating to food preparation and consumption within halal or kosher disciplines and secular folk tradition encompass measures that can be linked to prevention or limitation of the spread of diseases, including certain zoonotic infections.

Any infection stemming from an organism occurring in a foodstuff of wholly animal origin, present in the animal or its products at the time that it is 'harvested', is considered to be a food-borne zoonosis. In the past the risks associated with consumption of food were an accepted part of day-to-day living and dying. Today, with greater life expectancy, and the desire for and reality of a cleaner and safer environment, mortality associated with such diseases has become unacceptable.

In modern western society much traditional knowledge has been lost with social changes and fragmentation of family and social structures. A lack of knowledge among most of the population about basic food hygiene, coupled with our more extensive diet and demand for cheap and fast food, has led to the situation where the safety and availability of our food supply is not so much dependent on the turn of the seasons, as on specialised transportation, storage and the application of modern farming methods. Supply of foodstuffs is globalised, with fresh produce being air freighted and shipped by sea as well as by land. The supply chain for some products has lengthened dramatically, and the need for clean 'harvesting' and appropriately monitored transportation has never been greater. Storage of produce, as either raw material or processed product, at correctly maintained temperatures, has become essential in protecting the public from a whole range of pathogens, including some zoonoses.[15]

The changes in agricultural practice are particularly significant in relation to the re-emergence of certain zoonoses, because many modern animal varieties are bred to suit mass-marketing conditions and mechanisation of processing. The development of these breeds and the methods of feed and housing to optimise production often give rise to individuals with a decreased immunity, or a higher population of pathogens. The increased risk that such individuals pose to the wider animal population was addressed by the widespread use of antibiotics as growth promoters; however, after these products were banned across the European Union (EU), producers have had to review production methods and husbandry practice. Concern continues that the use of antibiotics in agricultural production, especially those moieties related to those used in human medicine, is leading to the emergence of resistant pathogens, although studies suggest that the major driver behind the development of resistance stems from antibiotic use/misuse in humans.[16]

Some of the more significant of these pathogens have a zoonotic potential, or are existing recognised causative agents of zoonoses. The organism with probably the most developed resistance to antimicrobials is *Salmonella typhimurium* DT104 R serotype. This had been found to be resistant to ampicillin, chloramphenicol, streptomycin, sulphonamides, tetracyclines, trimethoprim and the quinolones. A systematic review of the use of such agents was undertaken by DEFRA. This triggered changes in agricultural industry practice in the UK; however, it is unlikely to affect many other countries' use of these substances in agriculture. The previously mentioned globalisation of the food market may become increasingly significant in our attempts to manage antibiotic-resistant strains of bacterial pathogens.[17]

Much of the legislation in agriculture, and the food-handling industry, stems from the need to deliver a safe product to the consumer. Failures in systems or inspection procedures can lead to contamination of the production and supply chain. This in turn can lead to spectacular outbreaks, sometimes associated with fatalities, which serve as timely reminders of the need for care in handling and storing food. The Wishaw outbreak in November 1996 of E. coli O157 killed 18 people initially, and was the second most fatal incident ever recorded from this pathogen anywhere in the world. If we include the three people who died afterwards from complications caused by the infection, it becomes the most fatal. In the aftermath, the ensuing investigation into the outbreak and the subsequent report by Sir Hugh Pennington formed one of the political catalysts that motivated the UK government to establish the FSA. The report also highlighted the ignorance in a large proportion of the public of basic hygiene precautions relating to food storage and preparation, as have subsequent surveys.[12,17]

It is important to remember that, in agriculture, domesticated animals are tended for gain; they can contract zoonotic disease by its transfer from wild animal populations although sometimes links are difficult to prove, as in the possible transfer of TB from badgers to cattle. Farmers will often view zoonoses in solely monetary terms, which can have beneficial and detrimental implications for any control programmes, depending on the financial provisions of any compensation package. When contamination with a zoonotic organism downgrades a product in quality and associated value, the agricultural industry will spend much time and money in attempting to control not only the initial infection, but also the associated disease.

Present and past eradication campaigns, by either compulsory slaughter or vaccination, have massively reduced the incidence of brucellosis, TB, anthrax and tetanus, which were major causes of morbidity and mortality in previous decades. The massive slaughter of cattle carried out after the outbreak of BSE reduced the possibility of contaminated meat entering the food chain, and probably reduced the spread and incidence of vCJD in the human population. It also reduced the likelihood of breeding stock carrying the disease, so preventing possible recurrence.

In a wider context, most of the population in the UK now lives and works in urban areas, thus having no link with the countryside or its associated industries. Therefore most people's closest encounters with animals are with those species kept as companion or leisure species, in the domestic setting. The idea of our pets being a potential source of disease has also become more recognised.

Recommendations for pet owners on handling and caring for their animals stem from the need to control potential zoonoses and reduce infection rates. The appointment and use of dog wardens in urban areas, and campaigns by the Royal Society for the Prevention of Cruelty to Animals (RSPCA) in the UK and the Society for Prevention of Cruelty to Animals (SPCA) in the USA have reduced the number of stray dogs and cats, diminishing the possible reservoir for many animal diseases, including some zoonotic conditions.

Expanding interest in exotic animals as pets has generated its own problems. Snakes and reptiles are recognised as being the biggest population reservoir for certain unusual *Salmonella* spp. As a general rule, the more exotic the pet the more likely it is to carry unusual pathogens. Although there have been no proven clinical cases arising from a zoonotic source, it is known that armadillos are the only other species except humans that can suffer from leprosy.[18]

Responsible pet owners usually safeguard their pets through veterinary surgeon-led programmes to ensure comprehensive vaccination, worming and pest control of companion animals. Public awareness of animal welfare and the related animal health issues seems to increase with every episode of the currently popular television series involving real-life 'fly-on-the-wall' animal hospital documentaries.

Geographically, the UK is very fortunate. The temperate climate and physical isolation from continental Europe, coupled with the absence of large native predators and non-human primates, make many of the physical and legislational controls very effective and reduce the possibility of outbreaks of certain zoonoses. The current quarantine regulations for the movement of animals in and out of the UK prevent rabies in companion and other animals. The introduction of 'pet passports' linked to an effective vaccination programme, and the electronic tagging of vaccinated animals has proved very successful for both owners and their animals in disease prevention.

The continental USA is very different; it has a wide range of ecological and environmental parameters across a vast geographical area. Although it has no native primates, there are vast wild animal populations, including wild species closely related to domesticated animals, i.e. bison, mustang, and wild rodent and bird populations that provide a reservoir for many significant zoonotic diseases, including rabies and plague.

In both the UK and the USA, the social infrastructure offers protection from zoonoses and other diseases in many ways that are taken for granted or not recognised. The provision of high-quality, fresh, clean drinking water confers protection against disease, including some zoonoses. Current levels of public health and hygiene, with provision of safe sewage disposal and processing, reduce the risks from water-borne organisms and environmental contamination, reducing or preventing the spread of disease. The collection and safe disposal of domestic and industrial organic waste also offers a high degree of protection. All these measures form part of a protective umbrella that shields the populations from spectacular outbreaks of diseases such as cholera and typhoid – diseases that were endemic in the UK and the USA in the nineteenth century, and are still seen routinely in other places around the world.

Local authority responsibility for pest control forms an important part of public health protection, preventing rats, mice and other alternative hosts and their associated vectors from reaching sufficient numbers to precipitate a zoonotic epidemic.

Historically this was not always the case. The Black Death and the Plague of London were two memorable examples of epidemic zoonotic infection affecting the UK. The causative organism *Y. pestis*, still kills people every year in the south-western USA, Africa and Asia. We associate the spread of plague with rats; however, they are not the only associated host. Chipmunks, squirrels, dogs, cats, camels and rabbits can all act as alternative hosts, and their associated fleas as disease vectors.[19]

The understanding of causative organisms, their detection, classification and control have taken place only in the last century and a half. The emergence of BSE, a prion disease, is an object lesson that should teach us that, although our knowledge has advanced, we still have much to learn.

It is in the nature of human affairs that the response to control the spread, or threat of spread, of disease normally follows rather than pre-empts an epidemic or well-publicised outbreak. It is important that health-care professionals and society in general never forget that our infrastructure and legislation, although sometimes cumbersome, shield us from much morbidity and mortality associated with zoonoses and other diseases.[20]

Risk groups

Having discussed the threat that zoonoses pose, and the potential sources of infection, let us now turn to identifying those individuals most likely to contract disease on exposure to the pathogen. Most healthy adults with a competent immune system are unlikely to acquire a zoonotic infection at every exposure to the pathogen, even if an inoculum of potentially infective magnitude is present. Against an infective challenge, they are also likely to display better developed resistance to a range of possible causative organisms. This does not indicate that infection does not occur in this group – only that it is less likely than in the groups shown in Table 1.3, who are identified by the WHO as primarily 'at risk'.

In general, those most at risk are those individuals who come into daily contact with animals, are less resistant to infection or have less regard than normal for hygiene routines. Children and elderly people have traditionally been seen as more susceptible to certain of these infections. In addition,

Table 1.3 Main risk groups for zoonotic infection
Animal handlers
Neonates and children
Elderly and infirm people
Agricultural and food industry workers
Immunosuppressed or compromised individuals
Pregnant women

those individuals with a suppressed or damaged immune system stemming from whatever cause, be it infectious disease, chemotherapy or organ failure, are also at an enhanced level of risk. The realisation that animal handlers and food-industry operatives have an enhanced risk of infection or transmitting these diseases has led to health and safety legislation and recommendations on working practices to reduce risk.

Pregnant women are at risk from particular zoonoses. Information about *Listeria, Toxocara felis*, toxoplasmosis and chlamydial infection is now widely available from maternity services and special-interest groups such as the Toxoplasmosis Trust. Testing is not routinely carried out; however, individuals with particular additional risk factors, such as employment in agriculture or animal welfare, cat owners or food-industry operatives, would normally be screened for any infections likely to pose a threat to mother or baby.

Since the emergence of human immunodeficiency virus/acquired immune deficiency syndrome (HIV/AIDS), research has shown that individuals who are immunocompromised or immunosuppressed, for whatever reason, are more at risk from a range of pathogens, including some zoonoses. Patients who have had a total or partial splenectomy, are on high or prolonged doses of steroids, and patients undergoing chemotherapy or radiotherapy for treatment of cancer, also fall within this risk group. The diagnosis and recognition of the risk that cryptosporidial diarrhoea, psittacosis, toxoplasmosis and TB (whether avine, bovine or human) poses for immunocompromised patients have led to a process of risk reduction, and an extensive programme of education for patients and healthcare professionals.[21]

Risk factors appear to be additive in terms of associated risk from zoonoses. Any individual who falls within several of the identified risk groups has an increased risk of infection. An immunosuppressed agricultural worker, who keeps pet cats, and eats unpasteurised dairy products, while being licked by a pet dog, would be considered to be at a greatly enhanced level of risk.

Genetic susceptibility may also be an additional risk factor. The pattern of transmission demonstrated by the prion responsible for scrapie in sheep appears, on the best available evidence, to be a good model for the behaviour of BSE in cattle and vCJD in humans. It has been established that a sheep must have a certain amino acid sequence on its genes to be susceptible to acquiring a primary case of scrapie from environmental sources. The identification of clusters of human cases of vCJD in Leicestershire and Doncaster demonstrated the similarity in genetic make-up of the victims and offers a vital clue to unravelling the mystery of susceptibility and risk associated with exposure to the causative agent.

Implications for industry

In the UK and the USA, a developed system of legislation and mandatory inspection safeguards us from many zoonotic infections linked to animals and processes within our system of food production. To be effective these controls have to be enforced rigorously at all levels within the chain from the animal, through processing and distribution to the arrival at the consumer. At harvesting, routine inspection of meat, livestock slaughterhouse controls and the advisory work of DEFRA and the US Department of Agriculture (USDA) reduce transmission rates of many potentially dangerous pathogens. Further down the process of field to food, enforced regulation of food suppliers and vendors, sell-by dates, refrigeration and education of consumers all lead to lower levels of infection and associated illness or mortality.

Produce loss

Uncontrolled zoonotic disease can lead to produce loss caused by poor appearance or product contamination by pathogens. In the event of contamination or loss of quality, there will be an associated monetary loss, with destruction or downgrading of produce. Controlling the risk of zoonoses often requires increased inputs to achieve a higher quality in the finished product, so as to reach the standard required by processors, suppliers and consumers. Charging a higher price for the produce can often offset these costs; however, food pricing is a sensitive issue. In the quest for food cheap enough to compete in the global market, it may be very tempting for a producer to cut corners, and this can lead to outbreaks of disease stemming from inadequate or inconsistent standards of treatment or implementation.

Personnel loss

When zoonoses are present, personnel within the industry can suffer from anxiety, which may be as debilitating as the possible infection. Frank illness will often lead individual workers to change career path or employment.

Long-term effects due to prolonged exposure of pathogens may lead to disability and ultimately increased likelihood of morbidity and mortality, where appropriate measures to control spread of disease are not in place. This places additional health and safety requirements on employers to protect their workers from these risks.

The associated issues of compensation to individuals contracting zoonoses in the work place and the issues of recruitment and retention have encouraged producers and processors to put good working practices in place.

Public impact

The impact of zoonoses on the public (Table 1.4) can be profound, especially when the knowledge and understanding are mainly fuelled by adverse and dramatic media hype. Food scares are probably the most memorable of these manifestations. Eggs, beef, milk, cheese and pork have all suffered a bad press in their turn. In many of the cases reported by the media the causative agents of the outbreak were already well known, and the problem was already being addressed before the media chose to sensationalise it. In a population dominated by an appetite for sound bites, profound fear and anxiety can rapidly be generated by such reports. The only solution to the problem is education relating to the true likelihood of infection and its associated risks.

Media misreporting of zoonoses can be dramatic and misleading. During the recent outbreak of foot-and-mouth disease in the UK, there was an isolated news report stating that during the 1968 epidemic a man had died of the disease. An extensive search of reference books, archival material and other sources revealed no confirmation that there was any evidence of foot-and-mouth disease being a fatal zoonotic disease. Only two confirmed cases had been recorded in humans: one in the 2001 outbreak and one in 1967. There was overwhelming evidence that, although a wide range of animals were either susceptible to the disease or capable of acting as carriers, under normal circumstances humans were not liable to contract the affliction. No

Table 1.4 Public impact of zoonoses
Food scares with boycotts and dietary change
Increased legislation and consumer/producer costs
Public and private fear and anxiety
Morbidity and mortality
Political fallout

trace could be found of any report either in the UK or anywhere else in the world linking human fatalities with the disease.[22]

In desperation, a phone call was made to a friend and colleague who is a consultant epidemiologist. After he had finished laughing, he told me the following story:

> During the 1967–1968 outbreak, the British Army was employed to go on to some farms to kill and destroy the livestock. On one farm, night was falling as the troops carried on the work of building and lighting the funeral pyres. The farmer and his family had vacated the farmhouse and it stood empty with all the family's possessions inside. Some of the soldiers saw a man sneaking around the buildings and then break a window and enter the house. When he re-emerged clutching items he had looted from the house they were waiting for him. When called upon to stop by the now armed soldiers, the looter decided to try and run away and make his escape, so the troops shot him. He died, not of foot-and-mouth but of high-velocity lead poisoning. His death did much at the time to dissuade other opportunist criminals from looting deserted farmhouses.

The moral of this story appears to be that, when reading reports of zoonoses in the media, it is essential to remember the old adage 'Don't believe everything you read in the newspapers'. It could be argued that, although not directly responsible for the fatality, the infection was, at one remove, associated with the death, if somewhat apocryphally.

Long-term effects of food zoonoses on the public are usually confined to consumer avoidance of products perceived as suspect. Food retailers usually respond to such crises by demanding or imposing higher standards on their suppliers, which in their turn force producers to increase their inputs. Confidence in foodstuffs is easily lost, and takes a long time to be regained.

Morbidity and mortality arising from zoonoses are of particular public concern. The implications for the food industry of such events were explored earlier in this chapter; however, the public impact is not confined to those who work within the various stages of the food production and food-retailing chain. Individuals may become convinced that they are going to die, regardless of the true risk, from zoonotic infections; in the last few years in the UK, several individuals have committed suicide fearing that they were going to die of vCJD.

Reports of children dying from *E. coli* infection, following an educational visit to a farm, fuels and highlights the hysteria such cases are capable of generating. Many parents are extremely chary of allowing their children to go on organised agricultural visits or camping holidays. Although the statistical risk of infection is low, and the risk of mortality almost negligible, one of the less attractive facets of our society is a very obvious driver of political policy in this context. There appears to be a concerted desire within certain groups for risk reduction in normal everyday affairs to the point of absurdity. The complete absence of risk is unachievable, and would require restrictions to be placed on every aspect of human endeavour. This fallacy of a completely risk-free existence is an ever-present and all-pervading urban myth, which needs to be arrested.[23]

The realisation that education in both cerebral and physical skills is the most important factor in protecting individuals and society from the risks that these diseases pose needs emphasising by all involved in the day-to-day health of the nation. There is no substitute for knowledge, the provision and application of which could safeguard people far more effectively than legislation, and which would also ensure that future generations lead healthy, full lives.

In general, consumer pressure groups serve a useful purpose in encouraging government and others to be responsible when crises arise. In contrast, they can also increase public aversion or panic by unrestrained and ill-informed lobbying. This is especially significant where their agenda does not coincide with, or is diametrically opposed to, any of the other parties affected by the issue. The understandable aversion response of many members of the general public to the BSE/vCJD outbreak resulted in many people in the UK choosing to eschew meat, and become vegetarians. As a considered decision, based upon the known facts, this was a reasonable conclusion for people to reach. The less considered and sinister aspect was the declarations made by the more extreme groups and individual activists involved in the animal rights and extreme vegetarian movements, who informed the world that this was a judgement, or punishment, visited upon wicked people for their consumption of meat.

The more dramatic incidents associated with zoonoses can – especially if morbidity or mortality occurs – lead to significant political repercussions not only for entire governments and their departments, but also for individual politicians. Resignations over unwise utterances are not unknown. DEFRA or its various previous incarnations and USDA have been the graveyard for many an aspiring politician. Quick-fire legislation has peppered UK parliamentary proceedings over many decades and is often a knee-jerk response to zoonotic problems. As with many measures introduced rapidly, it can often be poor-quality law, being too draconian, too complex or unenforceable.

Much of the increase in regulations associated with animal husbandry has been the result of the perceived need to introduce new systems, rather than ensuring that existing schemes were made to work efficiently and comprehensively. Often the need to be seen to be doing something outweighs the more pragmatic approach, especially where this could lead to loss of votes or position.

This chapter has attempted to introduce zoonoses and place them in a wider societal context, and sets the scene for the more detailed examination in the remainder of the book. The following chapters aim to examine the more significant conditions in greater detail.

Once an awareness of these diseases is gained, it is remarkable how many chance conversations with patients, relatives or friends, snippets from radio or television, or newspaper and magazine stories become associated with these conditions. This disparate group of diseases and pathogens is of major significance in our day-to-day living and its associated processes, and it is not a matter that we should ever forget or ignore.

References

1. World Health Organization. *Ebola Haemorrhagic Fever in the Republic of Congo*. May 2005 and updates May and June 2005. Geneva: WHO, 2005.
2. Department of the Environment, Food and Rural Affairs. *Zoonoses Report UK 2006*. London: Defra, 2007.
3. Sechi LA, Mura M, Tanda E, Lissia A, Fadda G, Zanetti S. *Mycobacterium avium* sub. *paratuberculosis* in tissue samples of Crohn's disease patients. *New Microbiol* 2004; **27**: 75–7.
4. Hayes EB, Piesman J. How can we prevent Lyme disease? *N Engl J Med* 2003; **348**: 2424–30.
5. Palmer S, Brown D, Morgan D. Early qualitative risk assessment of the emerging zoonotic potential of animal diseases. *BMJ* 2005; **331**: 1256–60
6. Reiter P, Sprenger D. The used tire trade: a mechanism for the worldwide dispersal of container breeding mosquitoes. *J Am Mosq Ctrl Assoc* 1987; **3**: 494–501.
7. Taylor LH, Latham SM, Woolhouse ME. Risk factors for human disease emergence. *Philos Trans R Soc Lond B Biol Sci* 2001; **356**: 983–9
8. *Clostridium perfringens* gastroenteritis associated with corned beef served at St Patrick's day meals – Ohio and Virginia, 1993. *MMWR* 1994; **43**: 137–8, 143–4.
9. Geiter L, ed. *Ending Neglect: The elimination of tuberculosis in the United States*. Washington DC: National Academies Press, 2000.
10. Health Protection Agency. *Statutory Notifications of Infectious Diseases in England and Wales: MIDI Report for 2006*. London: HPA. 2007.
11. Prusiner SB. Prions. *Proc Natl Acad Sci USA* 1998; **95**: 13363–83.
12. The Pennington Group. *Report on the Circumstances Leading to the 1996 Outbreak of Infection with E. coli O157 in Central Scotland, the Implications for Food Safety and the Lessons to be Learned*. Edinburgh: The Scottish Office, 1998.
13. Chomel BB, Belotto A, Meslin FX. Wildlife, exotic pets and emerging zoonoses. *Emerg Infect Dis* 2007; **13**(1): E-edn.
14. Watson JT, Gerber SI. West Nile Virus: A brief review. *Pediatr Infect Dis J* 2004; **23**: 357–8.
15. World Health Organization. *WHO Global Strategy: Safer food for better health*. Geneva: WHO, 2002.
16. Teale CJ, Martin PK, Watkins GH *et al*. *VLA Antimicrobial Sensitivity Report*. Norwich: HMSO, 2004.
17. Advisory Committee on the Microbiological Safety of Food. *Report from the DEFRA Antimicrobial Resistance Co-ordination Group* (DARC). London: Defra Secretariat, 2005.
18. Public Health Laboratory Service. Salmonella infection and reptiles. PHLS press release. London: Public Health Laboratory Service, 2000.

19. Laudisoit A, Leirs H, Makundi RH *et al*. Plague and the human flea, Tanzania. *Emerg Infect Dis* 2007; **13**: 687–93.
20. Gratz NG. Emerging and resurging vector-borne diseases. *Annu Rev Entomol* 1999; **44**: 51–75.
21. O'Rourke K. Veterinarians' role in the AIDS crisis. *JAVMA* 2002; **221**: 764–5.
22. World Health Organization. *Foot and Mouth Disease: Consequences for public health*. Geneva: WHO (CSR), 2001.
23. Stirling J, Griffith M, Dooley JS *et al*. Zoonoses associated with petting farms and open zoos. *Vector Borne Zoonotic Dis* 2008; **8**(1): 85–92.

2

Zoonoses of companion animals

With a population, at the last recorded census in 2004, of 6.8 million dogs and 9.58 million cats, the UK deserves its reputation as a nation of animal lovers. Of the 25 million households in the UK approximately half own a

Table 2.1 Companion animal populations in the UK and the USA

Percentage of households	Pet type	No. of households	Pet nos
In the UK 24.6	Cats	6.1 million	9.58 million
21.1	Dogs	5.2 million	6.8 million
4.6	Rabbits		
2.5	Hamsters		
7.2	Birds (including parrots, finches, etc.)	1.39 million	
0.9	Horses/Ponies	975 000	
In the USA 31.6	Cats	33.2 million	70.8 million
36.1	Dogs	37.9 million	61.6 million
4.6	Birds	4.8 million	10.1 million
1.7	Horses	1.75 million	5.1 million

Sources:

Pet Food Manufacturers' Association. *UK Pet Population Statistics*, London: PMFA 2004.

The Henley Centre. *A report on research on the Horse Industry in Great Britain*. London: Defra and British Horse Industry Confederation, 2004.

Wise JK, Heathcott BL, Gonzalez ML. Results of the AVMA survey on companion animal ownership in US pet-owning households. *JAVMA* 2002;*221*:1572–3.

pet of some description. In the USA only about 34% of all households had pets of any description. These figures include only the accepted classes of companion animals. People also keep pets as diverse as bats, tarantulas, reptiles and sharks.

As the population of the UK has become increasingly urban, and families have become more fragmented, companion animals have gained importance. Studies show that there is a range of benefits in terms not only of health, but also in general well-being for individuals who keep pets. People who are bereaved, drug addicts, mentally ill or in long-term care settings have all been shown to benefit from animal contact.[1,2]

Under a scheme run by Pets as Therapy (PAT), part of the Pro Dogs Charity (PRO), there are over 10 000 dogs and their owners who visit hospitals, hospices and residential homes regularly as therapeutic support for patients. An equivalent scheme runs in Scotland called Therapet.

The benefits of pet ownership, or contact, do come at a price, in terms of healthcare, especially in people who have certain medical conditions. This chapter explores the more significant zoonoses associated with the main companion animal groups. Horses are also included in this chapter, as most of the 975 000 horses in the UK are not working animals in the accepted sense, being mostly kept for leisure purposes. This is not so true in the USA, although at least 6.6 million of the 9.2 million horses are designated in the American Horse Association survey as being kept solely for leisure.

Birds

Introduction

The species of birds kept as companion animals are extremely varied. Caged birds are often kept as pets, with budgerigars and canaries still being popular choices. There are many other species of bird as companion animals with everything from parrots, parakeets, cockatoos or cockatiels, to racing and fancy pigeons, rare poultry, hawks and owls. Most species have at least one breed society or a network of fanciers.

The main zoonotic diseases that birds can harbour are normally spread by inhalation of dried faecal material, often during cleaning out of cages or housing. Most infected people show no signs of disease; however, elderly, young and immunocompromised individuals are particularly at risk. *Mycobacterium avium* complex, *Cryptococcus neoformans* and psittacosis are particularly important in human immunodeficiency virus/acquired immune deficiency syndrome (HIV/AIDS) patients, where development of any of these diseases can be rapidly fatal. Recently, with the emergence of a strain of highly pathogenic avian influenza, H5N1, which has the potential to become a pandemic strain in humans, there has been an increased interest and awareness of the risks that avian zoonotic pathogens pose. The pathogens covered in this chapter are not the only zoonoses of birds; others can be found in the section on birds in Chapter 3, especially avian flu, and also in Chapter 7.

Cryptococcosis

This is an uncommon infection except in immunocompromised patients, especially those with HIV/AIDS. The causative organism is *Cryptococcus neoformans*, a yeast-like fungal agent that occurs worldwide. The organism is naturally found in birds, cats and dogs, cattle, sheep, horses, plants and soil. It is an uncommon pathogen and appears to have a predilection for pigeons because it is found most commonly in these birds or in their faecal matter. It has also been found in other birds, but less frequently.[3]

Disease in animals

Although it is rare in cats and dogs, it usually presents as systemic disease affecting the respiratory tract and central nervous system (CNS), and often animals present with enlarged lymph nodes. Occasionally distinctive skin lesions appear. It is seen as an opportunistic pathogen in cats that are immunosuppressed, particularly together with feline leukaemia virus (FLV). This is a disease that progresses in cats in a similar manner to HIV in humans.

Transmission

Transmission to humans is usually by inhaled dusts and aerosols; however, there is some evidence that inoculation of wounds can also initiate infection. Healthy individuals show no clinical signs of disease, although the organism can be grown from mouth swabs, skin scrapings and gut contents. Patients who are immunosuppressed as a result of organic disease, e.g. HIV/AIDS or leukaemia, or long-term steroid therapy are at a small but significant risk of catching the disease.[4]

Disease in humans

The disease usually presents as meningitis in immunosuppressed patients. As with animals, skin papules, usually with a necrosed centre, may be seen; however, this is rare. The disease may also be systemic, affecting the gut, lungs and nervous system.[5]

Treatment

Treatment for cryptococcosis is usually initiated in specialist units, using a variety of systemic antifungals. Therapy has to be closely monitored due to potential drug interactions and potentially life-threatening side effects, especially in immunocompromised patients. Women being treated for this condition are usually advised to use effective contraception due to the potential teratogenicity of the drug therapy.

Prevention

As the condition is rare, blanket prophylaxis to pre-empt infection is not recommended, especially as interactions with retrovirals can complicate therapy regimens. Widespread use of antifungal drugs could also lead to the development of resistant strains.

Complete protection from the organism is not possible due to the wide range of possible animal hosts and environmental sources. Immunosuppressed patients should avoid exposure to pigeons and their faeces, especially coops or roof spaces where birds roost.

Mycobacterium avium complex

Tuberculosis or TB is classically caused by *Mycobacterium tuberculosis (hominis)*, although M. *bovis*, a zoonotic pathogen, is responsible for a small percentage of cases. The term is often loosely used to describe a complex of infection states caused by a variety of aerobic bacteria of the genus *Mycobacterium*.

Several sections in this book deal with various members of this genus, some of which are associated with various diseases states that are often classified under this umbrella term. As the first section dealing with this family of microbes, there are some general remarks relating to these infections below.

General remarks

Mycobacteria are aerobic bacilli found widely in a variety of animal species, including humans, and also free living within the environment. They are intracellular dwelling and particularly capable of developing resistance to a variety of antimicrobial agents. The most significant members of the genera in terms of possible zoonotic infections are M. *bovis* (found in cattle, dogs and pigs), M. *avium* (found in birds, pigs and sheep) and M. *marinum* (found in seals, sea lions and fish).

M. *tuberculosis* is mainly found in humans and the infection circulates within that population. For this reason it is not seen as a zoonotic disease, although it has been isolated from primates, cattle, dogs, pigs and parrots.

In general, mycobacteria are transmitted from infected individuals, be they humans or animals, primarily by the aerosol route. Infection is also possible via contact with, or ingestion of, infected tissue, bodily secretions, or body fluids such as blood or plasma. Cutaneous inoculation is also possible via cuts or lacerations.

After infection there can be a short or long pre-patent period depending on the health of the individual and the strain and virulence of the organism. The disease progresses with the organism becoming disseminated throughout the body. Major sites of colonisation are usually the lungs, lymph nodes, circulatory system, liver, spleen and other major organs. Signs and symptoms vary depending on the main sites of infection. The classic tubercular lung disease usually presents as a persistent cough that does not resolve. As the condition worsens, quantities of mucus are produced which may contain traces of blood. As pulmonary damage worsens, coughing up of overt blood (haemoptysis) is seen. Other symptoms include loss of appetite and anorexia, fever that may be episodic, weariness and extreme fatigue. It is thought that the 'consumption' of the last centuries, immortalised in romantic fiction and drama by leaving the hero or heroine of the piece dying dramatically, was probably pulmonary TB. The disease can also manifest in a cutaneous form with ulcers and lesions progressing to persistent suppurative sores.

M. avium is endemic in wild and caged birds and, coupled with *M. intracellulare*, it can cause a form of TB with both pulmonary and systemic forms in susceptible humans. This is known as *Mycobacterium avium* complex or MAC. It is a major clinical problem in immunocompromised patients and is one of the marker infections in the progression of HIV infection to AIDS-related complex (ARC). There is some debate as to whether MAC is a zoonotic infection because the pathogen is widespread in the environment and some isolates display different serological profiles to classic bird-borne types. However, there is some evidence that infection may spread from birds in occupational and domestic settings. In addition to the well-documented manifestation of MAC in HIV/AIDS, there is continuing discussion about the possible involvement of *M. avium* in Crohn's disease. Any clinical links are as yet unproven.

Transmission

Transmission of *M. avium* usually occurs by inhalation of infected aerosols or dusts. Sneezing or coughing birds with subclinical cases can be prolific excreters of viable organisms. Ingestion or cutaneous contact has been postulated as an alternative route of infection; opinion is divided on the importance of this particular mode of infection.

Disease in humans

Infection usually starts with the development of foci in either the lungs or the gastrointestinal tract. Disseminated infection may develop from these foci, with an associated morbidity and mortality, especially in cases of advanced HIV.

Diagnosis

Diagnosis is often presumptive because *M. avium* can cross-react to skin testing for other mycobacterial conditions. Isolation and culture are difficult due to the intracellular nature of the bacterium; however, this does produce a definitive diagnosis and also allows drug-sensitivity testing.

Treatment and drug prophylaxis

There are specific problems with antimicrobial-resistant serotypes in this infection, which is especially important in immunodeficient patients. There are also additional complications relating to dose adjustments of other concomitant drug therapies when treatment or prophylaxis for MAC is necessary. For this reason patients with MAC are not normally initiated on drug therapy in primary care. Specialist secondary care practitioners initiate treatment.

Rifamycin has been used in the UK; however the adverse effects of the drug may mimic MAC infection and so the progress of treatment has to be monitored by culture and on serological findings.

By contrast, in the USA an alternative regimen is used with a macrolide antibiotic, either clarithromycin or azithromycin, being considered suitable alone or in combination with rifabutin. The premise for the use of this combination therapy is that it reduces the risk of producing drug resistance and also of secondary infections.[6]

Prophylaxis aimed at preventing the development of disseminated MAC is recommended for patients with a CD4 cell count < 50 cells/µL. There is some evidence that prophylaxis can be discontinued when the CD4 cell count tops 100 cells/µL. This is a decision that must be made carefully by secondary care agencies. The use of highly active antiretroviral treatment (HAART) has altered the prevalence and treatment of MAC and its prophylaxis in HIV/AIDS patients, and the latest recommendations should always be followed.

Psittacosis (ornithosis)

Psittacosis is the classic 'parrot's disease' of comedy, although clinical cases will not have patients splitting their sides with laughter. The disease is also referred to as avian chlamydiosis (AC). The causative agent is *Chlamydophila psittaci* (formerly known as *Chlamydia psittaci*) which typically, like all other *Chlamydophila* spp., is an intracellular parasite. It has a biphasic reproductive cycle, with only one phase being infectious. A closely related organism is an important zoonosis of sheep, although the pattern of disease and the transmission pathway are very different (see p. 91).

Disease in animals

C. *psittaci* is widespread in both wild and domestic birds. Parrots are the most frequently encountered hosts in a companion animal setting, and 1% of the population are estimated to have active disease at any time. Other potential hosts as zoonotic reservoirs include turkeys, ducks, geese, pigeons, starlings, pheasants and birds kept for competitive showing. Estimates have been made of the prevalence of infection in wild pigeon populations in the USA. These range from 50% to 100% of all feral pigeons within a population sample. The number of birds infected within a population increases where over-crowding or stress occurs. The associated levels of inadequate ventilation and cleanliness in poor and overcrowded commercial housing also promote the rate of infection with the disease in commercial flocks. Infection in birds is usually subclinical and may remain latent for a period of months or years. Apparently healthy birds can shed viable organisms and cause infection in others during the latent period. The pathogen can survive in the environment for extended periods following contamination with infected droppings or aerosols originating from the nasal discharge of infected birds. The organism is resistant to drying, and can be found in dust in hen houses, pigeon lofts and other roosting sites. Bird cages, pet shops, lofts or roof spaces inhabited by wild and feral species must be treated as possibly contaminated.

Transmission

Transmission to humans follows inhalation of dried bird faeces or nasal discharge from infected birds, direct contact with birds or their feathers and by bird bite (a rare but possible occurrence, especially in aggressive non-domesticated parrots). Once across the species barrier, human-to-human transmission may occur by the aerosol route. Poultry workers in the turkey industry, in either rearing or processing birds, show an increased incidence of the disease. Individuals who handle wild, pet or domesticated birds in any setting are at increased risk. However, obvious risk is not reliable as a diag-nostic yardstick, because 20% of cases reviewed in the USA could remember no overt contact with birds. Verification of the presence of C. *psittaci* may be difficult; as yet there is no rapid test available to differentiate serologically between this and other *Chlamydophila* spp.

Disease in humans

The infection may be subclinical, leading to under-diagnosis. Onset of the disease is gradual; an incubation period of 1–2 weeks is followed by a series of symptoms similar to influenza or a respiratory infection. Symptoms include malaise, fever, chills and headache, and associated photophobia and non-productive cough. An unusual feature is that, although the temperature is elevated, the pulse rate does not undergo an associated rise. Joint and muscle pain with weight loss and loss of appetite may also be seen. Occasionally a full-blown acute pneumonia may occur.[7]

Rarely seen in children, the infection is most severe in elderly and immuno-compromised individuals. In severe cases, liver and splenic enlargement with gastrointestinal symptoms, including vomiting, diarrhoea and constipation, may occur. Cardiac involvement with valve failure and endocarditis is possible. Spread into the CNS may follow with disorientation, depression or delirium followed by meningitis or encephalitis. Severe breathing difficulties can follow exacerbation of pulmonary symptoms. Death can follow pulmonary insufficiency and toxaemia. In clinical cases fatality occurs in approximately 1%.

Treatment

Treatment consists of tetracyclines as the antibiotic of choice, with supportive measures. Tetracycline is given at a dose of 250–500 mg three to four times daily for at least 7 days, with the treatment period extended as needed. Doxycycline has also been used at a dose of 200 mg/day, as has azithromycin and erythromycin, although their use is normally associated with *Chlamydophila* spp. which cause urinogenital infection or endocarditis. Early diagnosis is very important to reduce complications, and prolonged treatment may be required to prevent reinfection or relapse in some cases. It is recommended as good practice to inform a consultant in communicable diseases of cases of psittacosis where there could be a public health risk.

Prevention

Prevention depends on education of individuals in high-risk groups. Early detection of cases in birds is an important part of any prevention strategy. Reduction in stress and overcrowding is recommended to control infective spread. Placing birds suspected of having psittacosis in isolation until they can be tested, and subsequently treated or slaughtered in confirmed cases, is also recommended as good working practice. Treatment of imported companion birds with prophylactic antibiotics is important, especially before their sale as pets. Good flock management at agricultural sites can reduce infection, and feral birds should be excluded from feed mills and rearing sheds. No vaccines are available for either humans or birds.

Cats and dogs

Introduction

The population of cats in the UK was estimated as 9.58 million in 2004 (the latest survey). This figure shows a marked increase in the number over the previous decade, and has now outstripped the dog population. This is associated with changes in lifestyle: urban living, employment patterns and the number of single-person households have all altered the balance of ownership towards animals that require less care. The Pet Food Manufacturers' Association (PFMA: http://www.pfma.com) has estimated that 34% of households in the UK own at least one cat, with the greatest density in south-east England. A similar pattern is seen in the populations associated with Europe and the USA, with 47 and 75 million cats, respectively.

The reasons most frequently given for cat ownership are companionship and love, with many cat owners allowing their pets the run of their houses. Cats are capable of carrying a wide range of zoonoses and, as the pattern of behaviour of certain owners falls outside the normal realms of good hygienic practice, there are many opportunities for the transfer of infection to occur. As the companion animal of choice for large numbers of the population, the control and prevention of cat-associated zoonoses are particularly important.

Cats are especially significant in two well-recognised conditions – toxocariasis and toxoplasmosis – both of which pose a well-publicised risk to children and pregnant women. Cat Scratch Disease (CSD) is now recognised as a serious condition in immunocompromised individuals, and the effective treatment or prophylactic therapy of cat owners with HIV/AIDS has begun to reflect the importance of this and other potentially serious zoonotic conditions.

Dogs

The PFMA survey for 2004 shows an estimated 6.8 million dogs in 5.2 million households across the UK. However, dogs are not just kept as companions; working dogs are still part of farming and sheepdogs are still invaluable for managing sheep, especially on extensive upland farms. Dogs are also used by the police, and as drug and explosive detectors, not forgetting hearing dogs for the deaf and guide dogs for the blind.

Many of the zoonoses associated with cats may also be acquired from canines; however, there are pathogens that may have a species-specific subtype; although differentiation may be possible it is not necessarily useful in clinical terms.

The following zoonoses are associated with either cats or dogs or with both, and are particularly important because they affect the urban population, who are often more in need of education and assistance in understanding that their companion animals, however cute, may be the source of serious disease.

Cat Scratch Disease

Cat Scratch Disease is caused by a rickettsia, *Bartonella henselae* (formerly known as *Rochalimaea henselae*). Little recognised in the UK, it is widely documented in the USA and shows a worldwide distribution. Other *Bartonella* spp. cause a number of diseases in humans, including trench fever (*B. quintana*), which occurs worldwide. *B. quintana* is transmitted to humans via bites from lice or fleas associated with rats.

Transmission

Although CSD was recognised previously as a distinct infection and illness, it was not until 1992 that the causative organism was identified because of difficulties in culturing the slow-growing bacterium. Infected cats carry the pathogen and show no ill effects; however, they can shed viable organisms, especially in their urine, for prolonged periods. In-species transmission between cats occurs usually through physical damage sustained in fighting, i.e. bites and scratches. Recent research has indicated that a flea that sucks blood from an infected cat becomes infected. *B. henselae* replicates and colonises the flea's digestive tract; subsequently viable organisms are passed in the faeces. Cats may be infected by bacteria in flea faeces introduced into a flea-bite wound or other cuts and abrasions by either scratching or grooming. This mode of transmission, of the introduction of contaminated arthropod faeces into wounds, occurs in other diseases caused by *Bartonella* spp. and is especially important in the rodent reservoir for trench fever.[8]

Human infection follows either a scratch or a bite from an infected animal. Saliva contaminated with flea faeces from the cat grooming itself or nibbling at the site of flea bites is presumed to be one source of the infective inoculum. The role of fleas in the direct transmission of *B. henselae* from cats to humans has not been characterised yet. Humans may also be able to contract the infection in a similar manner to cats by introducing flea faeces into a wound; this hypothesis is currently under investigation.

Disease in humans

A primary lesion appears at the injury site, usually forming a single, circular, pink, flat lesion or plaque or series of plaques along the length of the scratch. The initial primary lesion appears in 50% of cases after 10 days. Transient lymph node tenderness and swelling with some discomfort may develop and then regress. In about 15% of cases progression to more serious disease occurs with serious sequelae, which may include CNS damage, osteomyelitis and involvement of the lungs and respiratory tract. Immunocompromised patients may develop liver damage and hepatic lesions.[9]

CSD can also cause bacillary angiomatosis, a vascular proliferative disease seen in individuals with established HIV or those who are immunocompromised for a variety of reasons. It can be fatal, progressing from skin lesions, which are the most common symptom, to lesions in the bones and bone marrow, gastrointestinal and respiratory tracts, lymph nodes and CNS. Fever, weight loss, and associated swelling and tenderness of various internal organs are commonly seen. It is also suspected of causing bacillary peliosis, a condition associated with relapsing bacteraemia and endocarditis. Cystic, blood-filled spaces develop in the liver, spleen or lymph nodes. Fever, abdominal pain and weight loss follow gastrointestinal disturbance. A febrile bacteraemic syndrome associated with *B. henselae* is also seen in immunocompromised patients. Symptoms include chronic or cyclical fever, joint and muscle pain, and severe headache. Patients with long-term asymptomatic infections may shed viable organisms in their urine.

Treatment

Treatments recommended in the US literature are reserved for complicated cases. Simple cases are not usually considered for therapeutic intervention. In cases with complications, azithromycin 500 mg daily for 1 week followed by 250 mg for 4 weeks is recommended. In bacillary angiomatosis erythromycin 500 mg once daily for 3 months or doxycycline 100 mg twice daily for 3 months may be required to prevent relapse and effect a full cure. In peliosis hepatitis the same drugs may be used for 4 months.

Prevention

Owners are advised to avoid rough play with cats to reduce the risks of scratches and bites. Any wounds inflicted by the cat should be washed and disinfected immediately. The common-sense precautions of preventing a cat licking any human wound and washing any exposed areas after petting or stroking the cat are strongly recommended. Children and adults, especially those who are immunosuppressed, should avoid stroking or touching stray or feral cats. Immunocompromised patients, especially those with advanced HIV (or ARC), may need to consider keeping their cat indoors at all times to prevent it associating with other cats that may be infected.

Echinococcosis
Hydatid disease or hydatidosis

Worldwide, echinococcosis is caused by a number of species of *Echinococcus* that belong to a subgroup of tapeworms known as tissue cestodes, because for part of their larval life cycle they encyst in body tissues. *Echinococcus granulosus* causes cystic echinococcosis, the most commonly seen form of the disease. Another species, *E. multilocularis*, causes alveolar echinococcosis. In the UK only *E. granulosus* has been found and is usually confined to areas where there is intensive sheep farming. *E. multilocularis* has been seen in other countries in western Europe, but as yet no clinical cases have been seen in the UK, although there is a theoretical risk that tourists or travellers could pick up *E. multilocularis* while abroad.

The disease state caused by *E. granulosus* is sometimes known as unilocular hydatid, because only a single site is initially colonised, whereas *E. multilocularis* colonises multiple sites simultaneously and therefore leads to more serious clinical disease. In humans these tapeworms cause a condition known as hydatid disease where cysts of great size may develop over long periods post-infection.

Luckily, human infections in the UK with the tapeworm larvae responsible for the condition are rare. Over the last decade there has been reporting of between 5 and 26 cases annually, although it would appear that reporting is incomplete. In 2005 there were 11 reported human cases in England and Wales, and none in Scotland.

In the continental USA the disease is considered to be rare at less than one case per million inhabitants a year. As the disease has a long pre-patent period of between 10 and 20 years before cysts become palpable, the numbers of people with the disease may be higher because many subclinical cases may go undetected where there is no postmortem examination after death from other causes.

Disease in animals

These species of tapeworm require dogs (or foxes) and sheep to be present in the same environment for their complete normal life cycle to take place. Humans, although they can suffer the unpleasant effects of infection by these organisms, are a dead-end host in which the tapeworm cannot complete its life cycle (Figure 2.1). In the UK, sheep are the most important intermediate host, although cattle, horses and pigs can also carry the encysted larval stage.

The normal life cycle of the tapeworm consists of the following phases:

- A sheep grazing on contaminated pastures ingests eggs in faecal matter from dogs or foxes.
- The sheep acts as the intermediate host and after ingestion the eggs hatch into larvae, which migrate through the intestinal wall and then encyst in the organs and tissues, where they can multiply.
- After death, dogs eat tissue from the sheep contaminated with cysts; after ingestion the encysted larvae emerge and progress to adult tapeworms in the intestine of the dog.
- Eggs are then produced and pass out with the faecal matter, and so the cycle starts once more.

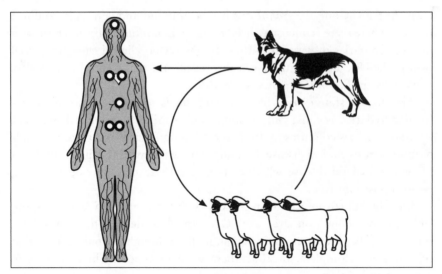

Figure 2.1 Hydatidosis in humans and the life cycle of *Echinococcus granulosus* in dogs and sheep. Open circles show probable sites for hydatid cyst formation.

In animals infection is often asymptomatic, although a heavy burden of developing larvae or adult worms may lead to diarrhoea. In dogs, segments of the adult worm or even the worm may become apparent either in the stools or in some cases protruding from the anus. Inspection of meat from infected sheep after slaughter can detect the cysts. Such carcasses will be condemned for human or animal consumption.

Transmission

Human infection follows consumption of food or water contaminated with viable eggs from dog faeces. In the USA, there is some evidence that infection may also occur by a hand-to-mouth route after stroking a dog with faecal contamination, or by handling objects contaminated with faecal matter.

Disease in humans

Following infection, the eggs hatch and the resulting larvae migrate and then encyst. The encysted larvae will then start a slow growth and multiplication process to form multiple hydatids, an infective larval form. Known as hydatid sand, this may consist of thousands of particles in a large cyst. Due to the slow growth, physical detection of the cyst may follow only after more than a decade. The most common site where the cyst forms is in the liver, with the mass restricted by a thickened membrane. Clinical signs and detection follow abdominal swelling and pressure on other internal organs or bile duct obstruction with associated nausea and pain. The retaining membrane may rupture into the abdomen, pericardium or pleural cavity with the possibility of anaphylactic shock, or severe allergic response to the fluid contained within the cyst or the hydatid particles. Death may follow, as can the formation of new cysts in other locations by the released hydatids.

Primary cysts may also form in other sites, with the lungs, kidneys, CNS and bone marrow being, in decreasing order, the most likely sites. Lung cysts are usually asymptomatic until they become large enough to block airways or they rupture. Persistent dry cough, pain or coughing of blood may occur.[10] Cysts in the CNS cause symptoms earlier than those in other locations, with epileptiform fits or paraesthesia. Spontaneous fracture and bone pain can be a result of cysts in the bone marrow, with the most common sites being the vertebrae. Compression of the spinal cord or dependent nerves may follow, with associated paralysis or weakness.

Diagnosis

Diagnosis is usually made by ultrasonography or serology testing. Exploratory or investigative surgery can be risky unless precautions are taken to avoid membrane rupture.

Treatment

Treatment traditionally was surgical to remove the cyst or cysts and the contents. After surgery washing out of the affected body cavity with ethanol, formaldehyde solution, hypertonic saline, iodine solution, hydrogen peroxide or silver nitrate solution has been recommended to destroy any hydatids that have escaped the cyst membrane and could start new cysts. Although surgery is still seen as the main option, prophylactic medication may be necessary to keep the cyst from recurring and drug treatment may be the only choice where cysts are in inoperable locations.[11]

Albendazole has been recommended for *E. granulosis* echinococcosis, with albendazole or mebendazole being used in cases of *E. multilocularis*.[12,13]

The World Health Organization (WHO) recommends albendazole 800 mg/day in divided doses for 28 days, followed by 14 drug-free days as a treatment cycle. Where surgery is impossible, the WHO suggests repeat treatments for up to three full cycles. As an adjunct in surgical treatment of hydatid cysts, before and/or after surgery, one cycle is suggested.

Prevention

Prevention strategies include the regular worming of dogs, especially working sheepdogs, with praziquantel. Stray dogs should be controlled by the usual methods of impounding or culling. Feeding dogs with sheep offal or infected meat should be avoided, with rigorous abattoir checks to prevent infected meat entering the food chain. Preventing human infection, as with other parasitic diseases such as toxoplasmosis, relates to implementation of strict hygiene measures and education. The condition is considered to be an occupational hazard for shepherds and others who work with sheep.

Although cases of echinococcosis associated with *E. multilocularis* have never been confirmed in the UK, a few notes are appended for the sake of completeness. Infection with *E. multilocularis*, also known as alveolar disease, follows the same pattern, with ingestion of eggs associated with faecal contamination from dogs, cats or foxes. The normal intermediate hosts are rodents rather than sheep. The cycle is completed when dogs, cats or foxes eat mice or other infected rodents. Unlike cysts associated with *E. granulosus* the cysts of *E. multilocularis* have no membrane and can therefore spread from the original foci more rapidly. Primary foci are usually in the liver or lungs and occasionally in other tissue sites. The associated hydatids are invasive and the condition can be rapidly fatal, with an estimated 90% of untreated cases dying within 10 years.

Hookworm
Ancylostomiasis; cutaneous larva migrans; creeping eruption

The hookworms *Ancylostoma duodenale*, *A. braziliense*, *A. caninum* and *Necator americanus* are associated with two clinical conditions affecting human beings: ancylostomiasis and cutaneous larva migrans. The adult worms are found in the gut of cats and dogs and the eggs are passed in the faeces to the soil. Under suitable soil conditions the eggs remain viable for considerable periods. Once hatched the eggs produce larvae that undergo two larval moults in the soil. On attaining the third larval stage they become infective. They can penetrate intact human skin, usually at the base of a hair follicle, or are ingested by consumption of contaminated food or water. The larvae then subsequently begin to migrate. The type of migration following infection is determined by the species involved and is classified by the clinical signs seen.

Ancylostomiasis

In ancylostomiasis, the larvae begin to migrate by deep tissue penetration, and by transit via blood vessels to the lungs. They then penetrate the alveolar sacs and migrate via the bronchi and trachea, where they are swallowed into the gut lumen.

The hookworm is named for the shape and structure of its mouth parts, which aid its attachment to the blood vessels in the gut of the host, from which they feed copiously. Once in the gut they grow to between 5 and 100 mm in length and in heavy infestations can cause anaemia. The worms produce and secrete hyaluronidase so that at their site of attachment they can continue to feed freely. Even after they lose their hold or are killed by use of an anthelmintic, continued blood loss can occur due to the presence of residual hyaluronidase and its anticoagulant effect. The worm matures in the gut and then produces eggs, which are passed in the stools. It is unclear if some species can or cannot complete their life cycle in humans, or if they can reach maturity only in other species.[14]

Disease in humans

Symptoms of infection in humans can include pneumonia related to damage caused by the migrating worms, anaemia, nausea, vomiting, abdominal pain, bloody diarrhoea or blood in the stools, and generalised weakness usually associated with anaemia.[15] Some larvae may penetrate other organs or structures than the lungs. Larvae have been found in the cornea, liver and spleen. In dogs maternal transfer to puppies is seen via the milk or through the placenta; this has never been documented in humans.

Treatment

As the anaemia produced by a hookworm infection is probably the most serious effect in humans there may be a requirement for iron therapy simultaneous with anthelmintic treatment. The *British National Formulary* (BNF) recommends the use of mebendazole at a dose of 100 mg twice daily for 3 days. In refractive cases, where a large population of worms across larval and adult stages is present, a repeat regimen may be needed to resolve the infestation.

Cutaneous larva migrans or creeping eruption

This condition is caused by the cat or dog hookworm *A. braziliense* and also, more rarely, by *A. caninum*. It is normally seen in tropical and subtropical areas; because of the nature of the infection and its aetiology it is often seen in travellers returning from beach holidays. Many of the public beaches in the West Indies, India and Sri Lanka are known to be sources of this infection. The presentation is very distinctive and diagnosis is based on the unusual appearance of the lesions.[16]

Disease in humans

The condition is most often seen in children, because their skins are softer, especially on their feet.[17] Clinical signs commence after penetration of the skin by the infective third-stage larvae, usually as a result of walking on contaminated sand or soil in bare feet. At the site of entry itchy reddened spots appear. After 2–3 days the larvae then start to migrate through the germinative layer of the skin, leaving a raised red and itchy track with localised swelling. The track extends by several millimetres daily. Although distressing, the condition is usually self-limiting because the larvae soon die. Although only one track is usually seen, multiple tracks are also possible. In the case of multiple tracks, or where the lesion continues to advance, and in cases where a secondary infection results from scratching, therapeutic interventions may be necessary.[18]

Treatment

Treatment uses anthelmintic preparations, with the use of ivermectin, albendazole or tiabendazole by mouth, all of which are available on a named-patient basis from IDIS Ltd (see Appendix 2).

Use of any of the broad-spectrum antihistamines by mouth or as a local application will help control itching. The choice of antibiotic in secondary infection follows the usual protocol for cutaneous or subcutaneous infection. Flucloxacillin has been used successfully with its ability to produce adequate therapeutic levels in deep tissue. Topical antibiotics such as fusidic acid have also been used.

Prevention strategies for both conditions

As physical contact with contaminated material is necessary for infection, wearing shoes on ground that could be contaminated with dog or cat faeces is recommended. If dogs are kept in closed areas the run should be disinfected with a chlorinated or phenolic disinfectant to ensure full decontamination and destruction of any egg cysts. In the UK the passing of bylaws and associated fines encourages dog owners to clean up after their pets when they foul in public places, thus reducing contamination of the environment. The exclusion of dogs from recreation areas frequented by children and the use of dog wardens to impound stray and feral dogs are useful measures to prevent this and other zoonoses arising from canine sources. Education of children in basic hygiene procedures helps prevent infection after exposure to the causative organism. In a holiday environment, wearing beach shoes and using beaches where dogs are excluded, and the sand is regularly raked and cleaned, reduce the chance of exposure. Dogs and cats should be regularly wormed to eliminate the adult parasite. The emphasis is on a programme of treatment, because one animal will often have not only adult worms present in the gut but migrating larval stages as well.

Vaccines to prevent hookworm infections are under development and may be of future importance for the health of animals and humans in developing countries, where the disease is more prevalent.[19,20]

Ringworm

Ringworm is a common dermatological affliction of cats, dogs, cattle and horses caused by the fungi *Trichophyton* spp. and *Microsporum* spp. The causative organisms of ringworm are so widespread in the environment that it is often impossible to determine the source of infection. Ringworm is also known as zoonotic dermatophytosis (or dermatomycosis). The lesions are commonly circular in form, and historically were believed to be caused by a worm, hence its common name. Defining the causative organism is very difficult even for expert mycologists, because there are at least four fungal species capable of affecting dogs that may cause clinical disease in canines and humans. Other carrier animals have as many or more species of causative organism, which may be host specific or shared between many species of mammalian host.[21]

The most commonly identified zoonotic organisms causing ringworm in humans are *Microsporum canis*, carried by dogs and cats, and *Trichophyton verrucosum*, carried by cattle. It is possible for pet animals to contract the disease from humans.

The picture of ringworm infection in humans is further complicated by a spectrum of organisms belonging to the genus *Tinea*. These are sufficiently ubiquitous for them to be classed as environmental pathogens. Differential diagnosis is often unnecessary before treatment begins, so it is sometimes difficult to determine whether or not infections are zoonotic.

Transmission

Fungal spores are shed by the animal host and then passed to humans either by direct contact with an infected animal, or by indirect contact with animal housing, fences and other contaminated fomites. Spores can remain viable for long periods of time, especially in unclean conditions. After infection the spores have an incubation period of approximately 10–12 days. After this time lesions may appear, with isolated plaques gradually forming the characteristic weals as the infection establishes. The circular appearance is caused by the healing of the central area, while the organism proliferates outward. The fungus establishes in the hair follicles and may cause the hair shaft to fracture at skin level. This leads to hair loss, which may be permanent in some cases.

Established infections gradually lose the circular appearance as they progress away from the initial site of infection. The lesions are red, scaly, itchy and inflamed, oozing and crusted, especially where secondary infection after scratching occurs. Autoinfection may also result from spores trapped beneath the fingernails. Ringworm can be serious in very young children, who are specifically at risk of scalp infection, which can lead to extensive and rapid hair loss.

Elderly patients and immunocompromised individuals are also at risk: dermatomycosis causes further complications in individuals who already have a spectrum of infections and afflictions.[21]

Incidence

M. canis can be carried by up to 89% of asymptomatic cats. Up to 50% of people exposed to infected cats, both symptomatic and asymptomatic, have serological markers for past or present infection. Infection is more likely from animals displaying overt signs of infection.

Diagnosis

Diagnosis in animals and humans may be assisted by the use of an ultra-violet light, because the lesions will often fluoresce. Definitive diagnosis requires culture of the organism; however, this is normally unnecessary or not undertaken.

Treatment

The condition is usually self-limiting, although use of topical and/or systemic antifungals may be required. Topical imidazole antifungal agents such as miconazole and clotrimazole are probably the most frequently used topical creams in mild cases. Terbinafine cream is usually reserved for more serious or resistant fungal manifestations. Ketoconazole shampoo may be used in scalp infections.

In persistent systemic infections, griseofulvin, terbinafine or fluconazole may be necessary. Therapy usually needs to be prolonged so that the therapeutic agent can penetrate to the dermis surface in the skin cells.

Therapy in immunocompromised patients is further complicated by significant drug interactions between imidazole and triazole agents and a spectrum of drugs including antiretrovirals, rifamycins, tacrolimus and certain cytotoxics. Expert advice and monitoring are essential with dose adjustments.

Prevention

Infected animals should be treated when clinical signs develop, and prophylactically where deemed necessary. Individuals identified as being particularly at risk should be encouraged to handle animals as little as possible, particularly where animals are wild or feral in habit. As the disease can arise from fomite transfer, animal pens, blankets, bedding, etc. should be disinfected and cleaned to prevent initial infection or reinfection.

Scabies

Scabies is caused by a burrowing arachnid mite, *Sarcoptes scabiei*, in humans. Recent work has demonstrated that each mammalian species has a specific species of the parasite. Zoonotic infection by mites other than of the human-specific species can be extremely irritant; however the organisms do not demonstrate the ability to complete their life cycle on a human host.[22]

Disease in animals

Sources of zoonotic scabies include dogs, foxes, cats, horses and, on occasion, pigs. Infection results from close direct physical contact and also fomite spread. After zoonotic infection the mite does not burrow under the skin surface and is believed to cause itching and an associated rash solely by causing a contact dermatitis.

Feline scabies caused by *Notedres cati*, also known as notoedric mange, causes intense itching on the face, ears and neck of the cat.

Disease in humans

Feline scabies is transmissible to humans. It presents with blisters, red papules and crusting. It appears rapidly, is intensely itchy, and when the lesions have been scratched, crusting may be seen. Lesions appear on the areas of the body in contact with the cat and are especially common on the arms, chest, legs and abdomen. Canine scabies shows a similar pattern in human infection.

Diagnosis

Diagnosis may be difficult, as in zoonotically acquired disease the distinctive burrows are absent. The usual techniques of the burrow ink test or skin-scraping examination will therefore not produce definitive results. The condition is usually of short duration, and it may be necessary to treat blindly and symptomatically. A more serious problem may be the secondary infection of the lesions by other opportunistic infections, especially in immunocompromised patients.

Treatment

Insecticides are the usual therapeutic choice for treatment, with both malathion and permethrin normally being effective; however, permethrin is preferred on safety grounds. When hyperkeratotic lesions are present repeat applications may be required. The itching and irritation normally associated with the condition can be treated with topical or oral antihistamine preparations. Oral ivermectin has also been used, but is not licensed in the UK.[23]

Toxocariasis (visceral larva migrans and optical larva migrans)

Disease in animals

Toxocara canis and *T. cati* are roundworms of the dog and cat, respectively, and are found in animals worldwide. The main zoonotic reservoir is latent infections in female dogs and cats that are reactivated during pregnancy.

Transmission

T. canis is mainly transmitted from dog to dog and from dog to human by the ingestion of material infected with encysted eggs. Indirect transmission via an intermediate host is also possible. Unusually in dogs, transmission from bitch to puppies is possible via the placenta and milk. The life cycle of *T. cati* is similar, although transmission across the placenta has not been demonstrated and is believed not to occur.[24] *Toxocara* spp. demonstrate both direct and indirect life cycles in dogs, whereas in cats only the indirect cycle is seen. In the direct cycle the eggs are passed with the dog's faeces; these eggs have a variable latent period before they become infective. Eggs of *Toxocara* spp. are extremely resistant to damage and desiccation and can remain viable and infectious in the soil for many years. The eggs may also develop into infective larvae under suitable conditions. Eggs are spherical and 75–90 μm in size.

Once mature eggs or young larvae are ingested on faecally contaminated matter, they hatch or mature through the first larval stage in the small intestine. The second larval stage (L2) penetrates the wall of the intestine into the lymphatic system and thence into the bloodstream. Migration continues through the heart and lungs. In the lungs the larvae moult to the third larval stage (L3). The L3 larvae migrate up the trachea and are ingested for a second time. Returning to the small intestine, the final moult occurs and the adult worms mate and produce eggs, and the cycle begins again.

In contrast, in the indirect life cycle there is a requirement for an intermediate host, which is normally small rodents in the case of *Toxocara* spp. These ingest viable oocysts that subsequently hatch in the small intestine. Once the larvae reach L2 they migrate and penetrate muscle tissue. A dog or cat that subsequently eats the infected rodent will become infected with the encysted larvae. Once in the gut the larvae will then migrate into the tissues of the dog or cat. They soon go back to a state of dormancy. In a bitch or queen, the dormant larvae become active during late pregnancy. Subsequently some larvae migrate to the small intestine and others migrate to the unborn pups in dogs. The cycle then starts over again, in either direct or indirect modes in the dog and in indirect mode in cats (Figure 2.2).

There has been some evidence in cats that reinfection may result from the cats grooming either themselves or their kittens.

Disease in humans

Infection is acquired by ingesting encysted eggs (oocysts) in soil contaminated with cat or dog faeces. The eggs hatch, and larvae penetrate the intestinal wall and migrate through body tissues. In most cases, toxocara infections are not serious and many people, especially adults infected by a small number of larvae, may not notice any symptoms. Annually approximately 20 cases a year in the UK are reported to the Health Protection Agency (HPA). In the USA, there are an estimated 10 000 cases of infection with *Toxocara* spp. in humans annually (approximately one case/27 000 people). Due to the nature of the disease and the lack of clinical signs, this figure does not represent a true picture of the number of people infected at any time. The most severe cases are rare, but are more likely to occur in young children who often play in dirt or eat soil. Humans are a dead-end host for *Toxocara* spp. in that the larvae that hatch from any ingested eggs cannot progress to full maturity.[25]

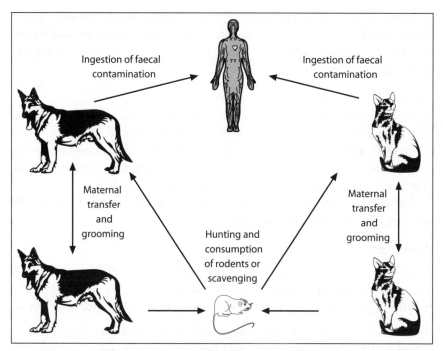

Figure 2.2 Toxocara transmission cycle with direct and indirect pathways from animal to animal and animal to human.

There are two conditions that are recognised as affecting human hosts: visceral larva migrans and ocular larva migrans.

Visceral larva migrans

Visceral larva migrans occurs when hatched larvae migrate through the body of the affected individual. The larvae may continue to migrate for up to 6 months. They finally lodge in various organs, particularly the lungs and liver and less often the brain, eyes and other tissues, where they produce eosinophilic granulomas up to 1 cm in diameter. Migration can result in multiple abscesses, hepatomegaly and pneumonitis. Symptoms include coughing, nausea, vomiting and fever, wheezing, splenomegaly and lymphadenopathy. The acute phase may last 2–3 weeks, but resolution of all physical and laboratory findings may take up to 18 months.

Ocular larva migrans

Ocular larva migrans is a rare form of visceral larva migrans that can cause blindness. The migrating larva enters the eye, encapsulates and causes a localised inflammatory reaction with the production of scar tissue (granu-loma) on the retina, which may be confused with retinoblastoma. In some cases the larva can re-emerge and move within the eye structure later in life.

Sufferers can experience permanent or partial loss of vision. Variable degrees of ocular inflammation occur, and more severe manifestations of ocular larva migrans may require aggressive therapy to avoid serious sequelae such as glaucoma and blindness.

Treatment

Treatment relies on anthelmintic therapy with tiabendazole, mebendazole and ivermectin at normal clinical doses for both adults and children. Corticosteroids, antibiotics, antihistamines and analgesics can be used concomitantly for symptomatic relief. The ocular form may require vitrectomy with adjunctive laser treatment if drug therapies are not effective.

The current BNF carries no recommendations, and treatment is usually initiated by secondary care specialists.

Prevention

Prevention of larva migrans in humans involves a combination of human hygiene and vigilance, stray dog and cat control (where possible), and parasite control in pets. The following hygiene measures should be adopted:

- Children and adults should always wash hands well with soap and water after playing with pets and after outdoor activities, especially before eating.
- Children should be taught not to eat soil or sand.
- Regular periodic worming treatment of puppies, kittens, and pregnant and nursing dogs and cats will prevent acquisition and shedding of the parasite.
- Play areas and sandpits used by children should be protected to reduce contamination from animal faeces.
- Areas that are believed to be contaminated with eggs may be disinfected using ultraviolet light or by scorching.

Toxoplasmosis

Toxoplasmosis is caused by an intracellular protozoan parasite, *Toxoplasma gondii*, which can infect any mammal and is found worldwide. It poses a well-publicised threat to human health, especially to pregnant women, and is also a significant pathogen in immunocompromised individuals. The causative organism is transmitted by contact with, and ingestion of, material contaminated with cysts or oocysts, especially food or water (Figure 2.3). The disease is notifiable in Scotland, but not in the rest of the UK. In 2005 there were 102 cases reported to the HPA in England and 11 in Scotland. There is believed to be a significant underreporting of cases because, in an extensive survey of blood donations, more than 40% of the residents of the

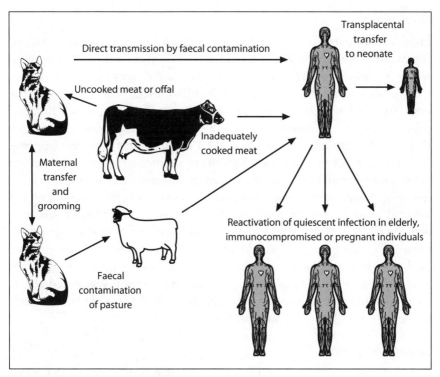

Figure 2.3 Toxoplasmosis transmission pathways.

UK had serological markers for having been at one time or another infected with *Toxoplasma gondii*. In the USA, it is estimated that 60 million people (22% of the population) are infected; however, few have symptoms.

Disease in animals

The major source of infection is cat faeces or food and water contaminated with faecal matter. The definitive hosts for *T. gondii* in which it can complete its life cycle and produce sexual oocysts are cats, either wild or domesticated. Feral cats are recognised as a significant reservoir because they hunt and consume rodents carrying the disease. Cats pass oocysts in the faeces; these become infective after a period of 24 hours, and can remain infective under suitable environmental conditions for more than a year. Sheep and goats are the main non-feline reservoir, especially pregnant or perinatal ewes, and their unpasteurised milk or cheese derived from the milk can be contaminated with the organism. Infection in sheep arises from grazing on pasture contaminated with cat faeces. Any other animal then infected acts as an intermediate host.

Transmission

In an intermediate host the organism will hatch from ingested oocysts, and the invasive form or tachyzoite will actively spread into cell structures, where it proliferates and invades the body via the blood supply. Cysts are then formed in tissues and organs, especially muscle, heart and brain. The cysts are filled with bradyzoites, a slowly maturing form, which if subsequently ingested by another susceptible animal can progress to disease. Dogs, cattle, pigs and rodents have been demonstrated to suffer from the condition and act as a reservoir. Meat from an infected animal may contain viable cysts; handling or consuming raw or undercooked meat may lead to infection. Thorough cooking is necessary to kill cysts before consumption of infected meat to prevent infection. Infection by fomite transfer has been demonstrated, and pregnant women should not handle overalls of people involved in lambing, nor should they handle perinatal ewes or neonate lambs. A live vaccine is available for sheep, and pregnant women are advised to avoid handling the vaccine or any recently vaccinated sheep. Contaminated material containing viable oocysts introduced into open cuts or wounds can also act as an inoculum.

Disease in humans

Although infection is common in humans (some surveys report that more than 50% of adults in the UK and 22.5% of the population in the USA over the age of 12 show immunological markers) serious disease is fortunately less common. Children or adults infected for the first time may well present with a generalised lymphadenopathy which is self-limiting, and resolves after a few weeks, leaving the individual resistant to infection, with possibly low numbers of encysted organisms in tissue or organs and persistent serological markers. Once infected, an individual can carry the cysts asymptomatically until reactivation occurs, especially in immunosuppressed patients. As with animals, the cysts are usually located in skeletal muscle, heart or brain tissue.[26,27]

If a woman has been infected previously (usually during childhood) with *Toxoplasma* spp., when she becomes pregnant, the fetus will be protected by the mother's immunity. However, if a pregnant women contracts toxoplasmosis shortly before or after conception, the unborn child runs a far greater risk of congenital infection following transplacental spread. In general, the earlier in pregnancy the disease occurs, the worse the outcome, with miscarriage, stillbirth, or visual and CNS damage, which becomes apparent after delivery, or later. The neonate may present with hydrocephalus or retinochondritis, which is an inflammatory condition of the retina and choroid in the eye. Nystagmus or squint may also be present, as may brain calcifications that can precipitate seizures and epilepsy.

Pregnant women in the UK are not routinely tested for toxoplasmosis. Testing is encouraged if they belong to a high-risk group such as cat rescue workers, those employed in agriculture, or those who have cats as pets. A concerned pregnant woman can also request a test, although the risks and limitations of the test should be explained. Testing can demonstrate whether infection is recent or historical, and may lead in some cases to either treatment of mother and unborn child, or termination of the pregnancy.

In immunosuppressed patients, toxoplasmosis can cause prolonged illness with acute episodes following either reactivation of an old infection or a new infection. Initially similar to glandular fever, symptoms include sore throat, swollen glands in the neck, armpits and groin, headache, fever, night sweats, and generalised skeletal and muscular aches. In HIV patients the development of clinical toxoplasmosis is one of the markers for transition to ARC. Reactivation can cause inflammatory lesions in the brain, leading to headache, impaired coordination, seizures, sensory loss, tremor, loss of vision, personality changes, disorientation and coma. Abscesses may also be present in the CNS. In a new infection, the disease is rapid and severe, requiring prompt and thorough therapeutic intervention.[28]

The pathogen may also cause severe pneumonitis, and can affect the retina with consequent loss of vision, and ultimately blindness.

Diagnosis

Diagnosis in pregnant women is usually made using pathogen-specific antibody testing of blood samples. Any positive findings are confirmed by a toxoplasma reference unit.

Polymerase chain reaction (PCR) tests on tissue and fluid samples have also been used. In AIDS/HIV patients antibody testing is not considered useful, because it only confirms that exposure has occurred and, as many cases are the results of reactivation of dormant cysts, other methods are needed to determine the status of the individual in relation to infection or active disease. Biopsy specimens of brain tissue can detect cysts, and the presence of tachyzoites is a sign of active disease.

Computerised tomography, magnetic resonance and radiographic imaging can also be used to detect cysts in the CNS, and monitor the effectiveness of therapeutic interventions.

Treatment

For most cases of toxoplasmosis, no therapeutic intervention is required. For pregnant women, HIV/AIDS sufferers and any individual with optical involvement, intervention is necessary. Treatment is particularly essential where evidence of encephalitis is seen.

The BNF recommends a combination of pyrimethamine and sulfamethoxasole given for a period of weeks, with addition of folinic acid if required; however, it is not the treatment of choice in pregnancy (see below). Combinations of pyrimethamine and clindamycin, azithromycin or clarithromycin have also been used. Expert advice is essential when drug therapy is initiated, and, with the toxicity of the agents used, constant monitoring is required, because pyrimethamine is a folate antagonist. Spiramycin, widely used in continental Europe for toxoplasmosis treatment, is available in the UK on a named-patient basis from IDIS Ltd (see in Appendix 2), and may reduce the risk of transmission of maternal infection to the foetus. Steroids are used as an adjunctive therapy to reduce intracranial pressure.

It must be borne in mind that, although the condition will respond to treatment, long-term therapy is necessary to prevent recurrence, and monitoring is essential. Individuals who have survived toxoplasmosis encephalitis (TE) should have lifelong prophylaxis. In some studies into the effectiveness of post-TE prophylaxis, relapse rates of between 20% and 30% have been seen. Non-compliance is a major problem, and relates to the complexity of dosing needed, as is the spectrum of adverse events associated with long-term use of these therapeutic moieties.

Dosage regimens vary depending upon complicating factors – including pregnancy – and adverse reactions, response to therapy, and age or weight of the person. Specialist units or consultants should make decisions about when to start therapy, monitoring and duration of therapy. Specific dosages are not given, because regimens change and alter rapidly with new research and trials being carried out.

Prevention

It is recommended that all individuals in high-risk groups eat only meat that has been thoroughly cooked, and avoid consuming raw cured meats such as Parma ham or cured venison. Unpasteurised goats' or ewes' milk and cheese should not be eaten. Good food hygiene should be routine: all fruit and vegetables should be washed before being eaten and all utensils should be washed well after raw meat has been processed. Personal hygiene routines and hand washing should be as frequent as necessary to prevent infection. Gloves should be worn when cleaning cat litter trays. This should be undertaken daily to remove the infective focus before any oocysts shed in the faecal matter can mature to an infectious stage. In HIV/AIDS patients it may be preferable for another person, who is not in a high-risk group, to carry out tray cleaning.[29]

Children should be encouraged in good personal hygiene habits, and wherever possible sandpits and other areas should be covered when not in use and cleaned to remove feline faecal material promptly. Patients in at-risk groups should wear gloves when gardening and clean both hands and gloves after use.

Pet cats belonging to people in at-risk groups should be kept inside and fed canned or dry foods to prevent infection from wild rodents or undercooked meat. Provided that adequate precautions are undertaken, there is no need to remove the cat from the domestic scene permanently.

Sheep may be inoculated against toxoplasmosis. This carries some risk to the operatives involved, and they should rapidly seek medical advice if accidental inoculation occurs. Swill fed to pigs should be heat treated to prevent infection.

Horses

Introduction

According to a survey carried out by Henley Research for the Department for Environment, Food and Rural Affairs (DEFRA) in 2004 endorsed by the British Horse Society, in the UK, approximately 2.4 million people ride, some occasionally, but many routinely as part of their lifestyle or work. In a horse population survey carried out in 1999 there were 900 000 horses in the UK, from shetlands to shires, via hunters, to cobs and racehorses.

In the USA, the American Horse Council, in a survey conducted in 2005, found that there were an estimated total of 9.2 million horses, with nearly 4 million being kept or ridden for recreation.

Horses and their riders participate in many events, from the Horse of the Year show, to the local gymkhana, and keeping horses as a leisure activity is becoming ever more popular. With this amount of human–animal contact, there is always some risk of medical problems. Luckily there are few zoonoses solely carried by equines; the likelihood of injury from other horse-associated activities is greater, with falls, kicks and occasional bites requiring the most acute medical care.

The diseases discussed in this section are, or have been, of major significance. Glanders was feared until the beginning of the last century, and has re-emerged as a significant zoonosis in other areas of the world. With the flooding that much of the country has experienced in recent years, the incidence of leptospirosis is increasing, and is likely to become more significant in future if the changes in weather patterns are sustained.

Tetanus is still a major issue in terms of public health measures, and the control of the disease requires constant application of a comprehensive vaccination programme.

Horses can transmit or carry other zoonotic diseases that are normally primarily associated with other animals. This is mentioned in other sections under the primary host animal. References to these conditions will be found in the index.

Glanders, farcy

Glanders or farcy is caused by the bacterium *Burkholderia* (formerly *Pseudomonas*) *mallei*. It is a notifiable disease of, in particular, horses but also donkeys and mules. Goats, cats and dogs have also been known to acquire the disease. Import of susceptible animals from countries where the disease has been reported is forbidden. In 2004, DEFRA issued a control notice that required increased control of horses imported from the United Arab Emirates (UAE) after the identification of clinical cases in native horses. It was deemed unlikely that bloodstock that enters the UK for racing or breeding purposes would have been infected; however, extra checks and procedures were put in place. Geographically, the disease is endemic in Africa, Asia, the Middle East, and Central and South America.[30]

The last recorded case in the UK occurred in 1928, but it is possible that many subclinical cases are not identified due to blind antibiotic use without sample culture. It is a notifiable disease under the Notification of Infectious Diseases System (NOIDS) regulations.

Historically it was very significant because it caused rapid fatality in horses and humans – this was a disaster in a society that was reliant on true horsepower for its transport of both people and goods. In 1902 many London boroughs closed their public animal water troughs because of an outbreak of the disease. In human patients, in the era before antimicrobial agents were available, 95% of victims with clinical signs would die. The use of antibiotics has reduced this toll dramatically.

Human infection is luckily now rare; however, it has been seen in pulmonary (glanders) and cutaneous (farcy) forms. It can affect stable personnel or people in close physical contact with horses in the course of their work. Infection in laboratory workers has also been seen. The inoculum necessary to cause infection is small, and the organism has been considered as a potential agent for biological warfare or terrorism.[31]

Transmission

The organism is spread by discharge from wounds and aerosols. Ingestion, inhalation or physical contact with the inoculum allows the bacterium to colonise the next victim. In several cases the initial inoculum has also occurred through the eye or nasal mucosa. Physical inoculation of wounds or abrasions with infected material has been shown to occur. In melioidosis, caused by a closely related bacterium, sexual transfer has been demonstrated and there is a single report of this also occurring in farcy, where human-to-human spread occurred. Once across the species barrier, patients' carers, especially where there is close physical contact, are at risk.

Disease in humans

Following inoculation, the incubation period usually ranges from 1–14 days. Symptoms in humans depend on the route of transmission. The cutaneous form is characterised by skin pustules that suppurate; localised lymph node swelling may then occur. Non-specific symptoms can include headache, with raised temperature, and aching muscles. If mucosal membranes are involved, excessive tear production or nasal discharge may be seen. The disease can then become systemic with an undulant fever, enlargement of the liver and spleen, an overwhelming septicaemia and a high associated mortality rate if left untreated.

The pulmonary form follows the same pattern in terms of early non-specific symptoms; subsequently pneumonia develops with copious mucus production. Abscess formation in the lung may occur with pleurisy and lung collapse. The bacteria may be shed in urine, blood, mucosal secretions and pus from skin lesions, leading to a risk of further infection.

Treatment

Human cases of glanders are rare so limited information is available about antibiotic treatment of the organism in humans. This also leads to problems with diagnosis, because serological assays are not reliable or readily available. Culturing the organism is time-consuming and, as the disease can be rapidly fatal, treatment usually starts on the presumption of illness. Sulfadiazine at an intravenous dose of 25 mg/kg four times a day has been found to be effective in experimental animals and in humans.

B. mallei is also usually sensitive to some or all of the following: penicillins (particularly amoxicillin either alone or in combination as co-amoxiclav), tetracyclines (especially doxycycline), ciprofloxacin, streptomycin, gentamicin, ticarcillin, azlocillin, imipenem, aztreonam, ceftazidime and ceftriaxone. Resistance to chloramphenicol has been reported. Streptomycin in combination with tetracyclines or chloramphenicol has been used historically in the USA but has been replaced by other agents. Where systemic infection with deep-tissue abscesses is present, therapy may have to be prolonged to resolve the infection; durations of more than 14 days have been reported.[32]

Prevention

No vaccine is available to prevent infection with *B. mallei*. Where the infection is endemic, prevention strategies consist of controlling and eliminating the disease in the animal reservoir. Any patient suspected of being infected must be carefully nursed to avoid infection, with appropriate measures including gloves, masks and gowns.

Leptospirosis

*Weil's disease, haemorrhagic jaundice (*Leptospira icterohaemorrhagiae*), canicola fever (L. canicola), dairy-worker fever (L. hardjo)*

Leptospirosis is caused by motile spirochaetes of the genus *Leptospira*. These organisms occur worldwide and are most common in temperate or tropical climates. They may be found associated with animals and humans, or free-living in water or soil. The most important zoonotic leptospires are *L. icterohaemorrhagiae*, found in rodents and dogs (specifically the organism responsible for Weil's disease), *L. hardjo*, associated with cattle and horses, *L. canicola* in dogs, and *L. pomona* in pigs and cattle, although there are other species that are occasionally seen, especially in cases affecting returning travellers. Incidence of the disease ranges from endemic in some areas to sporadic in others. More cases are seen in areas that have been flooded, because soil-living pathogens are released into the surface water and cause wider contamination of potable water sources.[33]

The disease is notifiable to the HPA in England and Wales and Health Protection Scotland in Scotland. It is considered by the Health and Safety Executive (HSE) to be a hazard at work and is subject to the Control of Substances Hazardous to Health (COSHH) Regulations 1994 in terms of provision of protective clothing and prevention measures for people at risk of occupational exposure. The disease is also covered by the Reporting of Injuries, Diseases, and Dangerous Occurrences Regulations 1995 (RIDDOR 95).

Disease in animals

The pattern of clinical signs in infected animals varies from species to species. Cattle often present with weight loss and a high fever, with mastitis in 'in-milk' heifers and declining milk yields. This disease is the most frequently diagnosed cause of bovine abortion in the UK: abortion occurs spontaneously in 'in-calf' heifers with afterbirth retention. Hepatic enlargement, anaemia and jaundice may also be seen. In dogs, acute haemorrhage, jaundice and hepatitis are seen with infection with *L. canicola*, and kidney damage in infection with *L. icterohaemorrhagiae*. Diarrhoea and gastritis may also be seen. Rodents are the only order of mammals that can show no sign of disease, yet are able to shed viable organisms throughout their lives, and are considered to be not only a reservoir for the disease, but also a vector. Organisms are shed in the urine of infected animals and contaminate soil or water.

Transmission

Transmission to humans usually follows either ingestion of water contaminated with infected animal urine, and particularly that of rodents, or contact with contaminated soil or food. The organism can also enter the body by skin abrasions or cuts, and also via the mucosal membranes of the nose, mouth or eyes. Bathing or swimming in infected waters appears to be a major route.[34] The disease is an occupational hazard for sewage, water and canal workers. Vets, aid workers and water-sport enthusiasts are also at a higher than average risk of contracting the disease. There are rare incidents of human-to-human transfer.

There were 3 confirmed reports of leptospirosis in humans during 2006 in Scotland, 3 in Northern Ireland and 44 in England and Wales, of which 34 were contracted in the UK, and 2 fatalities occurred. Of the 34, 18 were confirmed as *L. icterohaemorrhagiae*, 3 as *L. hardjo*, 1 as *L. saxkoebing*, 1 as *L. australis*, 1 as *L. autumnalis* and 1 as *L. javanica*, the other 9 not being serotyped. There is believed to be massive under-reporting of cases.

Disease in humans

After infection, there is a pre-patent period ranging from a few days to several weeks. Clinical signs vary from unapparent to severe acute manifestations with associated mortality. The onset may be sudden with high fever, headaches, aching muscles and fatigue. Vomiting may also occur.

Depending upon the causative organism and the severity of the disease there may be a second phase of the disease. After an apparent recovery the patient becomes ill again with declining kidney and liver function, mental confusion and delusion, meningitis, breathing difficulties and catastrophic hypotension. In the second phase, symptoms are continuous and do not regress until recovery or death occurs. This biphasic form is usually caused by *L. icterohaemorrhagiae* and is known as Weil's disease or icteric leptospirosis. The disease may last for days or weeks and untreated it can be fatal. Recovery can be prolonged, with an extended convalescence of months after clinical illness ends.

Diagnosis

Early in the disease, the organism may be identified by dark-field microscopy of a blood film or by culture. The organism is difficult to grow on conventional media and may require a period of weeks to establish identifiable colonies. More rapid diagnosis can be made using a dot enzyme-linked immunosorbent assay (DOT-ELISA) test. Recently a dipstick test has been developed using an immunoglobulin agglutination method and is now marketed under a number of trade names. This has allowed rapid diagnosis and enables early therapeutic intervention.

Treatment

Treatment is normally with penicillin at normal therapeutic doses or, in the case of penicillin allergy, tetracyclines at normal doses as alternative drugs of choice. Therapy should be initiated early in the course of disease and intravenous antibiotics should be used for people with severe manifestations.

Studies suggest that prophylaxis using oral doxycycline at a dose of 200 mg/week is effective in reducing infection in groups at high risk, due to either their occupational or their recreational pursuits.[35]

Prevention

Dogs, pigs and cattle may be vaccinated against the disease, reducing the infective reservoir. The vaccination is not necessarily routine in cattle because vaccinated cattle may be unacceptable for export to certain countries.

Wherever possible, individuals should avoid swimming in or drinking from potentially contaminated water. Workers likely to suffer occupational exposure should be supplied with adequate protective clothing. Rodent populations must be controlled wherever possible and prophylaxis with antibiotics should be considered for workers, especially where cases have been reported. Rodent carcasses should not be handled and cuts and abrasions should be covered with plasters or dressings.

Miscellaneous zoonoses of companion animals

All animals have diseases specific to species or genera. It is inevitable that some of the causative organisms of these diseases will be potential zoonoses. In general, the more unusual the animal, the more outrageous the possible zoonoses.

The fashion for keeping primates as pets has luckily almost disappeared because our closest cousins carry some very unpleasant pathogens. These may not cause clinical signs in the ape, but they are potentially fatal in humans. Apart from atypical mycobacteria and *Salmonella* spp., including *S. typhi*, simians can also harbour hepatitis A, herpes B virus (fatal in all recorded human cases), and other hazardous viruses such as Marburg (Green monkey). Primates can also become aggressive as they mature. Bites or wounds inflicted on owners or keepers can rapidly become seriously infected and pose a serious hazard.[36]

Reptiles such as turtles or terrapins, snakes and lizards have been identified as harbouring a variety of *Salmonella* spp. and are probably inappropriate as pets for owners who are not willing to become experts in their care and to devote sufficient time to appropriate hygiene routines.

Some of these diseases and conditions are covered in Chapter 8; however, there are many more zoonoses than it is possible to cover in a book of this size, and a decision has been made to exclude those that are not of major significance. To highlight the variety of pathogens that are potential zoonoses, it is enough to consider that armadillos are the only other known species in the world that can suffer from leprosy, apart from humans.[37] No cases have ever been attributed to zoonotic spread, and nobody in the UK keeps armadillos as pets because their importation is prohibited under the Convention on International Trade in Endangered Species (CITES) treaty. Other exotic species probably harbour novel pathogens that might also be zoonotic, and are probably best avoided as pets.

References

1. Charnetski CJ, Riggers S, Brennan FX. Effect of petting a dog on immune system function. *Psychol Rep* 2004; **95**(3 Pt 2): 1087–91.
2. Irani S, Mahler C, Goetzmann L, Russi EW, Boehler A. Lung transplant recipients holding companion animals: impact on physical health and quality of life. *Am J Transplantation* 2006; **6**: 404–11.
3. Yao Z, Liao W. Fungal respiratory disease. *Curr Opin Pulm Med* 2006; **12**: 222–7
4. Sánchez P, Bosch RJ, de Gálvez MV *et al.* Cutaneous cryptococcosis in two patients with acquired immunodeficiency syndrome. *Int J STD AIDS* 2000; **11**: 477–80.
5. Kim JH, Shin DH, Oh MD *et al.* A case of disseminated cryptococcosis with skin eruption in a patient with acute leukemia scan. *J Infect Dis* 2001; **33**: 234–35.
6. Benson CA, William PL, Cohn DL *et al.* Clarithromycin or rifabutin alone or in combination for primary prophylaxis of *Mycobacterium avium* complex disease in patients with AIDS: A randomized, double-blind, placebo-controlled trial. *J Infect Dis* 2000; **181**: 1289–97.
7. Eidson M. Zoonosis update. Psittacosis/avian chlamydiosis. *JAVMA* 2002; **221**: 1710–12.
8. Chomel BB, Boulouis HJ, Maruyama S, Breitschwerdt EB. *Bartonella* spp. in pets and effect on human health. *Emerg Infect Dis* 2006; **12**: 389–94.
9. Chomel BB, Boulouis HJ, Breitschwerdt EB. Cat scratch disease and other zoonotic *Bartonella* infections. *JAVMA* 2004; **224**: 1270–9.
10. Yilmaz A, Tuncer LY, Damadoglu E, Sulu E, Takir HB, Selvi UB. Pulmonary hydatid disease diagnosed by bronchoscopy: a report of three cases. *Respirology* 2009; **14**: 141–3.
11. Papathanassiou M, Petrou P, Zampeli E, Vergados I, Paikos P. Disseminated hydatid disease in a child: albendazole treatment of orbital cyst. *Eur J Ophthalmol* 2008; **18**: 1034–6
12. Adas G, Arikan S, Kemik O, Oner A, Sahip N, Karatepe O. Use of albendazole sulfoxide, albendazole sulfone, and combined solutions as scolicidal agents on hydatid cysts (in vitro study). *World J Gastroenterol* 2009; **15**: 112–16
13. Arif SH, Shams-Ul-Bari, Wani NA *et al.* Albendazole as an adjuvant to the standard surgical management of hydatid cyst liver. *Int J Surg* 2008; **6**: 448–51.
14. Tu CH, Liao WC, Chiang TH, Wang HP. Pet parasites infesting the human colon. *Gastrointest Endosc* 2008; **67**: 159–60.
15. Budhathoki S, Shah D, Bhurtyal KK, Amatya R, Dutta AK. Hookworm causing melaena and severe anaemia in early infancy. *Ann Trop Paediatr* 2008; **28**: 293–6.
16. Heukelbach J, Feldmeier H. Epidemiological and clinical characteristics of hookworm-related cutaneous larva migrans. *Lancet Infect Dis* 2008; **8**: 302–9.
17. CDC. Outbreak of cutaneous larva migrans at a children's camp – Miami, Florida, 2006. *MMWR* 2007; **56**: 1285–7.
18. Patel S, Aboutalebi S, Vindhya PL, Smith J. What's eating you? Extensive cutaneous larva migrans (*Ancylostoma braziliense*). *Cutis* 2008; **82**: 239–40.
19. Bethony JM, Loukas A, Hotez PJ, Knox DP. Vaccines against blood-feeding nematodes of humans and livestock. *Parasitology* 2006; **133**(suppl): S63–79.
20. Bottazzi ME, Brown AS. Model for product development of vaccines against neglected tropical diseases: a vaccine against human hookworm. *Expert Rev Vaccines* 2008; **7**: 1481–92.

21. Havlickova B, Czaika VA, Friedrich M. Epidemiological trends in skin mycoses worldwide. *Mycoses* 2008; **51**(suppl 4): 2–15.
22. Rabinowitz PM, Gordon Z, Odofin L. Pet-related infections. *Am Fam Physician* 2007; **76**: 1314–22.
23. Hu S, Bigby M. Treating scabies: results from an updated Cochrane review. *Arch Dermatol* 2008; **144**: 1638–40, discussion 1640–1.
24. Despommier D. Toxocariasis: Clinical aspects, epidemiology, medical ecology, and molecular aspects. *Clin Microb Rev* 2003; **16**: 265–72.
25. Fisher M. *Toxocara cati*: an underestimated zoonotic agent. *Trends Parasitol* 2003; **19**: 167.
26. Sukthana Y. Toxoplasmosis: beyond animals to humans. *Trends Parasitol* 2006: **22**: 137–42.
27. Chirch LM, Luft BJ. Cerebral toxoplasmosis in AIDS. *Handb Clin Neurol* 2007; **85**: 147–58.
28. Nath A, Sinai AP. Cerebral toxoplasmosis. *Curr Treat Options Neurol* 2003: **5**: 3–12.
29. Davis RG. HIV/AIDS and the veterinary practitioner – making a difference. *Compend Contin Educ Vet* 2008; **30**: 128, 130.
30. Chen AC, Dance DAB, Currie BJ. Bioterrorism, glanders and meloidosis. *Eurosurveillance* 2005; **10**: 1–2.
31. Srinivasan A, Kraus CN, DeShacer D *et al*. Glanders in a military research microbiologist. *N Engl J Med* 2001; **345**: 256–8.
32. Russell P, Eley S M, Ellis J *et al*. Comparison of efficacy of ciprofloxacin and doxycycline against experimental melioidosis and glanders. *J Antimicrob Chemother* 2000; **45**: 813–18.
33. Bharti AR, Nally JE, Ricaldi JN *et al*. Leptospirosis: a zoonotic disease of global importance. *Lancet Infect Dis* 2003; **3**: 757–71.
34. T Pavli A, Maltezou HC. Travel-acquired leptospirosis. *J Travel Med* 2008; **15**: 447–53.
35. Seghal S, Sugunan A, Murhekar M, *et al*. Randomized controlled trial of doxycycline prophylaxis against leptospirosis in an endemic area. *Int J Antimicrob Agents* 2000; **13**: 249–55.
36. Chomel BB, Belotto A, Meslin FX. Wildlife, exotic pets and zoonoses. *Emerg Infect Dis* 2007; **13**(1): E-edn.
37. Lane JE, Meyers WM, Walsh DS. Armadillos as a source of leprosy infection in the Southeast. *South Med J* 2009; **102**: 113–14.

3

Zoonoses of agricultural animals

There is a large and active indigenous farming and livestock operation in the British Isles and the USA. Eggs, milk and meat are currently produced in quantity for human consumption by domestic flocks and herds.

In June 2006, the Department for Environment, Food and Rural Affairs (Defra) estimated that there were 149 million poultry (hens, chickens, pheasants, ducks, etc.), 10.2 million cattle (dairy or beef), 34.7 million sheep

Table 3.1 Provisional figures for number of livestock for each country in UK, June 2006[a]

	England	Wales	Scotland	N. Ireland	UK
Cattle	5 378 028	1 326 300	1 929 990	1 635 700	10 270 000
Sheep	15 673 409	9 350 700	7 608 100	2 070 500	34 722 000
Pig	4 057 433	b	463 330	386 600	4 933 000
Poultry	114 905 849	b	12 119 320	16 297 900	148 929 000
Goats	82 774	b	4 130	3 400[c]	98 000
Deer	21 000[d]	b	6 380	3 397[e]	36 000
Horses	2 578 000	b	30 220	10 300	Note[f]

[a]Figures do not total due to rounding and data from different time period.
[b]Results for 2006 not available.
[c]2001.
[d]2002.
[e]2004 data.
[f]Equine database should give more accurate figures in future: figures relate generally to horses on agricultural land.
Figures courtesy of DEFRA.

and 4.9 million pigs in the UK. This probably represents a fairly accurate estimate of the numbers today (Table 3.1) broken down by region.

The Health and Safety Executive (HSE) estimate that there are more than 20 000 cases of zoonoses in agricultural and other associated workers annually. Many of these cases have been reported under the Control of Substances Hazardous to Health (COSHH) regulations, because the causative pathogens fall under the terms of reference for those regulations. Much has been done to reduce the risks associated with zoonotic infection while caring for domesticated animals or processing animals and their products from farm to table, but much remains to be done. The provision of protective clothing and equipment, the adoption of safe working practices and other safeguards protect not only workers but also the public at large.

Many of the diseases in this chapter have a long historical association with animal husbandry, probably dating from the first domestication of wild species. Many of the pathogens are almost household names and certainly maintain a hold on our collective consciousness, sometimes out of proportion to their current significance. Others are less familiar; nevertheless, they may still pose a risk.

One of the recent developments in agricultural enterprise has been the extended range of animal species kept for commercial purposes, as farms have responded to the changing market by diversifying. These changes in the spectrum of species, with which those employed in the industry come into close contact, can lead to different zoonotic pathogens becoming more important. The last section of this chapter deals with some examples of such diseases.

Birds

Birds currently kept for commercial purposes in agriculture come from a variety of species across the avian genera. It is hard to come to terms with an industry where not only do traditional poultry have a place, as providers of meat and eggs, but also other non-traditional species such as the ostrich and the Gressingham duck (a cross between traditional domesticated ducks and the mallard).

In recent years, while there has been a diversification within the poultry farm and other bird-based enterprises, the pattern of farming has also changed. Eggs produced by battery hens can still be seen on supermarket shelves, but in response to consumer pressure the free-range hen and its eggs are making a dramatic comeback on the basis of better animal welfare and improved flavour. Chickens and capons are again being reared solely for the table, rather than as a sideline to the industrial broiler unit.

These changes come at a price to healthcare. The implications for food and its consumption are discussed in Chapter 4; the importance for zoonotic

disease in poultry workers is slightly different. Any of the zoonotic conditions discussed in Chapter 2, which are capable of affecting companion bird
species, may also strike domesticated fowl. In addition there are a variety of
other conditions that tend to be seen only in commercial bird flocks.

The change in husbandry practice carries with it the exposure of the birds
to a wider environment and, with it, wild bird species. With the current risk
of pandemic bird flu, this has had some repercussions for commercial flocks.
In Northern America, the West Nile virus (WNV) is known to be established
in wild birds across the continent in endemic areas, acting as a reservoir for
the pathogen that may then infect domestic flocks, which do not act as a
reservoir for the virus, but are victims of it.

In the past, wild species were excluded from poultry housing by never
allowing birds out, and by controlling feral pigeons and other birds from
gaining access to feed mills and storage. This probably slowed the spread of
possible pathogens, be they zoonotic or not. There is a growing realisation
that new patterns of operation may require heightened vigilance and
monitoring.

Newcastle disease (UK)
Exotic Newcastle disease (USA) (pseudo-fowl pest)

Newcastle disease is caused by avian paramyxovirus type 1 (APMV-1), and
similar disease can be caused by eight other serotypes (APMV-2–APMV-9).
It is a notifiable disease in poultry and routine vaccination prevents major
outbreaks, which historically rapidly wiped out whole flocks. The organism
is classified under the Advisory Council on Dangerous Pathogens as a
Group 2 Hazard. It is also controlled under Part 7 of the Anti-Terrorism,
Crime and Security Act 2001 (Extension to Animal Pathogen Order 2005).
It is notifiable under the Animal Health Act 1981, the Diseases of Poultry
(England) Order 2003, and also the Animal Health Act 2002 and the Avian
Influenza and Newcastle Disease (England & Wales) Order 2003.

It was named for Newcastle upon Tyne in England, where the first cases
of clinical disease were seen following the feeding of dead chickens from a
ship that had arrived from the Far East to local poultry.

The last recorded outbreak in the UK was in 2006, in East Lothian. To
control the disease 14 000 birds, principally grey partridge, had to be culled.
In the previous year there was also an outbreak in pheasants near Guildford,
Surrey, which was controlled after the slaughter of approximately 10 000
birds. The natural reservoir for the disease is in wild birds, and the severity
of the infection varies from species to species, to such a degree that in some
species the disease can be unapparent.

This is insignificant in economic and casualty terms compared with
an outbreak of exotic Newcastle disease (END) that started in southern

California in October 2002. It spread from small non-commercial flocks into commercial flocks by mid-December 2002. By mid-January 2003, despite efforts to control the outbreak by culling, the disease had spread into Nevada. The resulting ban on exports of poultry and poultry products from California caused considerable economic loss.

The previous major outbreak of END virus in commercial poultry in the USA occurred in southern California during 1971–3. A total of 1341 infected poultry flocks were identified, and about 12 million birds were destroyed at a cost of $US56 million. Imported pet birds were the source of infection. There have been several other recorded small-scale outbreaks that were rapidly brought under control by the US Department of Agriculture (USDA).

Disease in animals

The clinical course of the disease is brief; following infection there is a brief incubation period averaging 5 days, but ranging between 2 and 15 days. Birds then often have catastrophic diarrhoea, breathing difficulties and copious mucus discharge from nostrils and mouth. The birds may become comatose and die, although in the most virulent form death is so rapid that few other symptoms are seen.

Transmission

Transmission occurs after inhalation of infected material, such as faecal matter, or direct contact with infected birds or their carcasses or live vaccine. Contamination of the conjunctiva can also occur via bird and plumage dusts. Fomite contact in intensive housing with high levels of infection can also lead to transmission.

Disease in humans

Individuals employed within the poultry industry are most at risk. Accidental infection during vaccination occurs occasionally. Slaughterhouse operatives and laboratory workers are also considered to be at risk if they are handling infected birds or clinical samples.[1]

The first clinical symptom of infection in humans is usually a painful self-limiting conjunctivitis. On occasions a debilitating low fever of up to 3 weeks' duration with spontaneous rapid recovery has been reported.

Treatment

Treatment is usually symptomatic. It may include antiviral or antibacterial eye preparations to treat either primary or secondary infection. Aciclovir eye ointment has proved effective in early primary infection, with either chloramphenicol or fusidic acid preparations for controlling any secondary pathogens.

Prevention

Prevention strategies involve thorough and comprehensive vaccinations of all poultry to prevent disease. Poultry workers should wear respirators and facemasks when working with flocks and in housing. Precautions should be adopted to prevent accidental inhalation of vaccine droplets during air-carried vaccination procedures, and all housing should be thoroughly cleaned when not in use.

Influenza
Flu, avian, swine and equine influenza, fowl plague

Influenza or 'the flu' is a familiar disease to most healthcare professionals and the public at large. Recently there has not been a pandemic outbreak associated with mass fatalities; however, the emergence over the last decade of a highly pathogenic avian strain of the virus brings the possibility of a pandemic, similar in nature to the one that occurred at the end of World War I, closer. That outbreak is estimated to have killed approximately 20 million people worldwide – more than the armed conflict itself. Subsequent pandemics in 1957 and 1968 led to many deaths. The causative agent, an orthomyxovirus, is categorised in three types – A, B and C – of which the A and B types cause the most serious disease. The virus is further characterised into subtypes according to the characteristics and proportions of the two main viral proteins – haemagglutinin (H) and neuraminidase (N), hence H5N5, H5N1.[2]

Influenza viruses are famous for their ability to mutate. In both types an antigenic drift following minor changes in the amino acid sequencing in the haemagglutinin portion can be observed, resulting in the structure of the virus altering gradually over a series of generations, either by endogenous re-sequencing or by exchanging blocks of amino acids with other influenza viral strains. This allows the virus to continue to be infective and avoid the development of an immune response and host immunity.

Type A viruses can additionally undergo dramatic sudden changes in structure called antigenic shift. The impact of this ability is the emergence of new strains overnight with an associated possible increase in virulence or pathogenicity. All the major pandemics are believed to have been caused by type A viruses capable of circulating within and between animal and human populations, that had undergone antigenic shift (Figure 3.1).

Viral subtypes are classified not only according to protein make-up but also by their place of origin and the year in which they were isolated. The 1918 virus, commonly known as Spanish flu, is believed to have arisen from an unholy union between bird and pig strains, with a few characteristics derived from human viral types completing the mix.[3] Until recently no animal reservoir of type B viruses was believed to exist; however, this type of influenza virus has now been found in harp seals.[4]

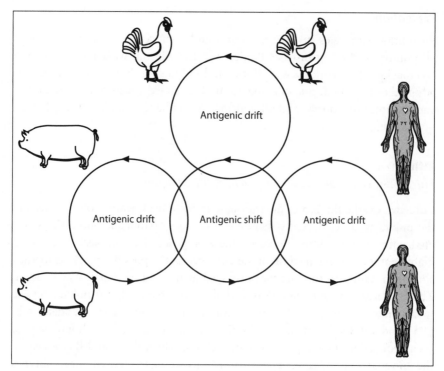

Figure 3.1 Antigenic shift and drift and the infection cycle in influenza.

Birds, pigs, humans and horses have been identified as reservoirs for the influenza viruses, most of which are species specific. The organisms cycle within the susceptible species, and remain within that population. Wild populations of these creatures can also maintain the virus, with wild boar carrying different viral types to the domestic swine in the same locality. Occasionally an outbreak of pure strain virus associated with another species, such as birds or pigs, has caused human disease.

It is more usual that infection in another species other than the normal host follows a mutation of the causative virus. Flocks of birds and herds of pigs can be decimated by outbreaks, which are seasonal, from viral subtypes particularly pathogenic to that species.

As stated above, in general, pure avian or swine-derived subtypes have a low potential to cause human disease and, although most workers in these industries can be demonstrated to have the antibodies to these families of viruses, clinical disease is rare. There are notable exceptions. In 1976, a type A virus arising from pigs caused anxiety when it was identified in army recruits at Fort Dix in the USA. Antigenically similar to 1918 Spanish flu, fears arose that a pandemic might occur. However, the outbreak was confined to the camp and did not cause any fatalities, although it was capable of transmission from person to person and caused severe symptoms.

The World Health Organization (WHO) states that a prompt response to the emergence of new strains is essential, especially where they have high toxicity potential. The pathogenicity of any subtype not only stems from its ability to cause severe symptoms but is also related to the potential for person-to-person spread. The identification of a new pathogenic viral subtype, now known as H5N1, led to a widespread cull of pigs in Hong Kong during October 1999.

The three conditions for a pandemic are that a new influenza subtype has to emerge, it must be able to infect humans causing serious illness, and it spreads easily and sustainably among humans. Currently the H5N1 virus does not spread easily from birds to humans and also person-to-person spread has been very rare (and as yet not fully substantiated) and seen only where continued close contact between victims has occurred, which could also be the result of a common source of exposure.

The first two conditions for a pandemic have been met. It awaits the last condition being met to see whether the current avian epidemic will escalate to a full human pandemic. Of concern is that there is no pre-existing immunity in humans to H5N1 and there is currently no vaccine, although many of the leading health organisations in the world are cooperating over vaccine research and development programmes together with vaccine manufacturers.[5]

As a result of concerns over a pandemic, most of the current focus on influenza centres on H5N1; however, there are a number of other pathogenic subtypes currently circulating. Serious clinical disease in humans in the Netherlands was caused by H7N7 in 2004.

Mexican Swine Flu (H1N1) – May 2009

As if to prove that with the influenza virus it is mandatory to expect the unexpected, in late April 2009, a new strain virus, now characterised as H1N1, emerged in Mexico, as this volume was going to press. Dubbed 'swine flu' by the media, as most initial cases had contact with pigs, it is an influenza A virus, with a mixture of elements of avian, swine and human-derived viruses. It has shown the ability to transfer from human to human, and this has led to the WHO Pandemic Index for this outbreak being raised to 6, following sustained human-to-human spread in more than two countries worldwide. This means that a worldwide pandemic is now in progress. The virus is currently susceptible to oseltamivir and zanamivir in most countries, but is resistant to amantidine. Some isolates in Denmark and Japan are now showing resistance to oseltamivir.

Initially blamed for over 100 deaths in Mexico, this has been revised downward reflecting only those cases confirmed by tissue sample (74 at 20 May 2009). Many (over 70) of the dead could not be tested. The picture may also be complicated by a possible concurrent outbreak of H3N2 in North America (USA, Canada, Mexico).

Carried by returning tourists and other air travellers, the virus had spread worldwide by mid-May, with the majority of the cases being in Mexico, the USA and Canada. The majority of the deaths outside of Mexico have been seen in patients who had other underlying health problems. The USA has declared a public health emergency, with cases reported across 48 states. In the UK, the approach to the outbreak switched in early July from a prevention to a treatment strategy, with prescribing of antivirals being restricted to serious cases.

Transmission

Infection in animals follows the inhalation of infected aerosols. There is often a fever of rapid onset, followed by cough and breathing difficulties. Copious quantities of mucus and nasal discharge are produced which, associated with the cough, produce further infected aerosols capable of continuing the infection in other individuals. Recovery is usually speedy, as is the only other possible outcome – death.

Disease in humans

The clinical pattern and treatment of H5N1 differ to other viral subtypes so the following section refers only to non-highly pathogenic (HP) H5N1 disease in animals and humans; for information on HP H5N1 see 'The current outbreak of HP H5N1'.

In humans infection similarly follows the inhalation of infected aerosols derived from infected individuals coughing or sneezing in the immediate vicinity. There are particular groups who are potentially more likely to catch the disease; the 'at-risk' groups are very young children because they have an immature immune response, elderly people, and those people with asthma, diabetes, kidney or heart disease. Individuals who are immunocompromised for whatever reason are also at higher risk of complications following infection. The incubation period is usually no longer than 2–3 days. Clinical onset is characterised by fever, with temperatures as high as 40°C that may last for up to 5 days. Associated with the fever are loss of appetite, headaches, lethargy, cough, generalised joint pain, sore throat and nasal discharge. Gastrointestinal disturbance may also be seen in children. Patients are probably infective from the time that symptoms appear up to about 5 days later. As the fever starts to subside nasal congestion sets in. Convalescence normally does not extend beyond a period of 2 weeks once the major symptoms resolve; however, in elderly people and other major at-risk groups bacterial or viral pneumonia may follow, with risks of mortality. Bronchitis can also arise in individuals with previous lung damage.

Diagnosis

Diagnosis is usually symptomatic, although for monitoring purposes swabs will be cultured to ascertain prevalent subtypes.

Treatment

Treatment in non-H5N1 cases in humans usually consists of simple symptomatic control. Patients are advised to rest and use suitable minor analgesics and anti-inflammatory drugs, preferably paracetamol or ibuprofen. Cough suppressants or mucolytics may also be useful. Dehydration is also a risk, so patients should be encouraged to drink copious quantities of fluids.

Amantadine is licensed in the UK as an antiviral for use against type A viral subtypes as an acute treatment or a prophylactic measure; however, it is currently not recommended by the National Institute for Health and Clinical Excellence (NICE). For acute cases in adults and children aged over 10 years a dose of 100 mg/day for 4–5 days is considered suitable. The same dose may also be used as prophylaxis in people identified as at risk but is not suitable for vaccination and healthcare workers. Prophylaxis may be extended, usually to 6 weeks or the end of an outbreak. Individuals who have been vaccinated can receive amantadine for 2–3 weeks until immunity develops. There are issues relating to the drug's use for treatment and prevention within the same household, arising from concerns over the possibility of viral subtypes developing resistance.

A therapeutic advance in the treatment of influenza (both types A and B) was the development of the neuraminidase inhibitors, zanamivir and oseltamivir. They are licensed for therapeutic use in the UK. Therapy has to be initiated as soon as possible after exposure and no later than 48 hours after the onset of clinical symptoms. The data available suggest that the duration of the infection can then be reduced by a day or several days, depending on how quickly it is used. The neuraminidase, an enzyme, prevents the virus from migrating from infected cells to the rest of the respiratory tract. Zanamivir is available as a dry powder inhaler with 5-mg blisters; the recommended adult dose is 10 mg twice a day for 5 days.

NICE currently recommends that they not be used for seasonal or post-exposure prophylaxis. They are also NOT to be used for the treatment of otherwise healthy individuals with influenza. NICE does recommend their use for post-exposure prophylaxis in at-risk adults, residents in care establishments and adolescents who are not effectively protected by vaccination; prophylaxis should commence within 48 hours of possible exposure. At-risk adults who show symptoms of influenza should be treated with these agents if they display symptoms of influenza, with treatment commencing within 48 hours of onset of clinical signs.

The current HP H5N1 outbreak

In 1997, a type A virus classified as H5N1 of avian origin with a high lethality was detected in Hong Kong. A comprehensive cull of all poultry (chicken, ducks and geese) was carried out in the region following the death of many chickens and several people. Of the 20 human cases recorded in this first outbreak, 6 died, and the 14 survivors were seriously affected and their convalescence was protracted. A subsequent outbreak in 2001 led to another cull. The source of this secondary outbreak is believed to have been the local wild bird population, because the primary cull of domesticated fowl was very complete.[6]

Since these first outbreaks, two forms of the virus have been identified: a low pathogenic type that causes only mild symptoms in birds, and a highly pathogenic type that causes dramatic rapidly and massively fatal outbreaks in wild bird and poultry flocks, with death following multiple organ failure, often within 48 hours of first infection.

The virus has spread rapidly across continents and is now viewed as being endemic in certain areas, with sporadic outbreaks with associated mortality in bird flocks. Its geographical spread has been unprecedented. The virus is now established in the wild bird populations and can move freely along migration routes.

H5N1 has also been seen in pigs, cats, dogs, civets and weasels. Some of the most dramatic cases were those in tigers in Bangkok Zoo where 141 animals out of a population of 447 died after ingesting infected raw chicken meat.[7,8] The virus is heat sensitive and can be destroyed by thorough cooking. This applies not only to meat but also to eggs.

UK animal cases to date

The only avian case of H5N1 at the time of writing in the UK associated with a wild bird was a case in Scotland. On 29 March 2006, a dead Whooper swan (*Cygnus cygnus*) was found at Cellardyke in Fife. In early April 2006, the swan was confirmed to have died from HP H5N1. There have been no further cases since identified in the wild bird population.

In February 2007, vets were called to the Bernard Matthews farm in Holton, Suffolk. Bernard Matthews is the largest provider to UK supermarkets of turkey products, and has extensive managed flocks of turkeys. Initial tests showed that 2600 of the birds had died of HP H5N1. A 3-km protection zone was established in a radius around the affected farm with a surveillance zone out to 10 km. Subsequently the rest of the flock were culled with 159 000 birds being gassed on site. The outbreak was linked back to imports of processed turkey meat from Hungary. No further outbreaks have occurred since.

The Department of the Environment, Food and Rural Affairs (DEFRA) have set up a series of protocols to control this and any future outbreaks. At the site of the outbreak all poultry have to be culled, visitors have to be disinfected and access is restricted. Within the 3-km zone all poultry have to be kept indoors and tested. Within the 10-km surveillance zone, there can be no movement of poultry to or from the area except for slaughter. No trains carrying live poultry can stop anywhere in the protection zone; all bird fairs and markets are banned. There is increased surveillance of wetlands for dead birds. Measures have to be made to isolate domestic from wild birds and prevent them sharing water – both for drinking and for swimming.

To prevent any risk of spread of H5N1, DEFRA introduced a ban on pigeon racing in July 2007. This followed the detection of the virus in wild birds in France.

So far in the USA only low pathogenic (LP) H5N1 has been isolated from wild birds in Michigan, Pennsylvania and Maryland, with no mass die-offs. The USA has imposed a comprehensive import ban on birds and bird products from all infected areas.

International surveillance and collaboration is happening on both a European and a global basis. Notification of outbreaks and statistics are shared as widely as possible, with human and animal case data being shared with organisations as diverse as the Organisation for Animal Health (OIE), the European Commission, WHO and many bodies involved in civil contingency planning.

Transmission of H5N1

The disease remains rare in humans; luckily, HP H5N1 has a low transmission potential, keeping the total number of cases and deaths relatively low. The virus seems to prefer to colonise the lower lung, hence the clinical symptoms and the current low transmissibility because infection requires a very narrow particle size, which does not cause deposition in the higher airways but is sufficiently large to give an infective inoculum.[9]

As of January 2009, there had been nearly 400 clinical cases of H5N1 in humans with an associated mortality rate of approximately 60% across the Near East, Middle East, Africa and south-east Asia. Unlike classic influenza, most cases have been in children and young adults younger than 40. Morbidity has been highest in 10–19 year olds. The most significant factor in contracting the disease is contact with sick or dead poultry (or wild birds) or their faeces, visiting a poultry market, or consumption of blood or meat from infected birds. Many of the cases in south-east Asia appear to relate to the close proximity of the population and their poultry in that area. Slaughtering, plucking, butchering and preparing birds for cooking have also led to infection.

The largest numbers of clinical cases of HP H5N1 to date in humans have been seen in Indonesia and Vietnam. There has been some evidence of human-to-human transmission with probable child-to-mother transfer in a Thai hospital. There have also been a numbers of clusters of cases seen in humans, mostly in blood-related family members living in the same household. It is not yet known if this reflects genetic susceptibility or is purely a common route of exposure to the pathogen.[10]

In human cases the incubation period is 3–4 days post-exposure with a range of 2–8 days. Initial symptoms include fever, sore throat, muscular aches, headache, lethargy and conjunctivitis. The H5N1 virus shows clinical symptoms similar to the 1918 Spanish flu of avian origin. Difficulty breathing with chest pains may rapidly progress to acute respiratory distress syndrome (ARDS) and multiorgan failure. Diarrhoea is often seen as a symptom, unlike in classic influenza.

Treatment of HP H5N1

In H5N1 cases the treatment regimen is very different. In Vietnam, Thailand and Indonesia resistance to amantadine has been seen in H5N1 cases.[11] This leaves the neuraminidase inhibitors oseltamivir (Tamiflu) and zanamivir (Relenza) as treatment options. The efficacy of these agents depends upon their early administration within 48 hours of symptom onset. The WHO recommends the choice of oseltamivir over zanamivir. Zanamivir has been effective against a small number of oseltamivir-resistant cases seen to date. There is also some evidence for the use of a neuraminidase inhibitor and amantadine in synergistic combination.[12]

In Vietnam, some cases of H5N1 demonstrate a rapid elevation of cytokine levels, which are associated with fatality. The rapid initiation of antiviral therapy can reduce this risk. Lymphopenia and thrombocytopenia have been seen in patients and have been linked to cytokine release, with increased fatality associated with the development of septic shock. This is the only reason for using corticosteroids in the treatment of influenza, and is not desirable but may be necessary as a life-saving measure.

Associated pneumonia should be treated with antibiotics only if necessary, and usually empirically with a β-lactam (cefotaxime, etc.) plus azithromycin or fluoroquinolones. Adjunctive therapy with oxygen may also be necessary.

Prevention of influenza (both classic and H5N1)

Due to the potential seriousness of an epidemic/pandemic, a new major public health monitoring scheme for influenza in the UK was introduced in late September 2006. A similar scheme is run in Scotland, called GP Flu Spotter, along with another scheme, the Scottish Enhanced Respiratory Virus Infection Surveillance (SERVIS). NHS Direct also has an analysed call data scheme that would allow epidemic monitoring, and is believed to offer an opportunity to monitor geographical spread. Given the name QFLU (QResearch Centre for Influenza), it monitors daily numbers of people being seen by general practitioners (GPs) with influenza and influenza-like illnesses, those suffering from respiratory infections, such as pneumonia, and the numbers being given antivirals. The Royal College of General Practitioners also collects data from GP practices. The Health Protection Agency (HPA) and Health Protection Scotland (HPS) have surveillance schemes monitoring types and subtypes currently circulating in the human population. This information, when collated for pathogenicity, case incidence and subtype, is passed to the Chief Medical Officer (CMO) and is used to drive campaigns aimed at increasing the uptake of vaccination in at-risk groups. Data is also fed into the WHO monitoring scheme.

The Medical Officers of Schools Association (MOSA) monitors infection in approximately 9000 children at 35 boarding schools. The Office of National Statistics also monitors deaths from respiratory illnesses such as bronchitis, pneumonia and influenza. All of these data are coordinated by the HPA Communicable Disease Surveillance Centres (CDSCs) in England and Wales, and Northern Ireland, and by the HPS.

The strategy for prevention is geared to the production and comprehensive uptake of an effective vaccine. The uptake of the vaccine is monitored by the HPA Centre for Infections (CPI), Colindale in England and HPS in Scotland.

In the UK and the USA, there is a major pandemic prevention and planning process being undertaken, involving an integrated approach across a large number of government departments. There is a programme of assistance for both domestic and international surveillance in both bird and human populations, and also support for clinical research into treatment and diagnosis. Stockpiles of vaccine and antiviral are being prepared for emergency use.[13]

As the circulating subtypes of influenza have the potential to mutate rapidly, preparation has to be predicted on emerging and current subtypes. The WHO makes the decision twice a year as to which subtypes should be used as the basis for the vaccine. This decision is based on the data that it derives from its monitoring laboratories in London, UK (the National Institute for Medical Research [NIMR]), Atlanta, USA, Tokyo, Japan and Melbourne, Australia, which are fed by a worldwide network of National Influenza Centres (NICs).

Following the decision, vaccine manufacture begins immediately, and is released as rapidly as possible. The effectiveness of the vaccine hinges on the sophistication and accuracy of the prediction and monitoring system. During the 2007–8 season, the UK Department of Health (DH) ordered 15 million doses of vaccine for administration in the UK.

In classic influenza, those individuals considered to be suitable and most likely to benefit from vaccination are elderly people, workers in social care and healthcare services, and those who are immunosuppressed. It is particularly important that elderly people in long-stay residential accommodation are vaccinated because a localised outbreak has the ability to spread rapidly. Physically fit adults under 65 years of age and children are not considered to need immunisation unless they are healthcare workers or carers, or they have chronic respiratory, renal, heart or liver disease.

In addition it was recommended for the first time by the HPA in 2007, for the 2007–8 season, for patients who have had a stroke or a transient ischaemic attack (TIA), have multiple sclerosis (MS) or a chronic degenerative neurological disease (i.e. Parkinson's disease), and all patients with diabetes. Individuals identified as at risk should be encouraged to stay at home rather than frequent public places during epidemics to avoid infection.

The decisions on classes of people requiring immunisation in the event of an H5N1 epidemic will be different, with essential workers across society being a major priority. This reflects anticipated mortality rates and the different pattern of infection that it displays.

Normally animals are not vaccinated against influenza; however, English zoos have been permitted to vaccinate their birds against avian influenza because of their vital role in global conservation. English zoos wishing to vaccinate their birds can now apply for permission, subject to meeting the eligibility criteria. During 2006–7, four zoos took advantage of the permission to vaccinate and proceeded to vaccinate their birds.

Vaccine development

A novel influenza vaccine is being developed by Immune Targeting Systems (ITS) in the UK. Their aim is to produce a 'universal vaccine' that provides protection against an emerging influenza subtype, including H5N1. ITS is not alone in trying to develop this type of vaccine, with companies across the world also attempting to develop a product that can be used against antigen families present across a spectrum of influenza A viruses. The resulting vaccine could be manufactured in advance of any pandemic and, although it would not offer complete strain specificity, it could give some protection until a strain-specific product could be manufactured.[14]

The vaccine contains immune response-stimulating complexes linked to antigenic proteins, giving a vaccine that is also capable of conferring immunity in the face of viral mutation. The technology may also be applicable to other rapidly mutating viral diseases such as HIV or hepatitis C.

In the USA, the government has set a challenge to the Defense Advanced Research Project Agency (DARPA) to develop new technologies for influenza vaccine technology and production.

Industry measures

In agriculture, importing poultry from areas where avian influenza is endemic is prohibited under the Animals and Animal Products (Import and Export) (England and Wales) Regulations 2000 and the Products of Animal Origin (Import and Export) Regulations 1996. All poultry, hatching eggs and poultry meat must be declared free of avian influenza and other notifiable diseases by the producer and the importer.

When the Ministry of Agriculture is informed of an outbreak, a declaration may be made by the Minister making it an offence to import specified animals and/or animal products from the affected country or region. This led to the banning of eggs and poultry from some regions of Italy during 2000.

Defra and the HSE's advice to poultry workers is that they should wear protective clothing, including respirators, wherever and whenever fowl plague is present in flocks. This is good practice at any time.

Cattle

Cattle are kept around the world for the production of meat, milk and cheese, and hides for leather. The zoonotic infections that cattle suffer are particularly important, not only because they are emotive (such as bovine spongiform encephalopathy/variant Creutzfeldt–Jakob disease [BSE/vCJD]), but also because of the widespread consumption of cattle products. Concerted efforts have been made over past decades to reduce the risks of particularly important zoonoses, such as brucellosis and bovine tuberculosis, and the success of the measures taken is demonstrated by the current low incidence of these diseases.

Prion disease is discussed further in Chapter 5, because its emergence is considered to be one of the most significant events of zoonotic transfer that has occurred recently in the UK. In the following section the diseases discussed are those that have either currently or historically been of significant healthcare importance.

Brucellosis
Mediterranean fever, undulant fever, Malta fever

Brucellosis was named after Bruce who, in 1887, identified the bacterium that caused Malta dog, a disease familiar to many generations of seafarers. He named this pathogen, which he isolated from goats' milk, *Brucella melitensis*. This is only one of the causatives of the group of diseases that are aggregated under the general name of brucellosis. They are caused by various species of *Brucella*, depending on source of infection and the associated animal host. As our knowledge and exploration of the bacterial fauna of other species have become more extensive, there has been the identification of varieties of *Brucella* associated with species as diverse as dolphins, seals and rats. Other species such as hares have been identified as carriers, capable of infecting other animals, particularly pigs, over wide geographical areas.[15]

The species responsible for most human infections are *B. abortus* from cattle, *B. melitensis* from sheep and goats, *B. canis* from dogs and *B. suis* from pigs. The diseases are distributed worldwide and are particularly prevalent in South America, Africa, the Mediterranean, Asia and eastern Europe, where large flocks of animals are tended, and eradication programmes are impracticable or unenforceable. The WHO has an ongoing programme of eradication by slaughter and vaccination aimed at controlling the disease in countries around the Mediterranean basin. A significant numbers of cases were seen in Malta during 1995, which led to cases in the UK in returning travellers. In England and Wales all cases seen in humans are known to have been acquired abroad, with 19 cases in 2004 and 8 in 2005. Some cases of *Brucella abortus* are seen in Northern Ireland; however, the rest of the UK declared eradication in 1993, and the use of pasteurisation, vaccination and slaughter inspection has been successful so far in preventing recurrence. *B. melitensis* has never been isolated from animals in the UK and is therefore not considered to pose a threat. Only a small proportion of dairy produce is derived from goats and sheep in the UK and there is a testing and screening programme in place, which constantly monitors for this pathogen.[16]

Disease in animals

In animals the main symptoms in all breeds suffering from the four main zoonotic strains previously mentioned are focal necrosis of the placenta, abortion and future infertility. The birth fluids and afterbirth are highly infective, and grazing cattle are infected by ingesting contaminated material from pasture. The disease is not apparent before the heifer aborts. Bulls may also be infected and can sexually transmit the pathogen, until ultimately becoming sterile. Cattle may be infected with any of the zoonotic strains, whereas horses appear to be resistant to all of the known zoonotic strains.

A new species of *Brucella* (tentatively named *Brucella maris*) has been identified in seals, cetaceans (whales, dolphins and porpoises) off the northern coast of England, in an otter from the south-western coasts of England, and in a bottle-nosed dolphin from California. It is unknown yet if this strain is zoonotic.[16]

Disease in humans

Disease in humans usually follows the ingestion of unpasteurised milk or milk products, contaminated with either *B. abortus* or *B. melitensis*. An alternative route for infection is by contact with contaminated bodily fluids, membranes or aborted young. In some countries where the disease is endemic, it may be spread at slaughter in abattoirs by direct contact with infected blood or meat. There is some evidence for aerosol spread by infected droplets or dusts. There have been isolated reports of human-to-human transmission by sexual contact, and also from mother to child by infected breast milk.[17,18]

Human disease presents with lymph node swelling, enlargement of the spleen, fever, testicular swelling, influenza-like symptoms, and lethargy, nausea and weight loss. Endocarditis or meningitis may follow, sometimes with fatal results.[19]

There is also a chronic undulant form that was often seen in people who work with cows and veterinary surgeons. Periodic bouts of high fever and clinical symptoms are interspersed with periods of remission with no clinical signs. This can persist for years or decades. The use of antibiotics quickly resolves most clinical cases; however, prolonged therapy may be necessary in refractory cases.

A septicaemic form is also occasionally seen. There is evidence that this is caused by the inhalation of infected aerosols in abattoirs and meat-processing plants where infected animals or their tissues are processed. It is characterised by an acute systemic disease with high fever.

Diagnosis

Diagnosis follows blood culture or using polymerase chain reaction (PCR) testing. The bacteria are relatively slow growing and successful culture in laboratories can prove difficult. Complement fixation is also now used in diagnosis.

Treatment

Treatment relies on the use of antimicrobials, usually in combination to prevent resistance. The *British National Formulary* (BNF) and the WHO recommend the use of doxycycline plus rifampicin or streptomycin. In the past co-trimoxazole was often used; associated toxicity has led to its replacement by more suitable agents. Therapy is usually prolonged; the WHO recommends 6 weeks as a minimum duration. The BNF recommends rifampicin 600 mg to 1.2 g daily in two to four divided doses with doxycycline 100–200 mg/day; the WHO recommendation is similar: rifampicin 600–900 mg/day plus doxycycline 200 mg. In severe cases streptomycin may be used in place of or in addition to rifampicin. Longer-term therapy may be required in the undulant form of the disease.

Quinolones in combination with rifampicin have undergone trials and been demonstrated to be as effective. Currently no effective vaccine for human brucellosis is available.

Prevention

Suitable protective clothing will reduce the risk from occupational exposure. The use of disinfectants, especially chlorinated or iodine- or ammonia-based products, can prevent environmental hazards. The mainstay of prevention is eradication by animal vaccination or slaughter programmes. On a personal basis, travellers to areas where the disease is endemic should be encouraged to avoid unpasteurised dairy products and undercooked meat.

Following the discovery of sea mammals infected with a variety of *Brucella*, which is not currently known to be zoonotic, the following advice had been offered by the HPA in the UK:

People who handle or work with seals or small cetaceans are advised to take suitable precautions to avoid any risk of infection although the new species of *Brucella* is not known to present any risk to human or animal health.

In domesticated animals, once *Brucella* is detected, often during routine testing and carcass screening, any infected beasts will be culled, and herds will be subject to a strict testing regime. Wild animals, such as deer that may be infected in the local area, will also be monitored *post mortem*.

Foot-and-mouth disease

It is questionable whether foot-and-mouth disease (FMD) is a zoonosis, although as a disease it has a huge economic impact for livestock farmers.[20] It does have a zoonotic potential, as a single case in the 1967 UK outbreak and one confirmed case in the 2001 UK outbreak demonstrated. However, the circumstances leading to human infection are usually extreme.[21]

The disease is found worldwide and all cloven-hoofed animals are affected. Caused by an aphthovirus, there are several different serotypes, of which the most virulent is serotype O (pan-Asiatic), which was responsible for the last UK epidemic.

Transmission

The virus can be transmitted by a number of routes, which include contact with already infected animals, infected aerosols (which can carry long distances downwind), fomites, and also uncooked or insufficiently cooked meat that is contaminated, especially where this is incorporated into animal feed.

Disease in animals

The first symptom of infection in animals is a high fever; blisters and ulceration develop on the mouth and the feet, leading to lameness and poor feeding ability. The disease spreads rapidly within herds, as infected animals are actively infectious and large amounts of live virus are produced before and after clinical symptoms start. Piglets are the worst affected, and the disease can cause high mortality.

Spread to other sites is believed to occur on the wind or by physical means, including vehicular, livestock or human movement. The virus can also infect wild deer which can then become a reservoir for infection.

Disease in humans

The WHO has recorded only about 40 confirmed cases of FMD in humans worldwide in the twentieth century, of which most were related to the O serotype. Transmission was first documented following deliberate ingestion of unpasteurised milk from infected cows by three German veterinary surgeons in 1834. In brief, very close contact with infected cattle or their products seems to be necessary for infection to occur.

Following an incubation period of between 2 and 6 days, clinical signs of infection commence. Blisters appear on the hands and sometimes on the feet and in the mouth and/or the tongue. Symptoms normally resolve spontaneously, usually within a week of the last appearance of blistering.[22]

Media misconceptions have much to do with the publicity that this condition has received. There is another, non-zoonotic, virus of the *Coxsackie* family that produces similar symptoms in children, called hand, foot and mouth disease, which leads to confusion, as may infection with other viral pathogens.

Diagnosis

Confirmation of the diagnosis is made by serology testing on clinical samples.

Treatment

There is no treatment except symptomatic support. Prevention of disease in humans is normally managed by protective clothing for personnel handling or culling infected animals, and the pasteurisation of dairy products. A vaccine is available for animal use; however, there is no provision or clinical need for its use in humans.

Prevention

Prevention of FMD in animals relies upon a host of organisations. Importation of infected foodstuffs, which then entered the animal food chain after inadequate heat treatment of swill, was probably the source of the latest UK outbreak. Customs services have the task of controlling this trade, but individual travellers may illegally import meat, meat products or contaminated dairy products into the UK in their luggage, making the task of control impossible. Importation of contaminated livestock has also been suggested as a means of spread, and outbreaks in continental Europe have been linked to infected livestock exported from the UK.

Locally, disinfectant in foot and vehicular baths helps prevent physical transfer. In the UK, DEFRA provides a list of disinfectants that are approved under the Diseases of Animals (Approved Disinfectants) 1978 as amended for use against FMD and/or in respect of General Orders (25 April 2001).

Case histories

The two confirmed human cases in the UK – the first in the 1966 outbreak and the other in 2001 – bear examination, if only to emphasise how difficult it is to catch the disease.

In 1966, a 35-year-old agricultural machinery salesman, Bobby Brewis, lived on a farm at Yetlington, Northumberland, with his brother. The cattle on the farm were slaughtered, having developed FMD. Mr Brewis took no part in the slaughter, but watched from some distance. Later he developed the symptoms of the disease. On being diagnosed he fainted, believing that he would be shot, like the infected cattle.

It is unclear how he became infected, but it is believed that he may have consumed milk deriving from the infected herd. As a result he was ostracised by the local community, lost his job and was last heard of as a fish-and-chip shop proprietor in Sunderland.

Details of the 2001 case are sketchier, with a confirmed case in a contract worker employed to cull cattle in Cumbria. From the details released, it would appear that the man was contaminated while dealing with a carcass. Material from the dead or dying animal sprayed the man copiously, and he later developed symptoms of the disease. As a spokesman for the then Public Health Laboratory Service (PHLS – now part of the HPA) so neatly put it: 'If you place a human being in contact with that size of inoculum, there is always a chance they will develop the disease.'

Pseudo-cowpox
Milkers' nodules, milkers' wart, paravaccinia, false cowpox

This is caused by a parapoxvirus, known as paravaccinia virus or milkers' nodule virus (MNV). It is endemic in cattle worldwide. The virus is closely related to orf and bovine papular stomatitis virus, both of which are capable of causing zoonotic infection.[23]

In cattle, horseshoe-shaped crusted lesions or erosions are seen around the mouth and nose, with papules or other lesions on the teats and udder.

Considered to be an occupational disease, human infection follows contact with infected cattle, especially the teats of infected cows; however, infection can also be via fomites because the causative agent is resistant to desiccation.

As it is usually self-limiting, most people involved in the cattle industry accept that they will be infected and, as immunity follows infection, most cases are not seen by, or notified to, healthcare workers.

Disease in humans

Following infection, there is a pre-patent period of between 4 and 21 days. The clinical presentation is usually a single painful or itchy nodule on the digits, hands or lower arms. This develops into a reddened, weeping and then crusted lesion, which heals, usually with little or no scarring.[24] In rare cases, where systemic infection occurs, there may be fever, lymph node swelling, skin rashes and secondary infection. Sometimes gastrointestinal disturbance may occur.

Diagnosis

Differential diagnosis may be difficult and is often based on patient history. Culture of the causative virus usually takes longer than the course of the disease. Differentiation between milkers' nodules and orf is impossible in most settings.

Treatment

There is no treatment, although use of antibiotics and local antiviral cream prevents secondary infection and may accelerate healing. Symptomatic treatment may also be useful in reducing fever and other symptoms.

Prevention

Gloves should be worn when handling animals suspected of being infected; however, due to the self-limiting nature of the disease, and its ability to survive on fomites, this may just defer rather than prevent infection and associated immunity.

Q fever
Query fever, Balkan influenza, abattoir fever

Q fever, first described in Australia in the 1950s, is a disease that stems from cattle, although it usually causes no symptoms in the host animal. It is caused by a rickettsia, *Coxiella burnetii*, an obligate intracellular bacterium. The causative organism has a global distribution and it is possible for many species, including ticks, fleas and lice, as well as many vertebrates, to carry the disease. The main significant zoonotic reservoir is considered to be bovines and also sheep. Once infected, the organism colonises and produces infective foci in the mammary glands and the placenta of pregnant animals. During birth large quantities of the organism can be found in the amniotic fluid and on the placenta. The organism is capable of forming an environmentally resistant spore form capable of forming the inoculum for delayed outbreaks. Surveys carried out on dairy herds in England and Wales suggest that up to 20% of all stock may be infected.[25]

The presence of the organism in milk results from the colonisation of the mammary system, and host animals can carry the disease for prolonged periods, with shedding occurring sporadically or constantly during lactation. The organism is resistant to heat but ideal pasteurisation conditions will remove it from milk; however, there is a risk from unpasteurised or incompletely pasteurised milk or milk products. It has been postulated that urine or faeces from infected animals may also be a carrier medium for the organism.

Seventeen cases of Q fever were reported in England during 2005, and six in Northern Ireland. Most cases were in male agricultural workers who were probably exposed to the pathogen in the course of their work.

Transmission

Transmission to humans usually follows exposure to infected material and DEFRA considers it to be an occupational zoonosis of agricultural and other workers closely involved with cattle and sheep. The people at highest risk are veterinary surgeons and stock people who assist at births, although the organism is highly resistant to desiccation and therefore can infect individuals working with hides, fleece or bones of infected animals. Transmission is by direct contact with contaminated materials, especially the afterbirth or material contaminated with amniotic fluid. There is some evidence that inhalation of dust from infected straw or bedding and even soil may also cause infection. Further down the food-processing chain, transport drivers and abattoir workers may also be at risk. Drinking milk or consuming contaminated milk products is also a possible route of infection, and transmission via ticks, lice or fleas has been demonstrated.[26]

Disease in humans

Most exposed individuals display no signs of clinical disease. Infection rates and recording of clinical cases correspond to lambing and calving cycles, allowing for the time lag associated with the organism's incubation period. After infection there is an incubation period of between 2 and 4 weeks followed by an acute onset with high fever, associated chills, profuse sweating and severe headache. Unlike other rickettsial diseases, in humans there is no skin rash. The patient may also present with anorexia, sickness and lethargy. The fever may last anything from 9–14 days and can recur at intervals, with a total duration of up to 3 months. A dry cough may be present, with pain in the chest cavity similar to pleuritic pain. 'Cracking' in the chest may also be heard during respiration. Lesions in the lungs may be apparent on radiographic examination. Liver enlargement or tenderness with associated hepatitis-type symptoms can be seen.

Untreated cases can resolve within 5–14 days, although symptoms may not regress for more than 7–8 weeks and relapses may occur. The untreated fatality rate is estimated at 1% of cases. Following severe infection there may be a need for prolonged convalescence. Elderly patients are particularly badly affected by this disease and may require prolonged supportive measures.

A chronic form also exists that causes a prolonged endocarditis leading to valvular damage, especially of the aortic valve. Recent figures show that damage is more common in patients with pre-existing valve damage. Symptoms can appear long after the disease has run its clinical course and may require replacement of damaged valves. The fatality associated with this form is estimated to be as high as 60% of cases unless corrective surgery is undertaken. Chronic hepatitis also develops in a small number of cases.

Diagnosis

Diagnosis follows serological testing, because the organism is slow growing and almost impossible to culture from clinical specimens. There are several techniques, of which the most reliable are indirect immunofluorescence, complement fixation, enzyme-linked immunosorbent assay (ELISA) and microagglutination.

Treatment

C. burnetii can be difficult to treat because it can show a lack of response, rather than true resistance to antibiotics. The BNF recommends the use of tetracyclines at usual clinical doses, and historically chloramphenicol has been used, although it is reserved for recalcitrant infections due to the incidence of major side effects. The length of the course may require adjustment so that therapy is extended for a period of days after the fever regresses to prevent relapse. Patients with endocarditis and valvular damage will need prolonged prophylaxis up to and beyond surgery, with valve replacement or repair. Studies have shown that the organism has a heightened susceptibility to combinations of drugs, which results in acidification of the intracellular vacuole. Chloroquine in combination with doxycycline has been used with some notable success, although there is a need for continued patient observation to prevent build-up of chloroquine in the eye. A minimum of 3 years' therapy prevents relapse.

Prevention

As with many other zoonoses, prevention strategies revolve around good personal and environmental hygiene. Bedding contaminated by postpartum material and the material itself should be carefully handled, with collection and subsequent burying or incineration. Disinfection of housing and other areas should be carried out with DEFRA- or USDA-approved products. Protective clothing, including respirators, overalls and gloves, must be worn wherever feasible. In the USA a vaccine for cattle has been developed; it is not licensed for use in the UK. Carrier animals have been subject to eradication by slaughter policy. Nevertheless, the organism is considered to be widespread in the environment and preventing animals from becoming infected is deemed to be practically impossible. All milk and milk products should be pasteurised, and monitoring of the process should be maintained in the normal manner to ensure that optimal temperatures and duration standards are met.

Tapeworm

The beef tapeworm (*Taenia saginata*, also known as *Cysticercus bovis*) and the pork tapeworm (*T. solium*), which is found in pigs and wild boar, are very similar in both overall appearance and life cycle. They are both members of the cestode worm family, and the definitive host for both worms is humans: the tapeworm reaches maturity only in the lumen of the human gut. The associated animal is an intermediate host, necessary for the larvae to infect humans after ingesting infected, inadequately cooked meat from a suspect carcass. Comparison with *Echinococcus granulosus* is of interest (see p. 36); this is also a cestode, but humans are blind intermediate hosts, and the usual cycle uses dogs as a host and sheep as a full intermediate host – the exact reverse of *Taenia* spp.[27]

In 2005 there were 72 reports in England and Wales made to the HPA of human infection with *Taenia* spp. Of the patients, three were travellers and were considered to have become infected while abroad. There have been no reported cases of *T. solium* in the UK since 1994. In the USA, most cases are seen in recent migrants, usually from Latin America, and specifically Mexico.

General parasitology and disease in humans

The adult worm is flat in cross-section and widens gradually from the head or scolex, through the proglottids or body segments. The scolex attaches to the gut wall of the host by means of suckers and/or hooks, depending on the species involved.

The body segments or proglottids are produced from just behind the scolex, and the oldest and most mature are at the opposite end of the worm. As the segments mature they develop both male and female reproductive organs, self-fertilise and produce eggs that are contained within the proglottid wall. The mature proglottids break away from the body (or strobila, consisting of all the proglottids and the scolex) and pass out of the gut via the anus. The secondary or intermediate host, in which the larvae can develop, is then infected by ingestion of either the eggs or embryos present in faecal matter.

The tapeworm absorbs nutrients from the gut of the host over its whole body surface, and has a rudimentary nervous and digestive system. The worms are host specific and exist as an adult solely in the gut of their preferred host. When eggs hatch in the gut of a host, either primary or intermediate, larvae penetrate the wall of the gut, and then migrate to a preferred site, usually in muscle tissue or other organs. In either pigs or cattle these normally migrate and encyst again in muscle tissue, where the cyst may develop daughter cysts with multiple internal scolices.

Alternatively they may migrate to other organs and cause a condition known as cysticercosis. The beef tapeworm rarely causes cysticercosis; however, the pork tapeworm can cause this condition in humans. In cysticercosis the migrating larvae encyst in sites as diverse as the brain or other areas of the central nervous system (CNS), eyelid and conjunctiva. The condition is seen mainly in intermediate hosts, but may also be seen in humans, where either eggs or larvae are ingested, or where the gravid proglottid (a mature proglottid full of eggs or embryos) ruptures in the gut before it can be expelled.

In cysticercosis, the cysts may be quiescent or active. Where active cysts are present they undergo a budding and proliferation process, called racemose cysticercosis, leading to a series of connected cysts with multiple scolices in the vacuole. When the cysts are sited in the brain, complications, including neurological disturbances, follow.[28] The intensity and type of symptoms seen in cases of neurocysticercosis depend upon the number of lesions present and their location, size and status. Live foci are usually asymptomatic; as the cysts degenerate and die there is a progressive inflammatory response causing encephalitis and swelling. Epileptic seizures are the most frequent symptom. Meningitis, raised intracranial pressure and paraesthesia may also occur.

Adult beef tapeworms can reach a size of between 12.5 and 25 m in length; the pork tapeworm is much smaller, only reaching between 2 and 7 m. They are usually solitary occupants of any infested gut as multiple worms can cause intestinal obstruction. The beef tapeworm differs from the pork tapeworm in having no hooks on the scolex. Both species are capable of producing a strobila of 1000–2000 proglottids, and can live for up to 25 years. There are few symptoms associated with the adult worm, except slight irritation of the site of attachment or vague abdominal symptoms with hunger pangs, loss of weight and general condition, indigestion, diarrhoea and/or constipation. Discomfort and embarrassment may be caused by migrating proglottids when they reach the anus. The proglottids may be seen with the naked eye, either grouped or as single segments in the stool. The proglottids may be mobile when moist, becoming quiescent as they become desiccated.

Diagnosis

Definite diagnosis of infestation either follows isolation of eggs or proglottids from the stool or protrusion of a portion of the strobila through the anal sphincter.

Serological testing using ELISA methods confirms diagnosis, and in cases of cysticercosis imaging by computerised tomography, radiology or magnetic resonance is usually necessary. Biopsy of subcutaneous cysticerci will also confirm other findings.

Treatment

For adult tapeworms treatment is undertaken using either niclosamide or praziquantel. The BNF states that niclosamide is available from IDIS Ltd (see Appendix 2) on a named-patient basis. It is solely active against adult worms and does not kill larval stages. Side effects are usually limited to gastrointestinal disturbances and itching with occasional rash. To prevent any risk of cysticercosis by autoinfection following emesis, an antiemetic should be given at the same time as the niclosamide, on wakening.

Praziquantel is available from Merck on a named-patient basis. It is deemed to be as effective as niclosamide, and should be given at a single dose of 10–20 mg/kg body weight after a light breakfast.

There is some controversy surrounding treatment of cysticercosis. Usually surgical removal of the cysts is advocated in humans before damage ensues, with concomitant administration of anthelmintics. This is very important in infection associated with the eyes.[29]

In CNS involvement, symptom control of associated epilepsy is achieved using the usual anticonvulsants. The BNF does not make any recommendations on the use of anthelmintics (or cestocides) in neurocysticercosis; however, elsewhere in the world praziquantel or albendazole has been routinely used. Albendazole is a benzimidazole anthelmintic and is approved for treatment of only hydatid disease and neurocysticercosis in the USA. It is teratogenic in animals, so a careful risk–benefit analysis must be carried out before it is used in women who are pregnant or of child-bearing years. It is hepatotoxic, and can also destroy bone marrow, so complete blood chemistry analyses and liver function tests should be routinely carried out before and during therapy. There are risks associated with the use of anthelmintics in neurocysticercosis, because they can cause serious adverse effects, so a risk–benefit analysis always has to be undertaken.[30]

To obtain a cestocidal effect praziquantel at an oral dose of 50–100 mg/kg per day three times daily for 30 days or albendazole at 15 mg/kg orally two to three times a day for 8–15 days, depending on radiological findings, has been shown to destroy viable cysts. Symptomatic treatment is also necessary to ensure good clinical outcome.

Prevention

Tapeworm infection is not common in the UK or the USA due to a strict system of meat inspection. This is not true of the rest of western Europe. Germany and France report significant numbers of cases annually, associated with the consumption of infected meat in national delicacies. In non-Muslim developing countries there is a high incidence of the disease, causing more than a third of all cases of adult-onset epilepsy. Due to the longevity of the parasite, immigrants from these countries could present with symptoms of the disease long after their arrival in the UK. In the USA there have been sufficient cases among migrant workers for the condition of cysticercosis to be routinely tested in cases of epilepsy among this sociological group. The numbers of tourists travelling to areas of risk, such as south-east Asia, the Indian subcontinent and Africa, have increased dramatically in the past decade, so tapeworm infestation should be excluded in any diagnostic path relating to persistent abdominal symptoms or seizures following such trips.

Suspect meat or meat products should be thoroughly cooked, avoiding wherever possible eating meat from dubious sources that is either raw or under-cooked. Suspect carcasses or meat should be frozen for at least 3 weeks to kill any larvae. Viable eggs or embryos may also be present in water contaminated by faecal matter; the usual precautions when drinking water of unknown quality should be applied.

Separation of human sewage and intermediate host animals is important in breaking the infective cycle. Sewage sludge should not be used to dress pasture where animals destined for human consumption are actively grazing or housed. Care should be taken after flooding where there is a possible risk of human sewage contaminating pasture.

Recent work on a vaccine to prevent animals from becoming infected has shown promise.[31]

Bovine tuberculosis

Although the prime cause of tuberculosis (TB) in humans is *Mycobacterium tuberculosis* (var. *hominis*), there are still some cases recorded annually of the condition being caused by the closely related zoonotic organism *M. bovis*. In England and Wales fewer than 1% of cases of TB are caused by *M. bovis*. Clinical signs and symptoms seen in the infection are identical regardless of which of the two mycobacteria is present. The disease can also infect a large number of other mammal species, and has become a source of bitterly contested debate between cattle farmers and wildlife groups in the UK over the role of badgers as a reservoir of infection. In the USA, the case rate of M. bovis is also approximately 1% of all TB cases. There is a connection to the consumption of dairy products sourced in Mexico; however, there are some cases linked to domestic cattle, with wild deer acting as a wildlife reservoir.

Disease in animals

The primary reservoir of M. bovis was historically cattle. Early control measures were focused on improving herd hygiene, culling infected beasts and preventing spread within herds. The most effective control measure was the development of reliable pasteurisation of milk, the primary source of transfer of infection from cattle to humans.

Within cattle herds the disease is transferred by aerosol inhalation with subsequent pulmonary infection, in addition, infection from cow to calf has been well documented, as has reinfection of TB-free herds by infected humans. Badgers suffering from the disease have long been suspected of infecting cattle. The hard scientific evidence is sketchy, and the mechanism of transmission is as yet unproven. The bacterium has also been found in many other species of animal, both in the UK and elsewhere in the world, with pigs, sheep, goats, horses, cats, dogs and foxes all being capable of carrying infection in endemic areas. In the USA, there is a monitoring programme in place to ensure that cattle herds are disease free and, except for some licensed producers, all dairy products are pasteurised. Deer and other wild animals act as a reservoir, so continual review of disease status in domesticated cattle is required.

In the UK, cattle have been compulsorily and routinely tested using the tuberculin skin test since the 1950s. Beasts with a positive test are slaughtered as a mandatory requirement under the Tuberculosis Orders (1984) and related Orders made under the Animal Health Act 1981. The provision within the legislation for agreed valuation and compensation payments to farmers has been a major asset in achieving farmers' agreement to the measures. Investigation of herds may also stem from veterinary slaughterhouse inspection of cattle and carcasses.

Testing frequency depends upon known regional prevalence, and has led to the UK achieving disease-free status. Devon, Cornwall, the West Midlands, South Wales and Northern Ireland have the highest current incidence of the disease in cattle; the level has risen since an all-time low in the 1980s. In 2006, a total of 50 327 tests were carried out across the UK. A total of just over 22 000 cattle were slaughtered as test reactors, contacts or inconclusive test reactors. The disease is only controlled, not eradicated, and could re-emerge if vigilance is not maintained.

Clinical signs in cattle are variable. Some animals rapidly lose condition and cough, and there may be udder involvement in dairy cattle. Other cattle may remain sleek and healthy; it was not unknown in the past for the best-looking beast in a herd to be the most infective. Ulcers may be seen in a cutaneous form of the disease that can affect some animals, usually with advanced disease. Generalised symptoms may be seen, with diarrhoea and enlargement of the liver and spleen. Pulmonary disease normally develops from a soft cough to haemoptysis. Physical examination of the walls of stalls for blood-stained mucus was a very primitive method of determining infection in animals, and fortunately this has now been superseded. Any of the other major organs can become affected, and persistent, extensive lymph node swelling may be present. Skeletal involvement can also occur. Paralysis of the hindquarters may occur in some cases.

Transmission

Transmission normally follows the ingestion of inadequately or non-pasteurised infected milk or dairy produce. Stock handlers are also at significantly elevated risk if their charges are infected. Transmission may follow inhalation of infected aerosols, or skin contact with cutaneous lesions on infected animals. In the UK only 34 cases of confirmed human infection were reported in 2006; in two of the cases multi-drug-resistant *M. bovis* was responsible. There was nothing to link any of the cases with diseased cattle, so these may represent reactivated disease contracted at an earlier date.

Elsewhere in the world control programmes have not been as effective in cattle, so there is a risk of infection following ingestion of dairy produce, especially in developing countries.

Disease in humans

Clinical symptoms vary depending on the source of contamination or route of infection, although this is not always associated. General symptoms include weight loss, pronounced fatigue and fever, all of which may gradually worsen. The classic pulmonary pattern of the disease may be seen with cough and haemoptysis. Ulcers or other lesions may be present in cutaneous disease. As with cattle, the organism can colonise any or all of the major organs or the skeleton, producing symptoms related to site and severity of infected foci. In the USA it has been found that TB patients infected with *M. bovis* are more likely to have extrapulmonary disease with organ or tissue involvement than those with *M. tuberculosis*.

Patients may be asymptomatic for long periods after infection. Activation and progression of disease may then occur when disease or age affects the immune system. Many of the current cases are among elderly people who were infected in their youth. The disease poses a considerable risk, along with other mycobacterial infection, to patients suffering from human immunodeficiency virus (HIV)/Acquired Immune Deficiency Syndrome (AIDS). Other people at an enhanced risk of contracting the disease are veterinary and animal workers. Migrant workers and members of other immigrant groups may also have the disease; however, as treatment of M. *bovis* and M. *tuberculosis* is similar, drug therapy of one will normally eradicate the other.[32]

In England and Wales, 25 cases of TB were caused by M. *bovis* in 2006, down from 28 cases in 2005. There were three cases in Northern Ireland, and six in Scotland in 2006. A cluster of six cases was seen between 2004 and 2006, in a socially closely linked group, with possible person-to-person transmission, because not all the cases, including one that was fatal as a result of M. *bovis* meningitis, could be linked to the consumption of unpasteurised dairy products.[33]

In the USA, there have been several studies into M. *bovis* infection. In New York City a cluster of cases was studied. Approximately 1% of all cases of TB seen were associated with M. *bovis* and the patients were mostly Mexican or Latino, either by ethnicity or by descent. The same pattern had previously been noted in a monitoring exercise undertaken in San Diego, California. Most infections were related to the ingestion of imported, unpasteurised, Mexican cheese. Studies have shown that 20% of milk produced in Mexico and 17% of meat are infected with M. *bovis*.

Diagnosis

Diagnosis follows positive skin reaction to tuberculin purified protein derivative (PPD). Bacille Calmette–Guérin (BCG) inoculation produces a positive test, so this must be excluded. Radiographic imaging, sputum testing or ELISA of samples supports the findings from skin testing. Differentiation of the causative *Mycobacterium* sp. usually follows growth of the organism; however, this can be difficult. PCR assay has been used to this end, with considerable success.

Treatment

The treatment of infection with M. *bovis* is identical to that for M. *tuberculosis*, and should be carried out by specialist centres. The regimens suggested by the Joint Tuberculosis Committee of the British Thoracic Society are normally used in the UK, and are regularly updated as data relating to prevalence of resistant serotypes are forthcoming. It is not appropriate for the regimens to be discussed in detail because these change rapidly.

In the USA, a standard four-drug regimen is used for the treatment of TB, consisting of isoniazid, rifampicin, pyrazinamide and ethambutol. Pyrazinamide-resistant isolates of M. *bovis* have been found. Since 2003, streptomycin is no longer routinely used in the treatment regimen due to both the emergence of resistant strains and safety concerns.[34]

Prevention

Prevention in animals revolves around the cattle scheme, as outlined above. Other animals may contract the disease and are usually destroyed if found to be positive for the disease.

Personnel at particular risk should wear protective clothing when handling suspect animals, and must be immunised whenever possible. BCG vaccine is made from a live attenuated strain of *M. bovis*, and is used to immunise people against contracting TB from both animal and human sources. In response to the reduction in the number of cases of TB seen in the UK, the immunisation programme has changed. Up to 2005, all children were routinely inoculated with BCG vaccine when they reached the age of 13. Since then, immunisation against TB has become targeted with vaccination being offered to babies living in areas of the UK where there is a high incidence of TB (i.e. 40 cases per 100 000 people per year, or more), or babies whose parents or grandparents lived in a country with a high incidence of TB.

Children (< 16 years) who have come to live in the UK from countries where TB is common (i.e. at least 40 cases per 100 000 people per year) who have not previously been immunised, and adults < 35 years who have come to live in UK from countries where there is a high rate of TB (> 500 cases per 100 000 people per year), or unimmunised contacts of patients with TB are also offered the vaccination.

In addition those people who are at a high occupational risk such as health workers, emergency service workers, prison staff and some public transport employees are routinely inoculated.

The vaccine should not be used in HIV-positive patients because it has been reported as causing cases of clinical disease. HIV-positive patients who travel to countries where *M. bovis* is endemic should be advised to boil all milk and abstain from any dairy produce that has not been pasteurised or cooked.

Sheep

Historically, the UK has always been a prolific producer of wool. In the seventeenth century, sheep were known as 'God's own animal', not only because of associated Christian symbolism but also because the sheep gave wool for textiles, meat for the table and milk or cheese. There are many varieties of sheep, and many have been specially bred for fleece or meat quality. Other breeds have been developed for hardiness in large areas of the UK, especially in upland areas in the North or in Wales where no other agricultural enterprise is possible due to the poor quality of the land and its pasture.

As a result of the numbers of animals involved, and the amount of human contact sheep receive, especially when lambing, there are a number of zoonotic conditions that are particularly important. It will come as no surprise that most cases of these diseases are reported from rural areas, and knowledge of these conditions is especially important in these regions.

Chlamydiosis (gestational psittacosis)

Infection with *Chlamydophila psittaci* has already been discussed in Chapter 2. Chlamydophilae are all intracellular dwelling parasites and have a strange biphasic reproductive cycle, in which only one phase is infective. Previously, it was not possible to determine if the *Chlamydophila* spp. responsible for infection in birds was the same as that seen in sheep and other species, because the serological and PCR tests used for diagnosis were not sensitive enough to produce species differentiation. Recently, the species have been differentiated and reclassified, and it is now known that the species of *Chlamydophila* responsible for infection in sheep and goats is a separate species, *C. pecorum*, and has been found in cattle, goats, sheep, swine and koalas, although it is not implicated in causing abortion. The species found specifically associated with cases of abortion in cattle, sheep and occasionally humans is identified as *C. abortus*. As it is difficult to determine the species present in animals from the clinical signs, the notes below provide general information. In addition to the main species mentioned above, there is another, *C. felis*, found in cats, which is also zoonotic, that is responsible for rare cases of conjunctivitis (see below).

Disease in animals

The species found in sheep, goats and occasionally cattle can cause a chronic infection, particularly in female animals. The disease in sheep is known as enzootic abortion, and in flocks with high incidence of infection is a major cause of economic losses due to low numbers of live-birthed lambs. It is usually isolated from the uterus and reproductive organs. In pregnant animals it causes placental insufficiency and abortion. The infection appears to be transmitted between animals by either the sexual or the faecal–oral route. Infected animals pass live organisms in the faeces, and after abortion or birth the organism is found plentifully in the uterus, vagina and placental material. Lambs may also be contaminated, especially while still wet and before maternal cleaning has occurred. The incidence rate in sheep is not known; however, in 2005, out of 1272 diagnoses of sheep abortion in the UK, this organism was implicated in 464 ewes. Numbers of cases of abortion in sheep related to *Chlamydophila* spp. in the last decade have ranged between 1000 and 1700 annually. No human abortions were attributed to *C. abortus* in 2005, although nine infected women were identified; luckily none was pregnant.

Transmission

Transmission to humans follows inhalation of dried faecal matter, direct contact with faeces, or contact with pregnant or postpartum ewes, lambs, birth fluids or placental tissue. The organism is capable of surviving desiccation and survives in dung or soil for several months.

Disease in humans

Following infection there is normally a 1- to 2-week pre-patent period. The disease usually then presents as an influenza-like illness with cough and congestion followed by high fever, aching muscles, and occasional back and abdominal pain. Respiratory symptoms are common, with dry cough and pneumonia. Anaemia and liver dysfunction with hepatic and splenic enlargement may also be present.

In pregnant women the disease may be life threatening. This form was first identified and reported in the UK in 1967, and is luckily rare. The disease can progress to give placental insufficiency, neonatal distress, and late term miscarriage or premature birth. In some cases, emergency termination may be necessary to save the mother's life. Disseminated clotting may occur in all major blood vessels.[35,36]

Diagnosis

Diagnosis is usually made using immunofluorescence techniques, ELISA or PCR tests.

Treatment

Tetracyclines or erythromycin is the drug of choice. Erythromycin is preferable in pregnant women because tetracyclines are contraindicated in pregnancy, although in resistant cases they may need to be used where the benefits of treatment outweigh the risks. Caesarean section at early term may also be necessary.

Prevention

Sheep may be vaccinated to reduce the incidence of enzootic abortion and shedding of organisms. Suitable protective clothing should be worn, including face protection, when handling pregnant ewes. Ewes that have aborted should be isolated until any vaginal discharge ceases.

Pregnant women should, wherever possible, avoid contact with pre-, peri- or postpartum ewes or goats, and kids or lambs. Contact with placental material or aborted lambs must be avoided. They should not handle unwashed overalls that may be contaminated with blood or secretions from ewes or lambs, or milk ewes. Any pregnant woman who has been in contact with sheep should seek medical advice if she has an onset of influenza-like symptoms or fever.

Additional notes

There is another species of *Chlamydophila*, *C. felis* (feline keratoconjunctivitis agent), which typically causes rhinitis, pneumonia or conjunctivitis in cats. This strain can also be transmitted to humans, but it is extremely rare. The resulting conjunctivitis responds to the use of antibiotic eyedrops or eye ointment, particularly chlortetracycline or fusidic acid.[37]

Giardiasis

Giardiasis is caused by the flagellate protozoan *Giardia lamblia*. It has a worldwide distribution and, although humans are one of the main reservoirs for the disease, it is considered to be zoonotic because sheep, cattle, pigs, dogs, birds such as budgerigars and parrots, and other species are known to harbour the parasite. It is a biphasic protozoan, having an encysted and a free-living or trophozoite form. The trophozoite is killed by gastric acid so only the encysted form poses a risk of infection to humans. The disease is endemic in developing countries where it is prevalent in most animals and children. Giardiasis is recognised not only as an issue for public health, but also as a traveller's zoonosis and as an infection of other risk groups domestically.[38]

Disease in animals

Infected animals may be asymptomatic; alternatively they may have weight loss with chronic diarrhoea and partially formed fatty stools. The parasite matures and reproduces in the host's intestine and is then passed with the stool. Once expelled, the cysts can survive adverse environmental conditions for prolonged periods.

Transmission

Faecal contamination of water or food and its subsequent consumption by humans is the most common route of infection. Water from wells or other ground systems can be contaminated with faecal matter, and when either unfiltered, or inadequately filtered, before consumption poses a significant risk. Tap water in countries with poor infrastructure support can also be a source of infection.[39]

The oral–faecal route of infection is also common, especially in children. The cysts are infectious virtually immediately they are passed in the stool, so person-to-person spread can occur as a result of poor personal hygiene. This can be of particular importance in care settings, such as day care, nurseries and other premises. Fomite spread by faecal contamination of surfaces or objects is well documented.

In addition to young children and elderly people living in communal settings, the other risk groups are travellers (especially those on a budget using poor-quality accommodation or eating in substandard venues), outdoor enthusiasts, sexually active homosexual males and immunocompromised individuals. Patients with HIV will often present with giardial infection; untreated this appears to adversely affect clinical outcomes and survival times.[40]

Disease in humans

The inoculum necessary to produce clinical disease has been estimated at as low as a single viable cyst, making it extremely infective. Following ingestion the cysts hatch in the small intestine. They can live free in the gut lumen or attach to the gut wall. The parasite reproduces rapidly and encysts as it progresses towards the large intestine. Infection may be asymptomatic; in other patients clinical signs appear after a pre-patent period of between 1 and 4 weeks.

The disease may present as diarrhoea of either chronic or acute nature, and of either mild or severe character. Unlike other organisms, the stools are associated with considerable gas and are usually fatty, frothy and foul smelling. They are usually free from blood or mucus. There is associated bloating, gastrointestinal spasm and abdominal pain. The patient may feel weary and nauseous, and report loss of weight and appetite. Dehydration may occur.

Untreated, the condition normally lasts for 1–2 weeks. Some individuals can develop a chronic form of the disease that may last for months or years, which leads to chronic malabsorption states with associated anorexia. Disaccharide intolerance may develop in almost 40% of any giardial sufferers during and for up to 6 months after infection. Once resolved, infection seems to confer some immunity against reinfection.

Diagnosis

Diagnosis has traditionally been by isolating viable cysts from faecal material of suspected sufferers. An ELISA test is now available, as is a fluorescent antibody test, which simplifies rapid confirmation of clinical findings.

Treatment

Metronidazole is the treatment of choice for giardiasis – either 2 g/day for 3 days or 400 mg three times a day for 5 days. Alternatively, tinidazole as a single dose of 2 g or mepacrine hydrochloride 100 mg every 8 hours for 5–7 days can be used. Mepacrine is unlicensed in the UK for this condition; however, it is available on a named-patient basis or as a special item from

BCM (see Appendix 2). As previously mentioned, rehydration therapy may be necessary as an adjunct to other therapy.

Chronic cases are often refractory, requiring repeated treatment courses to achieve elimination of the protozoan.

Prevention

The following general advice is applicable to many faecal-borne pathogens, and also forms a backbone of good practice for travellers. In countries where the disease is endemic or suspected, drink only bottled water and avoid drinking water or consuming foods that have not been washed in bottled water. Hot drinks, prepacked carbonated drinks and pasteurised items are usually safe. Ice in drinks made from local water should be avoided. Only fruit or vegetables that have a peel or can be peeled and then washed should be consumed. Any vegetables should be washed in bottled or boiled water and adequately cooked.

When consuming water from a suspect source is the only alternative, water purification tablets should be used or the water should be boiled before consumption.

Domestically, normal hygiene routines of washing hands after defecating and before handling food prevent spread. For care workers and others working where faecal contamination of patients or objects is commonplace, wearing gloves and ensuring that personal hygiene is observed aid prevention of infection and also spread.

Individuals with HIV should be encouraged to have their companion animals tested for giardiasis regularly and treated to eliminate the organism if present. Objects, areas and materials contaminated with animal faeces should be disinfected and cleaned. In severely immunocompromised individuals, pets may need to be housed permanently indoors to prevent reinfection.

Orf
Contagious pustular dermatitis

Orf is caused by a parapoxvirus of the *Poxviridae* family. It is endemic in sheep and goats and occurs globally; some herds are completely free of the organism. At present there is considerable discussion as to whether the incidence of the disease has been increased by the vaccination of herds where there was previously no history of cases.

Disease in animals

In sheep or goats, crusty lesions on or around the muzzle, eyelids, mouth, feet or external genitalia may be laden with virus. Necrosis of the skin of the gastrointestinal and urogenital tract can occur. The virus is shed by infected animals in secretions from lesions and also in faeces and urine. The virus is persistent in the environment and may survive for many years. The disease is under-reported because most farmers and veterinary surgeons recognise the condition and do not need to submit samples to confirm the diagnosis. In 2005, 27 incidents in sheep were recorded in the UK at government-associated laboratories. Since 1991 the number of recorded diagnoses of the condition in sheep has varied between 24 and 58 (average 40 per year).

Transmission

Orf is an uncommon disease in humans; however, it is easily transmitted by contact with lesions on animals or infected wool. Accidental infection with live vaccine during vaccination of sheep also poses a risk.

Disease in humans

After infection, ulcerative suppurating lesions on face, hands and arms appear. Shepherds, sheep shearers and others who handle live sheep, warm carcasses or unprocessed fleeces or wool are at risk.[23]

The low number of cases reported by laboratories is likely to represent a small proportion of the total number of cases seen by GPs in rural areas as diagnosis of human orf infection is often made on the basis of clinical presentation and history.

Cases of infection with parapoxviruses are generally under-reported. In 2005, one human case was reported in Scotland, and one in England and Wales occurred in an abattoir worker. There were no human cases reported in Northern Ireland in 2005. An annual average of 8 (range 1–25) cases of orf virus infection were identified between 1991 and 2005.

Treatment

Treatment is purely supportive, because no therapy is recommended. Lesions usually regress within 6–8 weeks with minimal scarring. Secondary infection of sores may occur and management using antiseptics or antibiotics may be required.

Prevention

Good hygiene practices and wearing rubber gloves when handling infected sheep helps to prevent infection in individuals at risk due to their occupation. Fomite contact may also be responsible for spread, and prevention strategies centre around good disinfection procedures. Care when using the live attenuated vaccine to vaccinate flocks is essential.[41]

Pigs

Introduction

Although the domestic pig industry has gone through a difficult period in the last decade, there are still approximately 4.94 million pigs in the UK, of which approximately 82% are in England. Much of the industry still focuses on the intensive pig unit, using selectively bred animals geared to the requirements of producers for rapid growth and of consumers for lean bacon and pork.

With the current increase in grain prices, and the programme of set-aside land coming to an end, it is unclear what acreage in the UK will be available for outside pig enterprises; however, there is an increasing demand by consumers for better welfare, and thus retailers are moving to require this from producers. This has the added advantage for producers that they are able to gain higher returns on their products while satisfying the demands for high welfare products by consumer lobby groups. It has also enabled producers to return to using older breeds of pig, with a reduction in the therapeutic interventions and medicated foodstuffs associated with intensive enterprises. It should also not be forgotten that some producers have switched to wild boar or boar/pig hybrids in an attempt to develop new products and tastes for the public palate.

The pig has always been considered to be the best and easiest option for xenotransplantation, and is considered to be closest of all our domesticated animals in biochemical terms to humans. Therefore it can be readily seen that diseases of pigs are likely to have a significant potential as zoonoses.

Ascariasis
Large roundworm

Infection with roundworm is estimated to affect at least 1 billion people worldwide. The intestinal nematodes of the genus *Ascaris* are common culprits. *A. lumbricoides* is usually deemed to be a human-to-human parasite transmitted by the faecal–oral route. The related worm *A. suum* is normally found in pigs; zoonotic cases have been seen. The infection is more common in areas where sanitation or hygiene routines are inadequate. Travellers to developing countries can return having been infected, as may immigrants or refugees. A previous infestation does not prevent reinfection, so patients who have been successfully treated can present with the same condition after subsequent exposure.[42]

Disease in animals

Parallel symptoms and signs are seen to human infection (see below). Migrating larvae can cause pulmonary symptoms. Symptoms of abdominal pain with diarrhoea or enteritis may be present. It is usually suckling pigs or weaners that show the worst effects. The condition is rarely fatal; however, larvae that migrate to sites other than the gut can produce unusual and severe symptoms. The cycle time from egg to adult is believed to be quicker in pigs infected with A. *suum* than it is in humans.

Transmission

Infection can be by one of two routes, either directly from ingestion of soil contaminated with eggs, or after the ingestion of vegetables or salad containing viable eggs adhering to it. The eggs hatch in the duodenum and migrate through the gut wall and then via the bloodstream to the lungs.

Disease in humans

The condition may be asymptomatic or initially there may be generalised symptoms of fever and headache. Symptoms derive initially from the immune response to the infestation from either the organism itself or its metabolic products. Larvae can cause pulmonary symptoms, with asthma, pneumonia, cough and wheeze. The larvae are usually coughed up or migrate up the bronchi and are then swallowed again.

Once they return to the gut the larvae will pass through their remaining larval stages. Adults will breed in the gut; the female worm is larger than the male. Females may reach up to 35 cm in length and 4 cm in diameter. They may migrate into the biliary or pancreatic ducts. Symptoms may include gastric cramps, vomiting and diarrhoea. Pancreatitis can occur, as may intestinal obstruction and malnutrition with weight loss. Jaundice may be seen if the common bile duct is obstructed.[43,44]

The whole cycle from egg to adult takes about 2 months. Eggs passed in the faeces become infective after 2 weeks. Some larvae may not migrate directly to the lungs and can cause complications arising from their travels or residence in the brain, eyes, liver or kidneys. The worm and its larva cause sensitisation. In some patients allergic reactions, some of which are severe, can be seen when reinfection occurs.

Diagnosis

Eggs may be identified in the stool; larvae or adults may be seen in faeces or recovered from the throat, mouth or nose. Larvae may also be present in sputum. Ultrasonography, computed tomography or endoscopy may assist the diagnostic process.

Treatment

The condition is usually treated with anthelmintics. The BNF states that levamisole (available from IDIS Ltd – see Appendix 2) is very effective against A. *lumbricoides* and is considered to be the drug of choice. Well tolerated, it can cause nausea and vomiting in approximately 1% of patients. A single dose of 120–150 mg in adults is normally sufficient to resolve the condition. Mebendazole may be used at a dose of 100 mg twice daily for 3 days. Piperazine has also been used but is considered to be less suitable due to the incidence of side effects. When used it should be given as a single dose of 4–4.5 g for adults as piperazine hydrate. Albendazole, metronidazole and pyrantel have all been used for human treatment in the USA.

Physical removal may be possible during endoscopic investigations. Larvae that migrate to sites other than the lungs during the invasive phase of development may require surgical removal. The use of anthelmintics may be associated with this migration, because it can cause larvae to flee the gut into other body organs in a random manner, leading to further complications. Early treatment of *Ascaris*-related pancreatitis usually results in complete recovery, although untreated cases can lead to a fatality rate of 3% in endemic areas.

Prevention

Vegetables and salads should be thoroughly washed before consumption to reduce or remove any contamination. Pig manure should not be used as a fertiliser or slurry on field, where produce is being actively grown.

Pasteurella
Shipping fever, fowl cholera

Pasteurella spp. form a group of well-recognised pathogens that are responsible for species-specific diseases. There are currently moves to rename at least some of this group of bacteria as *Mannheimia* spp. One member of the group, *P. multocida*, has particular zoonotic potential.

Disease in animals

The organism can cause pneumonia with concurrent pleurisy in pigs, often in a mixed infection with other *Pasteurella* spp. or mycobacteria. Infected pigs are feverish and display pulmonary insufficiency, with exaggerated gasping and panting. There will often be production of blood-flecked foam from the lungs, which can be seen in the mouth. Untreated cases can be fatal. A septicaemic form of the disease has also been seen in pigs and other mammals. Transmission between animals is usually by aerosol transfer.

In poultry the course of infection is very different. Turkeys, hens and other birds exhibit overwhelming diarrhoea, which is rapidly fatal in unvaccinated birds. This is normally due to *P. multocida*, although other *Pasteurella* spp. may be present and synergistic in the disease.

Transmission

In addition to pigs and birds, many dogs, cats and horses carry *P. multocida* as part of their oral flora, and can transmit it to other animals and humans via aerosols or saliva. These animals are often asymptomatic. Direct inoculation can occur through animal-inflicted bites or wounds. Ingestion of contaminated food or water can also lead to development of the disease.[45]

Disease in humans

Following transmission to humans there is usually localised inflammation around the infected bite or wound, followed by abscess formation and septicaemia. Pneumonia and meningitis may also occur, depending on the route of infection.

Infection by this organism is a serious risk, particularly to children, who tend to receive more bites from companion animals in rough play, to elderly people and immunocompromised individuals, in whom infection can be rapidly progressive and fatal. Septicaemic forms have been seen in patients with HIV/AIDS or liver cirrhosis, or who are on chemotherapy regimens.[46]

The disease is notifiable, and the HPA receives on average notification of approximately 200 cases annually, usually following bite injuries.

Treatment

Antibiotic therapy at standard therapeutic doses is normally sufficient to cure the condition, although in more serious cases supportive treatment may also be required. The drugs of choice are the tetracyclines, penicillins or cephalosporins; length of course and dosages are linked to age, weight, drug allergies and clinical response in the normal manner.

Prevention

Wounds, especially those inflicted by animals, must be thoroughly and rapidly cleansed and disinfected. Companion animals should not be allowed to lick patients' faces or wounds. Encouraging children to wash their hands and, if necessary, faces after playing with or touching animals is an important preventive measure. Vaccination is available and widely used in pigs and poultry to lower the incidence of the disease. Those involved in equestrian pursuits should recognise that bites from horses pose a particular threat from this organism.

Case study

In August 2006, a farmer's son in Suffolk died after catching *Pasteurella multocida* from dead rabbits. The 29 year old is believed to have been infected through a raw blister on his hand which became contaminated by infected body fluids from the rabbits. He contracted the bacterium on 1 August and died in Ipswich Hospital 4 days later. He initially displayed symptoms of flu, and then died from overwhelming septicaemia.

Streptococcus suis

Disease in animals

Streptococcus suis is a pathogenic streptococcus endemic in most countries that have domestic or wild swine. There are at least 35 different serotypes recorded, and of these the type 2 serotype is classically responsible for severe disease in swine, and also for the occasional cases seen in other animals including cattle, sheep, dogs, cats and birds. This serotype is also responsible for most cases in humans, although recently serotype 14 has been recognised as having the capability to be a human pathogen. The disease is prevalent in China, possibly due to the high density of pig farms and the number of swine processed annually.

Infection is often not apparent, with the pathogen being carried in the tonsils and nasal cavities; however, in clinical cases it can cause pneumonia, septicaemia, septic arthritis, endocarditis and meningitis, with behavioural changes, fever and ultimately paralysis. It may also cause abortion in pregnant sows. Infections in herds of swine can result in high rates of mortality and are often the result of poor husbandry or housing conditions.[47]

Transmission

Transmission to humans follows the handling of infected meat or carcasses, and it is therefore no surprise that most cases occur in abattoir workers, meat handlers, farm workers or veterinary surgeons where the disease is an occupational hazard. The annual case rate in humans is usually in low single figures, which suggests that the risk is low. In the UK, the disease is notifiable under the Statutory Notifiable Disease 1998 Notification of Infectious Diseases System (NOIDS) regulations, the Reporting of Injuries, Diseases, and Dangerous Occurrences Regulations 1995 (RIDDOR 95) and animal health legislation. It is also a prescribed industrial disease and reportable to the HSE if acquired occupationally.

Disease in humans

Following infection, usually through cuts or skin abrasions, the pathogen can cause severe infection in humans, with fever, septicaemia and, very occasionally, meningitis or endocarditis. Infection can lead to toxic shock syndrome, which may in turn lead to multiple-organ failure. Residual deafness and balance disturbances have been reported in patients after the infection has resolved. Asplenic or immunosuppressed patients are at a greater risk. *S. suis* infection is rare among humans in England and Wales: an average of two human cases are reported each year. In 2005, two cases were reported in England and Wales. There were no cases in Scotland and Northern Ireland. The last fatal case in the UK occurred in a farm worker in 1999, due to *S. suis* type 14. During 2004 a total of 112 isolates were found in pigs in England and Wales, of which 46% (51) were *S. suis* type 2.

Diagnosis

Diagnosis is confirmed by culturing the organism or using PCR assay. Treatment is usually initiated before identification.

Treatment

Treatment is usually oral penicillins or erythromycin with monitoring as to efficacy, because resistant serotypes have been identified in mainland Europe.

Prevention

Prevention revolves around good hygiene procedures and the use of protective clothing. All wounds should be covered and any occurring during handling of meat or carcasses should be disinfected thoroughly and dressed swiftly. An experimental vaccine has been developed for animals but the clinical efficacy has not yet been fully established.

Case History – S. suis *type 2 outbreak in China*

In south-west China's Sichuan Province, 215 people became ill, of whom 39 died between June and mid-August 2005. All the initial victims were from villages and towns across Yanjiang and Jianyang districts, and were farmers or butchers or had had contact with sick and dead pigs or sheep before becoming ill. Some also ate meat originating from the same beasts.[48]

Later cases were reported with a wider distribution across the region, including cases in Chengdu, Hong Kong and Guangdong. Media reporting of the outbreak was allegedly controlled, and the WHO did not gain access to the area. The WHO noted the 'disconcertingly high mortality rate' and said that it was monitoring the situation closely. Raw pork was impounded by officials in Nanshan, Shenzhen and Guangdong, and movement of live pigs was halted. People who had consumed cooked pork were monitored. Other provinces of China, Macau and Hong Kong halted sales of frozen pork from Sichuan, Shenzhen and Henan. Vietnam banned imports of all live pigs and pork products. Taiwan requested residents to refrain from travelling to Sichuan and its neighbouring areas following the outbreak. These precautions, which were endorsed by the WHO, prevented further spread.[49] Initially there was also concern that the cases could have resulted from infection with a Nipah-like virus, or by a porcine influenza; both of these possibilities were excluded through sample testing.

The disease onset was rapid, associated with high fever, fatigue, nausea and vomiting, followed by meningitis, the appearance of bruising, toxic shock, coma and then death. Initial cases were suspected of having haemor-rhagic fever with renal syndrome, but laboratory testing excluded this. The course of the disease and its high fatality rate have been linked to its short latent period and ability to cause multiorgan failure. The head of an expert panel set up by the Chinese Ministry of Health stated that some patients died within 10 hours of infection, and in one case a man died 2 hours after slaughtering a sick pig.[50]

Laboratory tests confirmed infection by *S. suis* serotype 2 of a particularly virulent and aggressive strain that produced a potent exotoxin. The pathogen was also isolated from pigs in the region. An emergency team from Beijing was deployed to Sichuan to assist in treating patients.

A complicating factor in this particular outbreak may also have been the presence of a tranche of population in rural areas in China who have been infected with HIV due to trading in human blood. Any aggressive toxin or infective agent could rapidly kill individuals with this underlying condition.

There was no reporting of person-to-person spread.

Trichinosis or trichinellosis

This condition is caused by a tissue nematode of the genus *Trichinella*. In the past most cases were associated with *T. spiralis*, but recently there have been cases of other *Trichinella* spp., such as *pseudospiralis*, *britovi* or *nativa*, causing human disease.[51]

The parasite is normally associated with pigs (*T. spiralis*, *T. pseudo-spiralis*) and dogs (*T. nativa*). Rats, cats and certain wild carnivores or omni-vores are also capable of acting as zoonotic reservoirs. It is an affliction that is worldwide in its distribution, but is luckily rare in the UK and the USA, often being associated with imported meat, or affecting returning travellers. The FSA carried out a survey on foxes in the UK for the presence of *Trichinella* spp. between September 2004 and March 2005. All tests were negative; however, since then, *T. spiralis* has been detected in a fox in Northern Ireland.[52] All carcasses of pigs and horses slaughtered in the UK are routinely tested for *Trichinella* spp. and no positive results have been found.

Disease in animals

Pigs fed on offal or swill containing meat (especially pork) that has not been sufficiently heat treated are at the greatest risk of contracting the disease, although there have been cases recorded after pigs have eaten the corpses of rats. The number of human cases seen in western countries has been dramatically reduced by changes in feeding practice for pigs and by meat inspection. A group of cases of *T. pseudospiralis* in 1999 was related to the ingestion of wild boar meat in the Camargue area of France,[53] and a further group outbreak was seen in October 2003, in southern France, related to the consumption of frozen wild boar meat, although the causative organism was characterised as *T. britovi*, which is not normally associated with swine.[54] Some of the largest outbreaks have been seen in Thai migrant workers in Israel who ate uninspected meat from wild boar killed in the Upper Galilee valley. In a large outbreak in 2005, 18 of 47 workers who had consumed boar meat presented with symptoms and needed treatment.[55] The organism was characterised as *T. spiralis*. Turkey holds the record for the largest outbreak yet. In Izmir between January and March 2004, beef meatballs adulterated with pork infected with *T. britovi* were sold; 1089 patients presented to local medical services with symptoms, of whom 418 were diagnosed with acute trichinellosis.[56] In France there have also been sporadic human cases linked to the consumption of infected horse meat.[57]

Encysted larval stages are ingested in animal tissue and then hatch in the gut of the host; these then develop into adults in the surface layers of the intestine. Eggs are produced by the female worms, and these hatch to produce larvae. The larvae pass through the intestinal wall and penetrate into the associated lymphatic or venous blood vessels. They can then be distributed around the rest of the host's body and will normally encyst in muscle tissue as a result of the host's immune response. The cysts may become calcified over time and can be detected in the muscle. The fibres of the muscle may be torn or damaged by the invasion of the parasite. The affected animal normally displays no clinical signs of infection. Infection with *T. pseudospiralis* does not evoke the same immune response and the cyst wall is normally not present.

Transmission

As with other mammals, infection in humans follows the ingestion of infected animal tissue.

Disease in humans

The severity of symptoms displayed is proportional to the number of viable encysted larvae ingested. The mildest cases are usually subclinical, with perhaps a small amount of muscle soreness being present. In heavy infestations there may be an abrupt onset of muscle pain, fever and swelling of the eyelids, followed by haemorrhages in the retina, conjunctiva and mouth with associated pain. An aversion to bright light (photophobia) may also occur. The most commonly seen sites for larvae to encyst are the diaphragm, ribs, biceps, larynx, tongue and jaw, or neck muscles. This may lead to difficulties in chewing and swallowing.

As the infection progresses, patients may display a profound thirst, with profuse sweating. There may be gastrointestinal disturbance with diarrhoea, stomach cramps and nausea. In 10–20% of patients showing severe

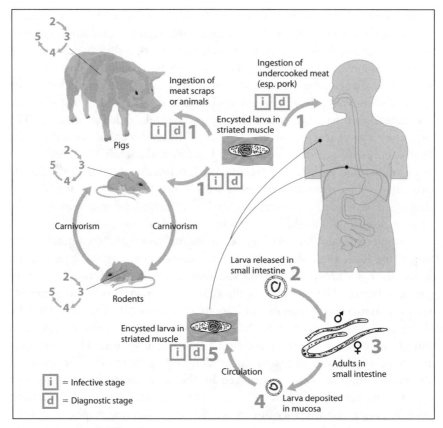

Figure 3.2 *Trichinella* life cycle.

symptoms there may be progression to cardiac, renal or CNS involvement. Fatalities due to myocardial failure have been recorded. Provided that patients do not succumb to the condition, it is normal for a complete recovery to be made over a period of months, although there may be residual damage with sequelae.

Between 1975 and 2005, 39 laboratory-confirmed cases of human trichinellosis occurred in the UK. All cases were believed to have contracted the disease abroad or from consumption of infected meat imported into the UK. The last recorded outbreak in UK was eight cases, reported in 2000. This also followed ingestion of infected meat or meat products imported into the UK. There were no human cases reported in England and Wales, Northern Ireland and Scotland in 2005.

Diagnosis

Diagnosis is made using serological testing or muscle biopsy. ELISA and PCR methods can be used successfully.

Treatment

Most cases resolve spontaneously, so purely symptomatic treatment and support are necessary. The BNF makes no recommendations, and specialist advice would be necessary in treating clinical cases of the disease. In the USA, tiabendazole anthelmintics such as mebendazole, tiabendazole or albendazole have been used to treat the condition. There is evidence, however, that once an infection is established these drugs only eliminate the adults and larvae in the gut, and prevent further egg and larval production, leaving any migrating or tissue-dwelling larvae intact.

Corticosteroids have been used to control the systemic inflammation caused by migrating larvae. The patients in the 1993 French case cluster of *T. pseudospiralis* were treated with albendazole at a rate of 800 mg/day for 10 days combined with prednisolone at a dosage of 30 mg/kg per day for the first 3 days. The outbreak among Thai migrant workers in Israel was treated with 5 mg/kg of mebendazole twice a day for 5 days.

Prevention

Ensuring that all swill or offal fed to pigs has been thoroughly heated at greater than 77°C prevents infection by ingestion of any infected animal tissue. Rats should be controlled in pig units and general hygiene measures, including the isolation and removal of sick individuals, should be enforced. There may be an issue relating to organic methods of pig rearing, and the possibility of infection being acquired from wild sources. This is also true of herds of domesticated or semi-domesticated boar, now extensively bred for meat in outdoor conditions. As *T. pseudospiralis* has now been identified as a possible human pathogen, there are some concerns that current meat inspection methods, which are geared to the detection of encysted forms, may not be sufficient, because this species does not evoke cyst formation response from the afflicted host. If more cases arise, there may be a need for alternative methods of detection.

Meat should be carefully inspected, and pork should be thoroughly cooked so as to reach more than 77°C in the centre. Suspect meat can also be rendered safe by prolonged freezing for more than 3 weeks.

References

1. Capua I, Alexander DJ. Human health implications of avian influenza viruses and paramyxoviruses. *Eur J Clin Microbiol Infect Dis* 2004; **23**: 1–6.
2. Bartlett JG. Avian influenza. *Medscape Infect Dis* 2006; 8(2): E-edn.
3. Tumpey TM, Basler CF, Aguilar PV *et al*. Characterisation of the reconstructed Spanish Influenza pandemic virus. *Science* 2005; **310**: 77–80.
4. Osterhaus AD, Rimmelzwaan GF, Martina BE, Bestebroer TM, Fouchier RA. Influenza B virus in seals. *Science* 2000; **288**: 1051–3.
5. WHO Update August 2007. Clinical management of human infection with avian influenza A (H5N1) virus. Geneva: World Health Organization, 2007.

6. To KF, Chan PT, Chan KF *et al*. Pathology of fatal human infection associated with avian influenza A H5N1 virus. *J Med Virol* 2001; **63**: 242–6.
7. Kaiken T, Rimmelzwaan G, van Riel D, *et al*. Avian H5N1 influenza in cats. *Science* 2004; **306**: 241.
8. Keawcharoen J, Oraveerakul K, Kuiken T *et al*. Avian influenza H5N1 in tigers and leopards. *Emerg Infect Dis* 2004; **10**: 2189–91.
9. van Riel D, Munster VJ, de Wit E *et al*. H5N1 virus attachment to lower respiratory tract. *Science* 2006; **312**: 399.
10. Nguyen TH, Farrar J, Horby P. Person-to-person transmission of influenza A (H5N1). *Lancet* 2008; **371**: 1392–4.
11. Hayden FG, Hay AJ. Emergence and transmission of influenza A viruses resistant to amantadine and rimantidine. *Curr Top Microbiol Immunol* 1992; **176**: 119–30.
12. de Jong MD, Thanh TT, Khanh TH *et al*. Oseltamivir resistance during treatment of influenza A H5N1 infection. *N Engl J Med* 2005; **353**: 2667–72.
13. McCullers JA. Preparing for the next influenza pandemic. *Pediatr Infect Dis J* 2008; **27**(10 suppl): S57–9.
14. Ilyinskii PO, Thoidis G, Shneider AM. Development of a vaccine against pandemic influenza viruses: current status and perspectives. *Int Rev Immunol* 2008; **27**: 392–426.
15. Abela B. Epidemiology and control of brucellosis in ruminants from 1986 to 1996 in Malta. *Rev Sci Tech* 1999; **18**: 648–59.
16. Godfroid J, Cloeckaert A, Liautard JP *et al*. From the discovery of the Malta fever's agent to the discovery of a marine mammal reservoir, brucellosis has continuously been a re-emerging zoonosis. *Vet Res* 2005; **36**: 313–26.
17. Mantur BG, Mangalgi SS, Mulimani B. *Brucella melitensis* – a sexually transmissible agent? *Lancet* 1996; **347**: 1763.
18. Palanduz A, Palanduz S, Güler K, Güler N. Brucellosis in a mother and her young infant: probable transmission by breast milk. *Int J Infect Dis* 2000; **4**: 55–6.
19. Miguel PS, Fernández G, Vasallo FJ *et al*. Neurobrucellosis mimicking cerebral tumor: case report and literature review. *Clin Neurol Neurosurg* 2006; **108**: 404–6.
20. David W, Brown G. Foot and mouth disease in human beings. *Lancet* 2001; **357**: 1463.
21. Prempeh H, Smith R, Muller B. Foot-and-mouth disease: the human consequences. *BMJ* 2001; **322**: 565–6.
22. World Health Organization. *Foot and Mouth Disease: Consequences for Public Health*. Geneva: WHO (CSR), 2001. Available at: http://www.who.int/emc/surveill/index.html.
23. Groves RW, Wilson-Jones E, MacDonald DM. Human orf and milkers' nodule: a clinicopathologic study. *J Am Acad Dermatol* 1991; **25**: 706–11
24. Strenger V, Müller M, Richter S *et al*. A 17-year-old girl with a black eschar. Cowpox virus infection. *Clin Infect Dis* 2009; **48**: 91–2, 133–4.
25. Tissot-Dupont H, Raoult D. Q fever. *Infect Dis Clin North Am* 2008; **22**: 505–14.
26. Raoult D, Tissot-Dupont H, Foucault C *et al*. Q fever 1985–1998: clinical and epidemiologic features of 1383 infections. *Medicine (Baltimore)* 2000; **79**: 109–23.
27. Garcia HH, Moro PL, Schantz PM. Zoonotic helminth infections of humans: echinococcosis, cysticercosis and fascioliasis. *Curr Opin Infect Dis* 2007; **20**: 489–94.
28. Kaiser C, Pion S, Preux PM, Kipp W, Dozie I, Boussinesq M. Onchocerciasis, cysticercosis, and epilepsy. *Am J Trop Med Hyg* 2008; **79**: 643–4.
29. Proano JV, Madrazo I, Avelar F *et al*. Medical treatment for neurocysticercosis characterized by giant subarachnoid cysts. *N Engl J Med* 2001; **345**: 879–85.
30. Garcia HH. Antiparasitic drugs in neurocysticercosis: albendazole or praziquantel? *Expert Rev Anti Infect Ther* 2008; **6**: 295–8.
31. Sciutto E, Rosas G, Hernandez M *et al*. Improvement of the synthetic tri-peptide vaccine (S3Pvac) against porcine *Taenia solium* cysticercosis in search of a more effective, inexpensive and manageable vaccine. *Vaccine* 2007; **25**: 1368–78.
32. Esteban J, Robles P, Soledad Jiménez M, Fernández Guerrero ML. Pleuropulmonary infections caused by *Mycobacterium bovis*: a re-emerging disease. *Clin Microbiol Infect* 2005; **11**: 840–3.

33. Evans JT, Smith EG, Banerjee A *et al.* Cluster of human tuberculosis caused by *Mycobacterium bovis*: evidence for person-to-person transmission in the UK. *Lancet* 2007; **369**: 1270–6.
34. CDC. Treatment of tuberculosis: American Thoracic Society, CDC, and Infectious Disease Society of America. *MMWR* 2003; **52**(RR11): 1–77.
35. Meijer A, Brandenburg A, de Vries J, Beentjes J, Roholl P, Dercksen D. *Chlamydophila abortus* infection in a pregnant woman associated with indirect contact with infected goats. *Eur J Clin Microbiol Infect Dis* 2004; **23**: 487–90.
36. Daniel M, Jorgensen DM. Gestational psittacosis in a Montana sheep rancher. *Emerg Infect Dis* 1997; **3**: 191–4.
37. Hartley JC, Stevenson S, Robinson AJ *et al.* Conjunctivitis due to *Chlamydophila felis* (*Chlamydia psittaci* feline pneumonitis agent) acquired from a cat: case report with molecular characterization of isolates from the patient and cat. *J Infect* 2001; **43**: 7–11
38. Adrabbo K, Peura D. Giardiasis: A review. *Pract Gastroenterol* 2002; 15–29.
39. Yoder JS, Beach MJ, Centers for Disease Control and Prevention (CDC). Giardiasis surveillance – United States, 2003–2005. *MMWR Surveill Summary* 2007; **56**: 11–18.
40. Aronson NE, Cheney C, Rholl V, Burris D, Hadro N. Biliary giardiasis in a patient with human immunodeficiency virus. *J Clin Gastroenterol* 2001; **33**: 167–70.
41. Health and Safety Executive. *Common Zoonoses in Agriculture 6/05.* Agricultural Information Sheet AIS2(rev). Sudbury, Suffolk: HSE, 2005.
42. Bethony J, Brooker S, Albonico M *et al.* Soil-transmitted helminth infections: ascariasis, trichuriasis, and hookworm. *Lancet* 2006; **367**: 1521–32.
43. Choudhury SY, Kaiser MS. Varied presentation of biliary ascariasis and its consequences. *Mymensingh Med J* 2006; **15**: 150–2.
44. Soomro MA, Akhtar J. Non-operative management of intestinal obstruction due to *Ascaris lumbricoides. J Coll Physicians Surg Pak* 2003; **13**: 86–9.
45. Freshwater A. Why your housecat's trite little bite could cause you quite a fright: a study of domestic felines on the occurrence and antibiotic susceptibility of *Pasteurella multocida. Zoonoses Public Health* 2008; **55**: 507–13.
46. Koch CA, Robyn JA. Risk of animal contact in immunocompromised hosts. *Arch Intern Med* 1998; **158**: 1036.
47. Segura M. *Streptococcus suis*: An emerging human threat. *J Infect Dis* 2009; **199**: 4–6.
48. World Health Organization. Outbreak associated with *Streptococcus suis* in pigs, China. *Wkly Epidemiol Rec* 2005; **80**: 269–76.
49. Huang YT, Teng LJ, Ho SW, Hsueh PR. *Streptococcus suis* infection. *J Microbiol Immunol Infect* 2005; **38**: 306–13.
50. Hashikawa S, Iinuma Y, Furushita M *et al.* Characterization of group C and G streptococcal strains that cause streptococcal toxic shock syndrome. *J Clin Microbiol* 2004; **42**: 186–92.
51. Gottstein B, Pozio E, Nöckler K. Epidemiology, diagnosis, treatment, and control of trichinellosis. *Clin Microbiol Rev* 2009; **22**: 127–45.
52. Zimmer IA, Fee SA, Spratt-Davison S, *et al.* Report of *Trichinella spiralis* in a red fox (*Vulpes vulpes*) in Northern Ireland. *Vet Parasitol* 2009; **159**: 300–3.
53. Ranque S, Faugère B, Pozio E *et al. Trichinella pseudospiralis* outbreak in France. *Emerg Infect Dis* 2000; **6**: 543–7.
54. Gari-Toussaint M, Tieulié N, Baldin J *et al.* Human trichinellosis due to *Trichinella britovi* in southern France after consumption of frozen wild boar meat. *Eurosurveillance* 2005; **10**: 117–18.
55. Hefer E, Rishpon S, Volovik I. Trichinosis outbreak among Thai immigrant workers in the Hadera sub-district. *Harefuah* 2004; **143**: 656–60, 694.
56. Akkoc N, Kuruuzum Z, Akar S *et al.* A large-scale outbreak of trichinellosis caused by *Trichinella britovi* in Turkey. *Zoonoses Public Health* 2008.
57. Boireau P, Vallée I, Roman T *et al. Trichinella* in horses: a low frequency infection with high human risk. *Vet Parasitol* 2000; **93**: 309–20.

4

Food-borne zoonoses

Food-borne zoonoses are defined as 'those diseases contracted from eating foods of animal origin'. This is a broad definition and covers a wide spectrum of pathogens, although the most important on a day-to-day basis are mainly bacteria.

The importance to our society of food-borne zoonoses must not be underestimated. In 2000, the Health Protection Agency (HPA) in the UK estimated that there were 1.4 million cases of food poisoning, not all of which had a zoonotic source, which led to approximately 21 000 hospital admissions and 480 deaths. It is considered by some healthcare organisations, that due to the likelihood of under-reporting the actual case figures are much higher.

Our domestic system of agricultural production is regulated to reduce transmission of disease into the food chain, and considerable sums of money are expended annually to make our food safe. Retailers have a statutory responsibility to handle food correctly and inspections should be carried out regularly by local and national enforcement bodies, to ensure compliance with the provisions of a wide range of regulations.

In the event of a profound failure in the system, by either an unforeseen emerging infection or a system or regulatory failure, the effects can be profound, e.g. bovine spongiform encephalopathy (BSE) or mass outbreaks of *Escherichia coli*. It can be very difficult after such occurrences to deal with ensuing public fear or panic, whether or not justifiable. The media have often been vilified, with some justification, for escalating some dramas into crises.

That said, food safety, the protection of the public, and addressing the concerns of consumers and their organisations are of paramount importance. The prevention of unnecessary disease, whether mildly inconvenient or fatal, has to be the concern of all individuals and organisations involved in food supply and public health and safety. Within the realm of healthcare professionals, those patients seen with infections acquired from food may have already been failed by some of the safety measures normally in place, although inability to store, handle or cook food correctly can also be a potential source of such infections.

Typical transmission pathway

An animal suffering from a disease, which may not be apparent, creates a product of either milk or body tissue in which the causative organism is entrained. This product is either further processed or directly passed to a final consumer who then either with or without cooking eats the contaminated item, and in susceptible cases develops the disease after a variable incubation period.

Food-borne zoonoses associated with fish

The most significant disease sometimes associated with fish is cholera, although as humans are one of the main reservoirs for the disease there is a continuing debate as to its status as a zoonosis.

Of more potential significance is a complex of diseases associated with certain types of planktonic algae called dinoflagellates. These produce toxins that accumulate in shellfish and certain other fish at a primary level, then moving up the food chain into carnivorous and predatory species of fish, and into the human food chain. Sporadic outbreaks may relate to weather, tidal, current and ambient temperature/sunlight, often with associated algal blooms, providing some predictive data for prevention schemes.

Ciguatera

This disease is associated with the consumption of farmed salmon, and also carnivorous species such as shark, barracuda, grouper and snapper, especially those found in tropical and subtropical regions between 35°N and 35°S. This disease now occurs worldwide due to transportation of fish to geographically distant regions for the gourmet restaurant trade.[1]

The toxin occurs in a dinoflagellate – *Gambierdiscus toxicus* – and then spreads into a variety of fish species. Transmission to humans occurs when contaminated fish is consumed, especially when it has been undercooked. Symptoms start with perioral numbness and tingling, which may become generalised. Tooth pain, nausea, vomiting and diarrhoea may follow as the condition progresses. Neurological symptoms include paraesthesia, arthralgia, myalgia, headache and acute temperature sensitivity. Vertigo and muscular weakness may also be seen. Cardiovascular involvement with bradycardia, tachycardia and hypotension can occur.

The condition is usually self-limiting, and symptoms regress within several hours or days. In isolated cases neurological symptoms can persist, although normally there is no permanent damage.

In the UK cases are normally seen on a sporadic basis, with farmed salmon or imported exotic fish being the source. In the USA, there were two recorded cases in Texas in 1998, and South Carolina in 2004; however, it is known to be massively unreported, with many fishermen aware of the symptoms, and prepared to accept them as part of their diet and way of life.

Contaminated fish are particularly prevalent in the Caribbean and Florida (on both coasts and in the Gulf of Mexico). Other areas where the problem occurs include Hawaii, Puerto Rico, Guam, the US Virgin Islands, Tahiti and the South Pacific generally.

There have been recent reports of cases in the Canary Islands, indicating that fish from West African waters may be contaminated.

Shellfish poisoning

In cases of poisoning following ingestion of shellfish a complex of afflictions is seen depending on the variety of toxins ingested. These vary depending on the different groups of dinoflagellates responsible. In general, saxitoxin derivatives cause paralytic shellfish poisoning (PSP), okadaic acid and yessotoxin cause diarrhoeic shellfish poisoning (DSP), brevetoxins cause neurotoxic shellfish poisoning (NSP) and domoic acid causes amnesic shellfish poisoning (ASP).[2]

In serious cases, if the individuals were to get all of the poisoning symptoms together, they would not be able to speak, they would be numb all over, the bottom would be dropping out of their world and they would not know why.

The last publicised case of DSP in the UK occurred in June 1997. Forty-nine people ate mussels or mussel-containing soups at two London restaurants. These mussels originated in UK waters. It was the first incident in 30 years attributable to domestic shellfish. DSP toxins were first detected in shellfish from the Thames estuary in 1991; no previous outbreak had occurred in the UK. No cases have ever been seen in the USA; however, the causative diatom is known to be prevalent in US coastal waters.

ASP can be a life-threatening syndrome, causing both gastrointestinal and neurological symptoms. Nausea, diarrhoea and cramps occur within 24 hours of the consumption of contaminated shellfish, with neurological symptoms appearing later (up to 48 hours). In 1987, four people died after consuming contaminated mussels from Prince Edward Island, Canada. Canadian waters are now monitored to prevent a reoccurrence. No cases of ASP have been reported in the UK. Where the disease does occur it is believed to be worst in elderly patients, and fatalities have occurred.

The last case report of PSP in the UK was in 1968. This condition is particularly dramatic as the toxins can cause respiratory paralysis within 24 hours and, unless supportive therapy is given, death follows rapidly.

The Department for Environment, Food and Rural Affairs (DEFRA) has a system of location warnings geared towards preventing dinoflagellate-contaminated crustacea and fish being harvested from affected sea and tidal areas. The warnings are generated by analysis of shellfish harvested from monitoring sites at a number of indicator sites around estuaries and coastal waters. Food protection legislation invoking emergency prohibitions are used to ban fishing in affected waters. Similar measures are in place around the USA, with the Food and Drug Administration (FDA), US Department of Agriculture (USDA) and local state authorities carrying out monitoring and enforcement.

Elsewhere in the world, especially in tropical waters where conditions are suitable for the causative dinoflagellates to multiply rapidly, these diseases are significant. Most international fish-trading nations have established similar monitoring and enforcement systems.

Food-borne zoonoses associated with meat

Most of the UK and US population still eat meat, although vegetarianism is on the increase. Meat may be consumed as discrete cuts, comminuted meat products, i.e. beefburgers or sausages, processed items such as spam or corned beef, and cured, smoked or salted products. The exact source of any outbreak can be linked to dietary preference which is usually set by cultural factors and prevailing religious belief. This can protect or expose populations to a variable spectrum of pathogens. The bacteria within this next section, however, form a universal threat to human health. The following section deals with probably the most serious pathogen of this group.

Escherichia coli

E. coli forms a part of most mammalian bacterial gut flora. It has a vast array of serotypes: some are benign, whereas others are dramatically pathogenic. This can vary from species to species; a benign form in one animal may be a deadly organism in another.[3]

The particular serotype of major concern is O157:H7, which was first identified as a major cause of serious outbreaks of food poisoning in the USA and Canada during the 1980s. This serotype is variously known as enterohaemorrhagic *E. coli* (EHEC), shiga toxin-producing *E. coli* (STEC) or verocytotoxin-producing *E. coli* (VTEC) O157. There are other serotypes that can produce similar clinical disease; however, this is both the most commonly seen in clinical cases and also the most severe. The Health Protection Agency (HPA) record approximately 1200 cases of *E. coli* O157 infection annually, of which approximately 50% are food borne. In 2006, minor UK outbreaks were linked to restaurants, schools, nursing homes, an open farm and a paddling pool. In the USA, there are an estimated 70 000 human cases of *E. coli* O157 per annum.[4]

Transmission

Disease in humans follows the consumption of food, usually meat or meat products, milk or water, that has become contaminated with faecal material. Direct contact with infected animal faeces has also been shown to be an efficient means of transmission. The organism is particularly associated with ruminant animals, especially cattle, sheep and goats, which remain healthy and asymptomatic, despite carrying the organism in significant numbers. It is also carried by horses, pigs, dogs, geese and wild rabbits, with viable organisms being shed in the faeces.

Contamination of carcasses with faeces at slaughter has also been demonstrated. Meat from such carcasses poses a considerable risk if jointed, sold and subsequently consumed undercooked. To prevent or reduce infection from this source, recommendations have been made that vets at abattoirs assess the faecal load of the animal's body surface before slaughter. Any animals likely to produce carcasses with high levels of possible contamination should be rejected, further cleaned and resubmitted, or processed with particular attention to hygiene procedures and additional precautions, as deemed necessary. Contamination may also occur following contact between cooked products and raw meat, or the instruments or surfaces used while processing raw meat. The inoculum necessary to initiate progression to clinical disease has been estimated at fewer then 100 viable organisms.

Outbreaks may be sporadic, and may affect only single individuals; these are often associated with animal faecal contamination of water or milk. Collective outbreaks with large numbers of cases usually stem from breakdowns in controls within catering establishments. During a widespread outbreak, there may be secondary spread from patient to carer, or other person-to-person transmission.

Disease in humans

Once in the gastrointestinal tract the organism adheres to the gut wall where it proliferates and produces a toxin that is capable of damaging the gut lining to a variable degree. Only 30% of those who become infected show symptoms. The effect of the toxin may cause solely fluid loss and diarrhoea; in more severe cases there is also haemorrhage into the gut lumen and this is known as haemorrhagic colitis (HC). The condition can progress to haemolytic–uraemic syndrome (HUS), especially in children, with kidney damage that may progress to full renal failure with associated haemolytic anaemia and occasionally death. HUS occurs in roughly 5–10% of clinical cases. The organism is now recognised as the main cause of HUS in children. Recently there has been some evidence[5] that the development of HUS may be linked to the use of antibiotics in patients, with the drugs rapidly killing the bacteria, and producing massive toxin release. In adults (especially elderly people), but also occasionally infants, the course may be slightly different. Neurological disturbances may develop in addition to the HUS symptoms; this complex is known as thrombocytopenic purpura, and fatalities follow its development.[5]

Treatment

Treatment is supportive, because there is no specific treatment that shortens or ameliorates the course of the disease. Rehydration is essential; dialysis may be necessary, especially where there is significant kidney involvement. If kidney failure occurs, short-term dialysis followed by later kidney transplantation is the only option. As previously mentioned, the use of antibiotics is considered to be inappropriate.

Incidence

The incidence of infection is currently decreasing, with 1002 cases in the UK in 2006, compared with 1429 in 1999. The major risk groups affected are infants, children, and elderly or immunocompromised individuals. There appears to be a seasonal pattern of infection – statistics show an increase in reporting during August and September. Within the UK there is also a characteristic geographical spread, with more cases being reported in Scotland and northern England.

Analysis of an outbreak

The largest outbreak of *E. coli* O157 in the UK occurred in November 1996, in Wishaw, Scotland (Table 4.1). The source of the outbreak was cross-contamination in the premises of a butcher, J. Barr, who also ran a bakery and catering business. There was an extensive supply and distribution network from his premises, with meat and meat products being supplied to 85 outlets in central Scotland. The outbreak was finally declared over in January 1997, but not before 969 associated incidents of food poisoning were reported, with 496 viewed as suspected cases, 272 confirmed, 60 probably and 164 possibly linked to consumption of contaminated food from the single source.[6]

A total of 127 people were admitted to hospital: 13 required dialysis and 18 died. Three further patients died later from complications associated with infection, giving a final figure of 21 fatalities for the outbreak. Of the dead, eight had attended a church luncheon, and six were residents of a local nursing home, to which cooked meats had been supplied. The 18 people who died in the initial phase of the outbreak were all over 69 years of age.

Table 4.1 Wishaw outbreak timeline	
17 November 1996	A pensioners' lunch is held at Wishaw Parish Church; the buffet is provided by J. Barr and Son, Butchers of Wishaw (initial infection)
22 November 1996	The possibility of outbreak of *Escherichia coli* O157 is identified after a history is taken from 9 of 15 confirmed or suspected cases. Eight of the nine consumed food directly or indirectly from J. Barr of Wishaw
23 November 1996	A birthday party is held at the Cascade Public House in Wishaw, with J. Barr as caterer. Outbreak control team established
24 November 1996	Barr's product chain is properly identified and its full extent mapped. There was an extensive supply and distribution network with meat and meat products being supplied to 85 outlets in central Scotland
26 November 1996	The first food hazard warning is issued
27 November 1996	The Wishaw premises of J. Barr are closed down
15 December 1996	The last case of infection linked to products from this source is reported
20 January 1997	The outbreak is declared over

Mr Barr was tried for recklessly supplying contaminated meat but acquitted and has since been privately sued for damages by about 120 people.

The significance of this outbreak cannot be underestimated. At the time this was the second-highest number of deaths associated with an *E. coli* O157 outbreak anywhere in the world. It was only surpassed by an outbreak in Japan in 1996 where nearly 10 000 people were infected, with an associated mortality in excess of 30 individuals.

Outbreak procedures

In any outbreak, it can be difficult to identify the focus. In the Wishaw case, as in many epidemics, it was difficult to identify the problem until people became ill. History taking becomes very important, because it is often the only key to identifying the source of the infection.

Once there is a presumption that an outbreak is occurring, an outbreak control team must be formed that meets daily during the outbreak until it is controlled. This allows successful coordination of health service matters with local and regional government environmental health agencies. It also forms a forum for epidemiology and other specialist support to be discussed and implemented in forming policy and strategy to control the outbreak.

In this outbreak it was of great significance that J. Barr was not solely a butcher. His premises also had a bakery and purveyed raw meat, cooked meat products and bakery items, which were sold from the premises, and also distributed as wholesale goods over a wide geographical area.

The records of the transactions involving sale and supply of products from the Wishaw premises were complex, and sometimes vague. It took a considerable amount of time and effort for health officials to ascertain their full extent. This allowed contaminated products to remain on sale for longer than was desirable. J. Barr and Son had more than 400 employees, including part-time workers, who lived in the local area, all of whom had to be tested, taking time and effort away from other areas.

For all of these reasons, this outbreak was serious and extensive. The lessons learned from this outbreak have informed later legislation and practice, with enhanced requirements for record-keeping and food hygiene.

Other outbreaks

In the USA, there have been several recent *E. coli* O157 outbreaks. Two of these were related to contaminated vegetable matter (spinach and lettuce), and two to meat products (beef patties and pepperoni). The lettuce outbreak in October 2006 was the worst, with 199 cases across 26 states; 102 patients were hospitalised, with 31 developing HUS and 3 deaths – 2 elderly women and 1 baby. The beef pattie-related outbreak between July and September 2007 resulted in 111 cases across 8 states, of which 21 were hospitalised; 2 developed HUS, but there were no deaths; 21.7 million pounds (approximately 10 million kg/10 000 tonnes) of frozen beef patties had to be recalled and destroyed.

In the UK, since the Wishaw outbreak, there have been a number of small outbreaks, usually associated with care settings such as schools, nursing homes and pre-school nurseries. Other outbreaks are associated with failures of food or environmental hygiene mechanisms, such as faulty pasteurisation, contact with raw sewage or consumption of contaminated water.

The Pennington report

Following the outbreak at Wishaw, Professor Sir Hugh Pennington was commissioned to investigate and make recommendations for future control of the disease. The group that he chaired produced a report that made 32 recommendations. The main points were that there should be enforced separation of cooked and raw meat at catering premises, a programme of lessons on food handling for children and an *E. coli* awareness programme for farm workers. In addition it was recommended that all butchers should be licensed, with one of the conditions of gaining and maintaining accreditation being mandatory staff training.[6]

The report's recommendations led to a media furore and, together with fears over *Listeria* and *Salmonella* and the onset of BSE/vCJD, formed part of the demand for the establishment of a Food Standards Agency (FSA) in the UK.[7]

Listeriosis

Listeriosis is an often serious infection, caused by eating food contaminated with the bacterium *Listeria monocytogenes*. In the UK during 2006 there were 210 clinically proven cases reported to the HPA; this was lower than the number of cases reported in the previous 3 years, which all showed a marked increase over case levels in the 1990s. In the USA, despite health warnings from various responsible government agencies, an estimated average of 2500 people become seriously ill with this disease annually, of whom in excess of 20% die. Refrigerated products can spread the disease, because *L. monocytogenes* is capable of slow growth at low temperatures.

Transmission

L. monocytogenes is found in soil and water. Vegetables can become contaminated from the soil or from manure used as fertiliser. Animals can carry the bacterium without appearing ill and can contaminate foods of animal origin, such as meats and dairy products. The bacterium has been found in a variety of raw foods, such as uncooked meats and vegetables, as well as in processed foods that become contaminated after processing, such as soft cheeses and cold cuts at the deli counter.

Unpasteurised (raw) milk or milk products made from unpasteurised milk may contain the bacterium. Humans and animals may also contract the disease by direct contact with infected faecal matter. A cutaneous form of the disease can occur from such contact. Transfer of the pathogen from mother to fetus or neonate has been well documented, as has infection following inhalation of infected aerosols, again in both humans and other animals. Venereal spread has been documented in cattle. It is estimated that 5% of the human population carries the bacterium asymptomatically in the gut.[8]

Risk groups

The main significant risk group is pregnant women. The disease can affect both mother and baby, and fetal or neonate death may follow maternal consumption of contaminated products. In an outbreak in north Carolina, USA, between late 2000 and early 2001, following the ingestion of infected Mexican-style soft cheese, of 11 women presenting with clinical signs, 10 were pregnant. As a result there were five stillbirths, three premature births and two infected neonates required treatment.[9]

Immunocompromised patients, from whatever cause, are also likely to suffer serious illness, with fatalities in serious cases. This is also true for elderly people or infirm patients. In otherwise healthy individuals, infection is possible; however, they are less prone to display serious or fatal sequelae. A study in the USA has also established that patients who use quantities of antacids or who take cimetidine may be at increased risk of contracting disease, due to the inhibition of gastric acid. It is not known whether this also applies to patients receiving proton pump inhibitors.

Disease in humans

In most cases, infection occurs following ingestion of contaminated food-stuffs. There is a pre-patent period of up to 10 weeks after infection. Clinical onset usually follows fever, headache, nausea and vomiting, and symptoms similar to a severe chill. Abdominal cramps, stiffness of the neck and photo-phobia may also be present. The condition may progress with organ involve-ment, including endocarditis, internal lesions, metritis, septicaemia and meningitis. As central nervous system involvement becomes more widespread, there may be convulsions, confusion and vertigo.[10]

Focal necrosis in the placenta may occur with spontaneous abortion, premature birth or infective transfer to the baby at birth. Babies may display a septicaemic infection within the first week after birth, or a septicaemic form with associated pneumonia within the first month of life.

A fatality rate of higher than 20% of clinical cases has been seen when treatment is not made, or is not started quickly.

Treatment

There is no vaccine available to prevent listeriosis in humans or animals. Treatment options are limited to the use of supportive measures and antibiotics.

Oral penicillins, especially amoxicillin at high doses by mouth, i.e. 500 mg three times daily for 5–7 days, have been shown to be effective. Erythromycin can be substituted in patients who are allergic to penicillin, at a dose of 500 mg four times daily for 1 week. In serious cases, penicillin or amoxicillin has been used successfully either intravenously or by mouth at high doses. Ampicillin plus gentamicin, or trimethoprim/sulfamethoxazole has also been used; however, this is normally reserved for secondary care usage under the control of expert opinion and monitoring. Even with prompt treatment some infections result in death. Use of recombinant DNA tests has undergone trials to speed diagnosis and treatment.

Prevention

Listeria spp. are killed by pasteurisation, and heating procedures used to prepare ready-to-eat processed meats should be sufficient to kill the bacterium; however, unless good manufacturing practices are followed, contamination can occur after processing.

The general guidelines recommended for the prevention of listeriosis are similar to those used to help prevent other food-borne illnesses, such as salmonellosis. Food from animal sources should be thoroughly cooked, especially beef, pork and poultry. Raw vegetables must be washed thoroughly in clean water before eating. Uncooked meats, vegetables and cooked or ready-to-eat foods should be stored separately or segregated. Unpasteurised milk or milk products should be avoided. General food hygiene precautions apply – knives, cutting boards and hands should be washed after each occasion of handling uncooked foods.

Recommendations for people at high risk, such as pregnant women and people with weakened immune systems are in addition to the recommendations listed above. In 1988 the following advice was issued by the Chief Medical Officer (CMO) in the UK:

> The CMO has established that the incidence of listeriosis in pregnancy stands at 1 in 30 000 live and stillbirths. Pregnant women should avoid certain ripened soft cheese, feta, Brie, Camembert, blue-veined cheeses such as Danish Blue, Stilton and Gorgonzola, and Mexican-style cheeses. Additionally they should not consume meat-based pâté. Cheddar and Cheshire-type cheeses, or soft fresh cheeses such as cottage cheese or fromage frais, do not pose a threat as they rarely contain *Listeria* or, if contaminated, carry insufficient organisms to cause infection. The same is true of processed cheeses, which have often undergone pasteurisation. Pregnant women should reheat chilled meals and ready-to-eat poultry thoroughly until piping hot. They should not assist with lambing, milk recently lambed ewes, touch the afterbirth or come into contact with newborn lambs. These recommendations also apply to immunodeficient individuals. Healthy children more than 4 weeks old are not at risk.

This advice is still current and valid.

In the USA similar advice has been issued by the Centers for Disease Control and Prevention (CDC), with general recommendations that reduce the risk not only from *Listeria*, but also from other food-borne pathogens:

- Thoroughly cook raw food from animal sources, such as beef, pork and poultry.
- Wash raw vegetables thoroughly before eating.
- Keep uncooked meats separate from vegetables and from cooked foods and ready-to-eat foods.
- Avoid unpasteurised (raw) milk or foods made from unpasteurised milk.
- Wash hands, knives and cutting boards after handling uncooked foods.
- Consume perishable and ready-to-eat foods as soon as possible.

The CDC makes further recommendations for people at high risk, such as pregnant women and those with weakened immune systems, in addition to the general recommendations listed above:

- Do not eat hot dogs, luncheon meats or deli meats, unless they are reheated until steaming hot.
- Avoid getting fluid from hot dog packages on other foods, utensils and food preparation surfaces, and wash hands after handling hot dogs, luncheon meats and deli meats.
- Do not eat soft cheeses such as feta, Brie and Camembert, blue-veined cheeses, or Mexican-style cheeses such as queso blanco, queso fresco and Panela, unless they have labels that clearly state that they are made from pasteurised milk.
- Do not eat refrigerated pâtés or meat spreads. Canned or shelf-stable pâtés and meat spreads may be eaten.
- Do not eat refrigerated smoked seafood, unless it is contained in a cooked dish, such as a casserole. Refrigerated smoked seafood, such as salmon, trout, whitefish, cod, tuna or mackerel is most often labelled as 'nova-style', 'lox', 'kippered', 'smoked' or 'jerky'. The fish is found in the refrigerator section or sold at deli counters of grocery stores and delicatessens. Canned or shelf-stable smoked seafood may be eaten.

Listeria *outbreaks*

Europe

During January 2000, after two deaths in France, Coudray, producer of a variety of meat products, was forced to disinfect its factory completely. In 1992 the same factory was the source of a listeria outbreak in which, of 279 cases, 63 people died and 20 women aborted their babies.[11]

In February 2000, the deaths of a 75-year-old man and a baby less than a month old followed consumption of pork-based coarse pâté by the pensioner and the mother of the baby. These deaths were followed by seven more, including two other infants.

Coudray exported widely within and outside Europe, so an extensive product recall and publicity campaign was mounted to stimulate consumer awareness. In France, health authorities were unable to identify the source of infection that left another 23 people ill across 19 regions of the country.

In August 2000, analysis of ice cream produced at a North Wales creamery was found to contain *Listeria*. Production was halted, and on investigation faulty processing was found to be to blame.

A cluster of five cases of listeriosis in pregnant women in Swindon, UK, was traced back to pre-packed sandwiches supplied at a hospital in Autumn 2003. There were no fatalities.[12]

The USA

A multi-state outbreak of listeria infection in the north-eastern USA was linked to pre-cooked turkey meat. Of 50 infected people, most were hospitalised, with 7 deaths, and stillbirth or miscarriage in 3 pregnant women. Six of the dead were immunocompromised. A widespread recall was instituted, with 27 million pounds (12.5 million kg/12 500 tonnes) of product having to be recalled.

A group of four cases of listeriosis, with two fatalities, in Massachusetts was traced back to contaminated dairy products supplied from a single dairy in summer 2007.

Salmonella

Famously, in 1988, in a statement made to the House of Commons, Edwina Currie (a then junior Health Minister) stated that 'most egg production in the UK is contaminated with *Salmonella*'. The resulting media frenzy and reaction from the public forced her to resign from her post. An investigation was launched in response to her statement and, in 1989, a cull policy was introduced to try to control the incidence of the disease. Two million chickens were slaughtered – with no detectable effect on disease incidence. The monitoring and testing for *Salmonella* spp. and other food-borne pathogens in the UK were tightened after this debacle.

On the basis of the outbreak data available from the HPA it is believed that the majority of all *Salmonella* infections affecting humans in the UK are derived from food, with 14 000 laboratory-confirmed cases of salmonellosis in 2006, half the incidence in 1997 (30 000 cases). It is believed that only one in four cases is confirmed, giving a true figure of 56 000 cases per annum. In the USA, there are believed to be approximately 1.4 million cases a year, with 15 000 hospital admissions and 400 deaths.[13]

Salmonella enteritidis is the main culprit in eggs and poultry, with 12 800 of the total cases (84%) in the UK in 2006 being this serotype, of which almost half were phage type 4 (PT4). In the USA, since the identification of epidemic *S. enteritidis* in eggs between 1978 and 1996, the introduction of egg quality assurance programmes (EQAPs) has led to significant reductions in infection rates, with current estimates that only 1 in 20 000 eggs is infected with *S. enteritidis*.

S. typhimurium is primarily associated with cattle but has also spread to pigs, sheep and poultry, and represented 12.5% of the total cases in the UK during 2006. Other *Salmonella* spp. are also clinically significant, with certain of the approximately 2300 serotypes so far identified being particularly invasive, specifically *S. virchow* and *S. paratyphi* var. *Java*. Reported cases of salmonella poisoning show a distinct consistent seasonal pattern, with a peak of infection observed in late summer and autumn, although with modern agricultural practice, and food supply patterns, cases may occur at any time.[14]

Comminuted meat products and eggs have been identified as a major source of infection, especially sausages and burgers, although the microbes have also been found in beef, pork, chicken and other meats. Contamination of other foodstuffs by faecal matter can result in some *Salmonella* spp. being isolated from foodstuffs as diverse as cereals, spices, vegetables, peanut butter and fruit.

Disease in animals

Animals may be asymptomatic carriers of *Salmonella* spp. They may also suffer clinical disease with intestinal disturbance, septicaemia and death. Spread within herds or flocks can be rapid, with disastrous results. *Salmonella* spp. are also an issue in companion animals: dogs, cats and particularly reptiles can act as carriers.

Transmission

Transmission usually follows ingestion of infected food, or direct or indirect contact with animal faecal material.

Disease in humans

Symptoms include sickness, diarrhoea, abdominal pain and fever. The infection can also not be apparent and present as unexpected overwhelming septicaemia. Susceptible groups include the usual individuals, with elderly, very young, infirm and immunocompromised individuals being at most risk. In the USA, recurrent salmonella septicaemia is used as a marker for progress from human immunodeficiency virus (HIV)-positive status to acquired immune deficiency syndrome (AIDS).

The most significant serotype in terms of mortality is *S. typhimurium* DT104, which shows a 3% mortality rate. It is especially dangerous in elderly people. There is also a threat from resistant serotypes, with more than half the isolates of *Salmonella* DT104 being multi-drug resistant to ampicillin, chloramphenicol, streptomycin, sulphonamides and tetracyclines. The R-serotype of this pathogen is, in addition, resistant to trimethoprim and quinolones. In the USA there has been increasing resistance to fluoroquinolones and cephalosporins in a number of *Salmonella* spp.[15]

Treatment

Treatment is usually symptomatic, using rehydration or antimotility agents such as loperamide. In severe or invasive cases, ciprofloxacin or trimethoprim is used at doses related to the age and weight of the patient and the severity of disease.

Prevention

There is now statutory surveillance for all breeding flocks of poultry, and voluntary monitoring for all other flocks in the UK. Under the Zoonoses Order 1989, *Salmonella* spp. isolated from animals must be reported to the

Minister responsible for DEFRA. In breeding flocks, under the provisions of the European Directive 92/117/EEC, any confirmed *Salmonella enteritidis* or *typhimurium* infection results in comprehensive slaughter to protect the food chain, with two flocks having to be culled in 2007. This ensures that chickens used for egg production start their working lives free of *Salmonella* spp. Industry codes of practice have also been established to complement the statutory *Salmonella* control programme. There is a vaccine available that can be used in laying flocks, and is used by many suppliers to the super-market trade to ensure clean egg supply. These measures have resulted in a reduction in the number of human cases associated with poultry and eggs. In the USA, EQAPs have had a similar impact.

Animal feed and its ingredients are routinely tested for *Salmonella* spp. and contaminated batches are rejected. Domestic precautions should be based on good hygiene practice in the kitchen, and ensuring that food is adequately cleaned and cooked.

The British Egg Information Service has issued the following guidelines for consumers relating to the consumption of eggs:

Consumers should avoid eating raw eggs; refrigerate unused or left-over egg-containing foods; discard cracked or dirty eggs; avoid cross-contamination of food by washing hands, cutting surfaces and plates after contact with uncooked eggs; and look for the lion logo and best-before date stamped on eggs. (The lion logo indicates that the eggs have been produced according to guidelines laid down by the Egg Marketing Inspectorate, a department of Defra with inspection and enforcement powers.)

Case histories

UK
Eggs
In 2007 there were two outbreaks of salmonellosis in the UK and Channel Islands, probably linked to pasteurised egg products imported from France.

The UK outbreak in October 2007 followed a formal dinner with 7 of 59 guests becoming ill, and *S. enteritidis* was isolated from pasteurised egg yolks and whites used in preparing the dessert.

Another outbreak, in which 10 of 83 diners became ill in the Channel Islands after a dinner also in October 2007, was linked to the same products.

These products had been supplied across most of the UK, and there was a possibly related cluster of cases in the East Midlands. The distributor recalled the product and the producer was informed and has taken measures to prevent future contamination.

Lettuce
In 2001 across the UK, and in 2004 solely in Northern Ireland, there were outbreaks of *S. newport* related to contaminated lettuces.

Chocolate

Cadbury, a major manufacturer of chocolate bars in the UK, had to recall more than 1 million chocolate bars after *Salmonella* was detected in some products between January and March 2006. Forty-two people became ill after eating the bars, with three requiring hospital treatment. The firm was fined £1 million.

USA

Outbreaks related to eggs

South Carolina, February–March 2001: 688 of 2317 inmates in 4 prisons in South Carolina were infected with *Salmonella enteritidis* by eggs obtained from a single source. Discontinuing supply resolved the outbreak.[15]

North Carolina, June–August 2001: 82 people became ill after consuming eggs from an unidentified source or sources, with the pathogen being identified as *S. enteritidis*.

Oregon, September 2003: 18 people were diagnosed with *S. typhimurium* infection following consumption of egg salad kits that were prepared using inadequately cooked processed eggs.

Tennessee outbreak from raw milk, 2002–3

Unpasteurised (raw) milk from a single dairy in Tennessee led to the infection of 62 people with *S. typhimurium*. The dairy stopped supplying raw milk and switched to pasteurising all of its product.

Multistate outbreak related to pet rodents December 2003–4

This was an outbreak of multidrug-resistant *S. typhimurium* associated with pet rodents (including rats, hamsters and mice) obtained from pet shops.

Multistate outbreaks related to reptiles

Between 1998 and 2002, there were a number of cases of salmonellosis linked to a variety of lizards (iguanas, bearded dragons, frogs, toads and skinks) kept as pets across the USA.[16]

Thirty cases of *S. kingabwa*, which rarely causes human disease and is normally confined to the area of Africa previously known as the Belgian Congo, were detected between 1995 and 2004 across the USA. All patients had had contact with lizards or other reptiles.

In 2006–7 a multistate outbreak of *S. pomona* related to reptiles led to 19 confirmed case and 1 fatality. A year later there was another multistate outbreak of 103 cases with 56% of patients being below 10 years of age of *S. paratyphi* var. *Java* (a particularly invasive species of *Salmonella*) related to small turtles (defined as turtles less than 4 inches in length). Although sales of small turtles have been prohibited since 1975, they are still available in some pet shops, flea markets and street stalls. There were no fatalities in the latter outbreak. It would appear that the turtles had become infected from a common source, probably at a wholesale market.[17]

Outbreaks linked to contaminated foodstuffs

There have been several large outbreaks of *Salmonella* spp. related to a variety of contaminated foodstuffs in the USA – fresh fruit salad (especially cantaloupe and honeydew melons) in 2006 (41 cases across 10 states), raw tomatoes between 2005 and 2006 (459 people across 21 states), and peanut butter in 2006–7 (628 people in 47 states). Each of the incidents stemmed from different routes of contamination, and illustrates the need for control, quality and tracking systems to be thorough and maintained to prevent recurrence.

Milk-borne diseases

Some of the zoonotic diseases that may be acquired from drinking infected milk will already be familiar from other chapters of this book. Brucellosis was discussed in Chapter 3. There are still occasional cases of infection caused by *Brucella abortus*, but *B. melitensis* has not been responsible for any cases of disease in the UK since case recording began. Surveillance for this organism is continually carried out by Defra.

Tuberculosis caused by *Mycobacterium bovis* needs no introduction. Human-to-human spread of resistant serotypes of *M. tuberculosis* is now more significant than the bovine form acquired from dairy products.

Q fever can also be spread by milk, and is deemed to be a serious zoonotic infection (see Chapter 3).

The usual suspects

In addition to the previously mentioned organisms, cases of food poisoning may relate to a selection of the 'usual suspects'. They are all guilty as charged, and constitute a threat to consumers of badly or inadequately prepared food.

Clostridium spp. *perfringens* and *C. botulinum*

Clostridium perfringens, the causative anaerobic bacterium of many cases of gas gangrene, may also cause a food-borne disease. Widespread in the environment, and an inhabitant of the gastrointestinal tracts of humans and animals, it is often found in foodstuffs as a result of faecal contamination.

As with other forms of clostridial disease, it is the production of exotoxins by the pathogen that causes the main damage, especially where the ingested food carries a large inoculum, or heavy toxin load. The usual pattern of disease is linked to the ingestion of a number of viable *C. perfringens* organisms that may produce clinical symptoms of abdominal cramps, diarrhoea and fever. The symptoms begin within 24 hours of ingestion and the clinical course is usually of short duration. Elderly patients and young children are most affected by this pathogen.

The more serious form, known as enteritis necroticans or pigbel, is linked to ingestion of a massive inoculum of *C. perfringens* type C. This form of the disease can be fatal, and is usually a result of inadequate cooking or slow cooling of cooked meats or meat products, with inadequate reheating, allowing the bacteria to multiply and produce quantities of exotoxin.

The clinical signs are linked to the effect of the exotoxin on the gut wall. Cell death and invasive necrosis lead to overwhelming septicaemia and circulating toxin levels that are toxic to major organs, including the heart, liver and kidneys (compare gas gangrene). Diagnosis is often presumptive, confirmed by isolation of the organism or the exotoxin from a stool sample. Treatment is usually solely supportive.

Large outbreaks are usually associated with communal events or places and mass catering, from either professional or domestic sources, especially where food prepared in advance is not correctly stored. One of the largest thoroughly documented outbreaks occurred at a factory in Connecticut, USA in 1985. An employee banquet prepared for over 1300 people resulted in 600 cases, linked to previously prepared gravy, which had been incorrectly stored and inadequately reheated.[18]

Nothing as dramatic has been seen since, although there is a continued sporadic number of cases in both the UK and the USA every year.

Botulism

Botulism as a complex of disease state arises from contact with *C. botulinum* or its associated neurotoxin. As with other species of *Clostridia*, it is an anaerobe that forms spores, which can survive desiccation and heat until conditions alter to those allowing their growth. There are seven types of botulism toxin associated with the bacteria, designated by the letters A–G. Only the A, B, E and F toxins are known to cause illness in humans.

Often associated with ducks, geese and some other types of poultry, it can also be found in cattle and horses, which can act as hosts and amplifiers for some strains. The organism is found in the environment, and also in the gastrointestinal tract of infected mammals that may be asymptomatic carriers and amplifiers, although certain strains of botulism can affect them also. In the UK, during August 2006, there were concerns that a prolonged drought and the stagnation of lakes and ponds could encourage *C. botulinum* to grow, with water birds becoming infected.

There are no specific risk groups for botulism. It can affect anybody, anywhere, at any time under the right circumstances. There are several distinct recognised types of botulism. These are food borne, infant and wound associated. Luckily there is a very low incidence of all three forms in the UK and the USA.[19]

In the UK, there have only been two cases of infant botulism and four cases of food-borne botulism in the last decade, with the food-borne cases being predominantly from home-preserved meat brought in from outside the UK. There has been a large increase in the number of wound botulism cases associated with injecting or intravenous drug users (IDUs).

In the USA an average of 110 cases of botulism are reported each year. Of these, approximately 25% are food borne, 72% are infant botulism and the rest are wound botulism. Annually there are incidents of food-borne botulism often caused by eating contaminated home-preserved foods. The number of cases of food-borne and infant botulism has changed little in recent years, but, similar to the picture in the UK, wound botulism has increased because of the use of black-tar heroin, especially in California.

There are two other forms of botulism, but one is extremely rare and the other has never been detected in practice. Inhalation botulism has occurred in laboratory workers after inhalation of the toxin, with symptoms similar to those of the food-borne form. In theory, the toxin could also be water borne; however, as western water treatment processes inactivate the toxin, the risk is considered to be negligible.

Food borne

The food-borne disease has to be differentiated from other types of botulism because it is not caused by an infective form, but solely by ingestion of botulinum toxin, and is normally associated with products such as duck pâté, sausages and seafood, including smoked fish, that have been inadequately heat treated, sufficient to kill the organism but not enough to destroy the neurotoxin which is destroyed at high temperatures. The amount of toxin necessary to cause clinical signs is measured in nanograms, so, although foods ingested may contain no active bacteria, the residual toxin content can be sufficient to produce symptoms.[20]

The disease usually begins 18–36 hours after the ingestion of the toxin. Early signs include gait difficulties, dysphagia and impaired vision. Respiratory distress, muscle weakness, and abdominal distension and constipation may appear progressively. In severe cases assistance to maintain breathing by mechanical ventilation is required to prevent death.

Many cases of food-borne botulism are believed to go undiagnosed, because the symptoms may be transient and clinical signs may be confused with Guillain–Barré syndrome (see p. 134).

In the USA, between 1990 and 2000, there were 97 cases of food-borne botulism, of which 91 (over 90%) occurred in Alaska. Alaska has the highest incidence of food-borne botulism due to the native foods consumed by native Alaskans, with most being prepared from marine mammals, such as whales or seals, by processes that do not kill the causative organism, i.e. dessication or fermentation. In July 2002, a cluster of 12 cases occurred after Alaskan Eskimos consumed meat and blubber from a beached beluga whale, which had died some time previously. All the victims tested positive for type E toxin, and were treated accordingly. There were no fatalities.[21]

Case number and fatality rate reduction in Alaska have been reduced since by the implementation of an education programme, which has also meant that patients or their families can rapidly access evacuation services, bringing sufferers to hospital rapidly. All local hospitals hold stocks of antitoxin, which, administered rapidly, can limit the consequences of the infection or intoxication.

Botulinum antitoxin is used to treat the condition and, provided that respiratory support is maintained, most cases will make a full recovery. The antitoxin may be obtained from locally designated centres throughout the UK, and in emergencies through the Department of Health Duty Officer on telephone number +44 (0)20 7210 3000. There are cautions related to its use, because hypersensitivity reactions are not uncommon. Therapy should start only after specialist advice has been obtained.

In the USA, it is illegal to use any drug product that is not licensed by the FDA; however, the FDA can approve drugs or biological products as investigational new drugs (INDs) and will permit treatment for a serious or immediately life-threatening condition, where no comparable or satisfactory alternative drug or therapy is available. IND status is maintained by the CDC Drug Service for certain products; most are manufactured by foreign drug companies and are commercially available in countries outside the USA, and the demand for them in the USA is so limited that commercial licensure is not practical or profitable, so these products are available in the USA if needed.

In the case of botulinum antitoxin, there are two products available through the CDC, the first being for toxin A and B, which has a full licence, and the second being an IND product solely for toxin E. The latter is only for concomitant administration with the anti-A and -B toxin product where contaminated fish or marine mammal material has been consumed. The CDC will release the products only for suspected or clinically confirmed cases of botulism, and where requests are made through state or local health departments, allowing the CDC to maintain effective surveillance and rapidly detect any outbreaks. It is stored around the USA at CDC quarantine stations within airports, so that it can be delivered wherever it is required rapidly. Requests should be made to the CDC on +1 (0)770 488 7100.

As a final note on the food-borne form of the disease, it should be noted that it has also been associated with non-animal-derived foodstuffs. In two outbreaks in the USA, one in 1985 and the other in 1989, chopped garlic in olive oil was the source of the toxin. This has been resolved since by the FDA insisting that such products be acidified using phosphoric or citric acid, thus destroying the toxin. There was also a case with two victims who ate home-prepared soya bean tofu, which had become contaminated.

Infant botulism

The disease stems from contamination of food with spores of C. botulinum, usually from environmental sources. In September 2007, an 8-month-old infant was admitted to a London hospital and later diagnosed with botulism (type A toxin). The source of the infection was never determined.

In the UK, there have only been six other cases since 1978, and the last case before 2007 was recorded in 2001 in a child aged 6 months during July 2001 which resulted in a recall of batches of formula baby milk. Confined to children aged under 1 year, the disease follows ingestion of viable spores. These become active, and over a period of days to weeks colonise the gut, producing the neurotoxin. This causes constipation and muscular weakness; the inability to control head movement is a particularly marked symptom, as well as a weak cry. There is marked lethargy and a disinclination to feed.[22]

As the loss of muscle tone and coordination progresses, the child may become floppy, with respiratory distress. Diagnosis is made by isolating the organism from stool samples or by toxin testing of faecal matter.

Treatment with the adult antitoxin is not suitable and antibiotic therapy has to be carefully initiated, because this can cause massive death of the organism with subsequent overwhelming toxin release. Respiratory support may be necessary. Over time, even in severe cases, the paralysis lessens and there is usually a full recovery with no major sequelae.

A human-derived botulinum antitoxin (Baby BIG) has been available for the treatment of infant botulism since October 2003 from the Californian Department of Health Services Infant Botulism Treatment and Prevention Program, and was used for the first time in the UK on the child in the 2007 case. The infant recovered fully.[23] The Californian Department of Health Services Infant Botulism Treatment and Prevention Program can be contacted on +1 (0)510 231 7600 (24 hours a day, 7 days a week, including public holidays). More information can be found at http://www.infantbotulism.org.

One of the major food sources of C. botulinum is honey, and fears relating to infant botulism have led to advice that children under 1 year of age should not be fed honey. The gastrointestinal tracts of older children and adults have sufficiently robust bacterial flora to prevent the colonisation, even if active bacteria are ingested.

In September 2006 the Advisory Committee on the Microbiological Safety of Food (ACMSF), a statutory committee set up in 1990, providing expert advice to the government on questions relating to microbiological issues and food, published a report on chilled and frozen baby foods, and concluded that there was no evidence to suggest that these foods had caused any cases of infant botulism, and that jarred or tinned baby food also carried a low risk.

The study had been prompted by concerns that the cooking processes used in chilled or frozen products might not be adequate to prevent *C. botulinum* growth. The manufacturing and process controls used in the production of chilled and frozen baby foods were examined and found to be safe.

Wound associated

Wound-associated botulism follows the inoculation of an open wound with material containing either viable spores or active bacteria. The progressive production of toxins causes systemic paralysis radiating from the inoculation site. Treatment is usually with antibiotics and antitoxin as necessary. Previously seen as a rare disease, the incidence has increased recently, associated with IDUs, especially where they use the intramuscular or intradermal administration route. The contamination seems to stem from the material used to 'cut' (adulterate) the drugs. First seen in New York City in 1982, it was not reported in the UK until 2000. There have been a total of 134 cases with 8 fatalities up to the end of 2007, and it is now the most common clinical presentation of botulism in the UK. It has also been seen in Europe, with 12 cases in Cologne, Germany during October and November 2005.[24]

Most cases have been associated with type A toxin, some with type B and in a few cases both type A and type B. A laboratory confirmation should not be awaited. If clinical symptoms indicate botulism, antitoxin therapy should be initiated as soon as possible to gain the greatest clinical advantage, once consideration has been given to possible adverse reactions. *C. botulinum* is sensitive to benzylpenicillin and metronidazole. It may also be possible to undertake surgical debridement of wounds to reduce organism load.

Clinical uses of botulinum toxin

Purified botulinum A toxin continues to be used in spasticity. In an extremely diluted form, it is also currently used for cosmetic use to reduce facial wrinkles. Although well tolerated on the whole, there have been incidents where side effects and toxicity have been seen.

Yersinia enterocolitica

Of the same bacterial genus as plague, it is transmitted to humans by ingestion of foods as diverse as meat (pork, beef and lamb), oysters, fish and raw milk. It causes an acute-onset gastroenteritis with diarrhoea and vomiting, marked fever and abdominal pain. The pain can be so severe that it mimics appendicitis and has also led to misdiagnosis of Crohn's disease. It is capable of producing clinical complications which include septic arthritis, colonisation of existing wounds, bacteraemia and urinary tract infections. Luckily it is rarely fatal. The inoculum is usually traced to environmental sources, including soil and water; however squirrels, pigs and rodents form an animal reservoir.[25]

Cryptosporidiosis

Cryptosporidium spp. are spore-forming parasitic protozoans found widely in the environment in an extensive variety of foodstuffs, including salad and vegetables, raw meat and meat products, offal and milk, usually associated with contamination arising from animal faecal matter. *Cryptosporidium parvum* is considered to be a particularly significant pathogen. Calves, lambs and deer have been identified as asymptomatic animal reservoirs, capable of shedding viable organisms in their faeces.[26]

Transmission

Human infection follows either direct contact with animal faeces or consumption of inadequately cleaned or cooked products. There have also been recorded incidents of individuals contracting the disease after swimming or otherwise undertaking water-based recreational activities in contaminated water, often where disinfection routines have become compromised. Person-to-person spread has been recorded, and is a particular risk in care settings.

Disease in humans

An inoculum of fewer than 100 encysted organisms can cause clinical disease. Following a pre-patent period of between 2 and 14 days, and in individuals with no underlying risk factors, there is profuse self-limiting watery diarrhoea, with abdominal pain and cramps, and a low fever that may last up to 7 days. Loss of appetite and anorexia can follow with severe weight loss, especially in immunocompromised patients. There is also a high probability of relapse, with many patients having another bout of diarrhoea within 14 days of apparent cure.

In patients with HIV/AIDS the disease may progress chronically, spreading to the bile duct, central nervous system and lungs. Unless treated swiftly, death will follow.

Treatment

In low-risk patients, treatment is purely supportive. Severe cases may need intensive care; however, treatment is difficult and as yet there is no specific therapy for conquering the pathogen. The strategy employed in HIV/AIDS patients centres on boosting the already damaged immune system with optimal retroviral therapy. There are some indications that those patients receiving clarithromycin or azithromycin, with or without rifabutin for prophylaxis against *Mycobacterium avium* complex, show less incidence of this disease.

Prevention

The pathogen can be destroyed by freezing, drying, heating materials to greater than 65°C and irradiation. It is resistant to many disinfectants in common use.

Campylobacter spp.

Campylobacter spp. is a much under-rated cause of food poisoning. The pattern of infection in the UK is very different to that in the USA for this pathogen. In the UK, 80% of clinical cases are linked to contaminated food, whereas in the USA most cases are water borne, although there have been clusters of cases associated with the consumption of unpasteurised milk.[27]

This particular pathogen is widespread and present in many farm animals. In particular, poultry are very susceptible to heavy bacterial loading. Under normal circumstances, the animals show no sign of disease, although there have been cases of abortion in sheep being linked to *C. jejuni*. The bacterium has been isolated from pigs, birds, cattle, dogs, cats, unpasteurised milk and water supplies. The measures in place to control *Salmonella* spp. have had little or no impact on the prevalence of *Campylobacter* spp. The two species considered significant in human disease are *C. jejuni* and *C. coli*, with the infective dose considered to be fewer than 100 viable organisms.

In 2003, a survey of animals at slaughter point across the UK indicated that 54.6% of cattle, 43.8% of sheep and 69.3% of pigs carried *Campylobacter* spp. This has led to the FSA initiating a control strategy (see Prevention below)

Transmission

The main route of infection is faecal contamination of carcasses *ante* or *post mortem*, or of milk.[21]

The organism is capable of surviving freezing and has been shown to survive for several months in frozen poultry, minced meat and certain chilled foods. Thus cross-contamination could be a factor in infectious spread.

Disease in humans

The most immediate symptom of campylobacter infection is a self-limiting diarrhoea of 2–10 days' duration, sometimes with bloody stools. *Campylobacter* mainly affects babies and young children, and immunocompromised and debilitated individuals. Other symptoms include fever, nausea and abdominal cramps which may vary from mild to severe, with occasional misdiagnosis as appendicitis, similar to *Yersinia enterocolitica*. Symptoms may regress and reappear over a period of weeks. A septicaemic form has been seen in HIV/AIDS patients. Clinical cases of *Campylobacter* infection are associated with 20–40% of cases of Guillain–Barré syndrome. The triggering of reactive arthritis has also been associated with the disease. After infection it is estimated that less than 1% of the population may become asymptomatic carriers.[28]

In 2006, 463 339 cases of *Campylobacter* infection were reported in England and Wales to the HPA (up over 2005 by 4.5%). During the Infectious Intestinal Disease (IID) study[29] in England during 1993–6 it was estimated that there were 870 cases per 100 000 head of population annually, with only 1 in 8 cases being reported, which has been confirmed in other epidemiological studies. This would give a total of 370 000 cases in 2006.

Treatment

In most cases the disease is controlled without resort to antibiotics. However, as it may be life threatening in immunocompromised patients, antibiotics may have to be used.

Campylobacter spp. display high levels of resistance to fluoroquinolones, so any of the macrolide antibiotics are preferable; there are now some isolates that are dually resistant to both antimicrobial groups, which is a cause for some concern. In acute cases where resistance is suspected, tetracyclines, chloramphenicol and gentamicin have all been used. This is usually only initiated in secondary care settings after sensitivity testing has been done.

Prevention

The main control measure is the reduction of faecal contamination of carcasses at and after slaughter. Hazard analysis critical control point (HACCP) measures (see below), including keeping raw and cooked meats separate and ensuring that temperature-controlled processing of products is correctly undertaken, are effective in controlling spread through the food industry. In the home, using pasteurised milk and thoroughly cooking meat and poultry are recommended for everybody and especially for members of high-risk groups. Pets can carry and spread the organism and should be excluded from kitchens. The organism is sensitive to heat and drying, so thorough cooking acts as an effective control measure.

Campylobacter and Guillain–Barré syndrome

Guillain–Barré syndrome can affect any individual, and is often associated with diarrhoea. It is an acute inflammatory episode in which demyelination of multiple neurons occurs. This can affect large portions of the peripheral neural network, and muscle weakness and paralysis may affect motor function, including breathing. Patients often require intensive care, especially if lung function is significantly impaired. Most patients recover, although convalescence may be prolonged. Luckily, fewer than 5% of cases are fatal. Some theories suggest that this may be an autoimmune disease triggered by bacterial or viral pathogens, of which *Campylobacter* spp. is only one of several possible culprits. As yet there is no clear scientific evidence, although research is currently being undertaken.[30]

Food Standards Agency inspection and enforcement

In the UK, the FSA was established in response to the Pennington report. It is responsible for monitoring safety and standards of all food for human consumption, advising on diet and nutrition, and enforcing the law pertaining to food. It is also tasked with commissioning research into food safety. The FSA is directed by an executive board, appointed to act in the public interest, and is established so as not to represent particular sectors of industry or government. Its members come from a wide and varied background, and bring to their work a range of relevant skills and experience.

The stated aim of the agency is to 'protect public health from risks which may arise in connection with the consumption of food, and otherwise to protect the interests of consumers in relation to food'.

The FSA has initiated a campaign called 'from farm to fork', aimed at making food less contaminated and safer for the ultimate consumer. Initiatives have also been launched for clearer labelling, and to educate the public on food safety, nutrition and diet.

The FSA is accountable to Parliament through the Minister of Health. As a safeguard for its independence, it has the unique distinction of being given by statute the legal power to publish the advice that it gives to the government. The Meat Hygiene Service is now accountable to the FSA.

At a local level, environmental health inspectors from local and county councils conduct inspection visits, and enforce standards at producer, supplier and retail levels.

In the USA, the Food Safety Inspection Service of the USDA acts in a similar role, in consort with the FDA, and public/environmental health departments across counties and states.

Reducing zoonotic risks in food

Reducing the risks of zoonotic disease from foodstuffs is not just a process that begins and ends with the final consumer. Legislation and other physical measures to reduce or exclude pathogens from food are applicable to every step of the food chain, from field to table. Examining the process step by step gives some knowledge of the systems in place and, when considered against the information given in this chapter, allows some insight into the system failures that enable outbreaks to occur.

HACCP (Hazard Analysis Critical Control Points)

One of the major food industry schemes for recognising and identifying risk and its remedies is the HACCP process, derived from an engineering quality control and production model, with wide application in other industries. This is now internationally accepted as the preferred system for the management of food safety in food businesses, and is used in the UK, the USA and Europe.

HACCP analysis identifies hazards and allows risk reduction and mitigation at all stages of production, distribution and retailing. It has seven principles that provide a structured format for food safety by controlling hazards inherent in the food handling and production process:[31]

1. Conduct a hazard analysis
2. Determine the critical control points (CCPs)
3. Establish critical limits
4. Establish monitoring procedures
5. Establish corrective actions
6. Establish verification procedures
7. Establish record keeping and documentation procedures.

Food producers as well as government bodies, such as the Advisory Committee on the Microbiological Safety of Food, have endorsed it as the gold standard. The HACCP also applies to retailing and catering premises through current legal measures. From 1 January 2006, Regulation 852/2004 of the European Parliament came into force, making HACCP mandatory for all food producers and associated industries.

This reinforces the stepwise approach to infection control that previously existed and was used by the most conscientious.

Stepwise prevention strategies

Knowledge of zoonotic infections is the key to producing an effective stepwise programme that informs the HACCP process. Understanding the likely routes of infection and the life cycle of the pathogen allows selective measures to be applied in a focused way, breaking the transmission route at its weakest point. The following generic points are used as an illustration only; a full case-by-case examination of all possible pathogens and their control is outside the scope of a book of this size. The references at the end of this chapter offer scope for deeper exploration of any or all of the topics raised.

Some of these measures may not be familiar or fully comprehensible to healthcare professionals as they relate to industrial processes. However, they do form a non-medical system for prevention of disease, and are no less valid than more therapeutically oriented methods.

Step 1: control the disease in the animal

The incidence of zoonotic disease in animals may be reduced by the use of vaccination, clean foodstuffs and water, and good housing and husbandry. Overcrowded or unsanitary conditions can often lead to overt disease or unthrifty animals, requiring more therapeutic support for them to maintain sufficient health to attain slaughter weight or to continue to be productive. A reduction in infection rates has a dramatic effect on the incidence of infection further down the food or product chain. The associated lower levels of inoculum produce a lower likelihood of illness. The difficulties in implementing strategies at this point in the system are often economic; although the measures may be available, there may be little or no economic benefit to using them. Good housing and intensive staffing of livestock units are expensive, not only in capital outlay, but also in continuing infrastructure costs. In some cases those costs can become offset by higher prices for produce, but that is not always the case. The lobby for animal welfare and organic produce has improved the willingness of producers and consumers to follow this route, and it has been proven that there is a portion of the public who will willingly pay more for their food if it is of better quality. The converse is that there is also a need for food at the lowest price, and a bulk producer for a large supply contract may need to cut corners to stay in business, increasing perceived, if not actual, risks.

Step 2: reduce contamination at harvesting

When eggs are picked out, or cows milked, the application of sensible hygiene precautions is essential. Eggs should be free of droppings and cleaned and date marked. In dairies, the udder of the cow and the milking machinery should be as clean and hygienic as possible, with subsequent disinfection after each milking. Pipework and items such as clusters should be maintained and replaced as necessary to maintain adequate operating parameters. Milk should pass to a bulk tank and be subsequently chilled rapidly for later transport and pasteurisation.

At abattoirs, tight veterinary inspection both pre- and post-slaughter must be practised. Animals that display heavy faecal contamination should be cleaned or rejected. Slaughterhouse controls should prevent or reduce onward transmission into the food chain, with rejection of suspect carcasses. Prompt refrigeration of meat and careful cleaning of the carcass can reduce bacterial contamination drastically.

Step 3: retailing controls

Disinfection of working tools and areas, along with personal and premises hygiene procedures, protect consumers and workers from zoonotic infection. Sourcing products from assured suppliers, temperature and environmental monitoring, and the separation of cooked and raw products reduce the possibility of amplification and transmission of infection. The tight control of 'use-by' and 'sell-by' dates is mandatory, as is periodic inspection by public health officials, and the implementation of monitoring of refrigeration and freezer plants.

Step 4: domestic precautions

In the home, consumers should use common-sense measures, including disinfection of surfaces and equipment, personal hygiene procedures and thorough appropriate cooking techniques. Using a refrigerator correctly and observing sell-by dates would prevent many cases of food poisoning.

It is perceived that the public in general has an acute need for education related to such matters, and the Health Education Authority and the FSA are to start a campaign aimed at addressing this problem.

General food hygiene recommendations

In the UK, the FSA, the Food and Drinks Association and other public bodies have made various recommendations regarding food handling. These measures are designed to prevent cross-contamination of raw and cooked foods, and also to reduce the risk of consumers eating products that are raw or undercooked. Similarly in the USA, the CDC, Food Safety and Inspection Service (FSIS) and other public bodies run education campaigns, and issue guidelines in an attempt to cut infection rates. In the UK, the advice is that people should clean surfaces, equipment and containers that have come into contact with raw meat. They must wash their hands after handling raw meat and before handling other utensils. The same plate should not be used for cooked and raw meat without washing the plate in between. Meat should be cooked until the juices run clear; this especially applies to burgers. Barbecues are considered to be particularly risky as meat may not be fully cooked and, if previously chilled or frozen, may be raw or undercooked in the middle.

These recommendations were made after surveys had shown that public awareness of food hygiene was lamentable. Figures obtained from the Food and Drink Federation survey in 2002 indicated that:

- 23% had never been taught to cook or prepare food
- 50% do not follow cooking instructions

- 15% admit not cooking meat fully or properly
- 25% do not always wash hands before cooking
- 10% do not separate raw meat from other foods
- 8% do not keep perishable items in a refrigerator.

It appears from these figures that the general public has a profound need for education and information related to basic food safety and hygiene.

In 2006, when the latest survey was carried out by the same organisation, things had not improved. Of 1000 people questioned:

- nearly 50% did not cook burgers and sausages thoroughly
- 33% admitted to eating food past its use-by date
- of those with pets, 14% said that they washed their pet's bowl with their own washing up; food storage was also found to be a big area of confusion
- nearly 50% did not know that they needed to keep their fridge at 0–5°C to store food safely
- 16% store raw meat on the top shelf of the fridge and a further 8% would store it anywhere – risking the chance that juices could drip onto ready-to-eat foods below.

Miscellaneous items

Food sterilisation

Provision of appropriate information and an understanding of likely infections in risk groups form part of the support role of many hospital pharmacists. Knowledge of prevention strategies and animal handling guidelines is a valuable tool in the non-drug management of many patients.

Among the measures that may be needed in secondary care to manage the seriously ill patient is the non-technical issue of food provision. Sterilisation of foodstuffs, the education of food handlers and their screening as carriers of resistant organism serotypes may be necessary in certain care contexts, especially where immunocompromised patients are routinely treated.

Lower-input animals and higher-priced food

The continued debate over price as the sole arbiter of food supply, and the use of organic and high-welfare systems in agriculture, has a direct impact on zoonotic disease and antibiotic resistance. The use of older breeds of animal with lower input requirements in terms of therapeutic intervention and their higher innate resistance to infections, including zoonoses, is becoming increasingly important in agriculture.

This option for control of all zoonoses, and in particular those that are food borne, will impact on the consumer. It will require considerable political will and willingness on the part of consumers to reach deeper into their pockets to make such initiatives commonplace.

The globalisation of food production and trading also has the potential to affect any country's domestic situation, and pathogens previously unknown in a country may easily be introduced on foodstuffs. There is still a debate raging over whether or not the epidemic of foot and mouth in the UK in 2000–1 followed the importation of infected meat, which was fed in inadequately treated swill to pigs.

Farm visits

Over the past decade, there has been considerable adverse publicity surrounding cases of illness following farm visits, especially as there have been some fatalities in young children. In the UK, Professor Sir Hugh Pennington, the eminent microbiologist who carried out the Wishaw enquiry and who has since advised government on zoonotic infection risks, has suggested that very young children should not visit farm premises because of the risk of infection.

The Health and Safety Executive has issued guidance to farmers under the Control of Substances Hazardous to Health (COSHH) provisions and there is a useful information sheet.[32] The CDC issues similar guidance in the USA.[33]

Farmers must consider that visitors may be exposed to contaminated faeces and other materials. Any farm open to the public should ensure that there are adequate washing facilities for visitors, with warm running water, soap and clean towels adjacent to all areas where the visitors may contact animals. Signs should be erected advising visitors to wash before eating, drinking or smoking, and also advising parents to check that their children do not put dirty hands or fingers in their mouths. Provision should be made for separate eating areas, close to washing facilities. After the visit, teachers and parents should notify health authorities or their GP of any illness, especially gastrointestinal.

References

1. Lewis RJ. The changing face of ciguatera. *Toxicon* 2001; **39**: 97–106.
2. Todd ECD. Domic acid and amnesic shellfish poisoning: a review. *J Food Protn* 1993; **56**: 69–83.
3. Tarr PI, Gordon CA, Chandler WL. Shiga toxin-producing *Escherichia coli* and haemolytic uraemic syndrome. *Lancet* 2005; **365**: 1073–86.
4. Rangel JM, Sparling PH, Crowe C, Griffin PM, Swerdlow DL. Epidemiology of *Escherichia coli* O157:H7 outbreaks, United States, 1982–2002. *Emerg Infect Dis* 2005; **11**: 603–9.

5. Wong CS, Jelacic S, Habeeb RL *et al.* The risk of the haemolytic–uremic syndrome after antibiotic treatment of *Escherichia coli* O157:H7 infections. *N Engl J Med* 2000; **342**: 1930–6.

6. The Pennington Group. *Report on the Circumstances Leading to the 1996 Outbreak of Infection with E. coli O157 in Central Scotland, the Implications for Food Safety and the Lessons to be Learned.* Edinburgh: Scottish Office, 1998.

7. Advisory Committee on the Microbiological Safety of Food. *Report on Verocytotoxin-Producing* Escherichia coli. London: HMSO, 1995.

8. Lorber B. Listeriosis. *Clin Infect Dis* 1997; **24**: 1–11.

9. Anonymous. Outbreak of listeriosis associated with homemade Mexican style cheese. North Carolina October 2000. *MMWR* 2001; **50**: 560–2.

10. Varma JK, Samuel MC, Marcus R *et al.* Dietary and medical risk factors for sporadic *Listeria monocytogenes* infection: a FoodNet case-control study: United States, 2000–2003. International Conference on Emerging Infectious Diseases, 29 February–3 March 2004, Atlanta, USA.

11. Dorozynski A. Seven die in French listeria outbreak. *BMJ* 2000; **320**: 601.

12. Health Protection Agency. Cluster of pregnancy associated *Listeria* cases in the Swindon area. *Communicable Disease Report 50.* London: HPA, 2003.

13. Schroeder CM, Naugle AL. Estimate of illnesses from *Salmonella enteritidis* in eggs, United States, 2000. *Emerg Infect Dis* 2005; **11**: 113–15.

14. DEFRA. *Zoonoses Report.* London: DEFRA, 2006.

15. Voetsch AC, Van Gilder TJ, Angulo FJ *et al.* FoodNet estimate of the burden of illness caused by nontyphoidal *Salmonella* infections in the United States. *Clin Infect Dis* 2004; **38**: S127–34.

16. Mermin J, Hutwagner L, Vugia D *et al.* Reptiles, amphibians, and human *Salmonella* infection: a population-based, case-control study. *Clin Infect Dis* 2004; **38**(suppl 3): S253–61.

17. CDC. Turtle-associated salmonellosis in humans – United States, 2006–2007. *MMWR* 2007; **56**: 649–52.

18. Anonymous. *Clostridium perfringens* gastroenteritis associated with corned beef served at St Patrick's day meals – Ohio and Virginia, 1993. *MMWR* 1994; **43**: 137–8, 143–4.

19. Cherington M. Clinical spectrum of botulism. *Muscle Nerve* 1998; **21**: 701–10.

20. Sobel J, Tucker N, Sulka A, McLaughlin J, Maslanka S. Foodborne botulism in the United States, 1990–2000. *Emerg Infect Dis* 2004; **10**: 1606–11.

21. McLaughlin JB, Sobel J, Lynn T, Funk E, Middaugh JP. Botulism type E outbreak associated with eating a beached whale, Alaska. *Emerg Infect Dis* 2004; **10**: 1685–7.

22. Brett MM, McLauchlin J, Harris A *et al.* A case of infant botulism with a possible link to infant formula milk powder: evidence for the presence of more than one strain of *Clostridium botulinum* in clinical specimens and food. *J Med Microbiol* 2005; **54**: 769–76.

23. Arnon SS, Schechter R, Maslanka SE, Jewell NP, Hatheway CL. Human botulism immune globulin for the treatment of infant botulism. *N Engl J Med* 2006; **354**: 462–71.

24. Brett MM, Hallas G, Mpamugo O. Wound botulism in the UK and Ireland. *J Med Microbiol* 2004; **53**: 555–61.

25. Lindsay J. Chronic sequelae of foodborne disease. *Emerg Infect Dis* 1997; **3**: 443–52.

26. Dillingham RA, Lima AA, Guerrant RL. Cryptosporidiosis: epidemiology and impact. *Microbes Infect* 2002; **4**: 1059–66.

27. Allos BM. *Campylobacter jejuni* infections: update on emerging issues and trends. *Clin Infect Dis* 2001; **32**: 1201–6.

28. Lee W, Mijch A. *Campylobacter jejuni* bacteremia in human immunodeficiency virus (HIV)-infected and non-HIV-infected patients: comparison of clinical features and review. *Clin Infect Dis* 1998; **26**: 91–6.

29. Committee on the Microbiological Safety of Food. *Report of the Study of Infectious Intestinal Disease in England.* London: Food Standards Agency, 2001.

30. Schmidt-Ott R, Schmidt H, Feldmann S, Brass F, Krone B, Gross U. Improved serological diagnosis stresses the major role of *Campylobacter jejuni* in triggering Guillain–Barré syndrome. *Clin Vaccine Immunol* 2006; **13**: 779–83.
31. Notermans S, Gallhoff G, Zwietering MH, Mead GC. The HACCP concept: specification of criteria using quantitative risk assessment. *Food Microbiol* 1995; **12**: 81–90.
32. Health and Safety Executive. *Avoiding Ill Health at Open Farms: Advice to Farmers* (with Teachers' Supplement). AIS 23. Sudbury, Suffolk: HSE, 2002.
33. CDC. Compendium of measures to prevent disease associated with animals in public settings, 2005: National Association of State Public Health Veterinarians, Inc. (NASPHV). *MMWR* 2005; **54**(RR-4): 1–12.

5

Prion diseases

For centuries sheep and goats have suffered from a condition of until recently unknown aetiology called scrapie, which is not zoonotic. All attempts to identify or classify the causative agent had failed, although infectivity had been demonstrated by using an inoculum of brain tissue from sheep to sheep in the late 1930s. Until the last decade of the twentieth century a 'slow virus' was suggested as the most likely cause, although no viral particle was ever isolated. The causative agent was known to be resistant to almost all methods and materials known to destroy or inactivate viral particles.

Research workers in the 1990s identified a protein fragment apparently responsible for the affliction. These fragments were designated prions, and defined as 'small proteinaceous infectious particles which resist inactivation by procedures that modify nucleic acids'. In 1997 Professor Stanley Prusiner won the Nobel Prize for Medicine for his discovery of prions (proteinaceous infectious particles), which contain no DNA or RNA. He postulated that prions may play a part in Alzheimer's disease, Parkinson's disease and other degenerative neural diseases. Most scientists now believe prions to be the causative agent of scrapie, bovine spongiform encephalopathy or variant Creutzfeldt–Jakob disease (vCJD) and a variety of other transmissible spongiform encephalopathies (TSEs), which affect most mammalian species, although other factors, such as manganese deficiency and bacterial infections, may be moderators in the rate of disease progression.[1]

Prions are unconventional as an infectious agent. Consisting of protein alone, with no nucleic acid, the diseases that they cause are also different to any other infection or disease, because both infective material and hereditary factors that give genetic susceptibility have to be present for disease to occur. It is now believed that, after infection by a sufficient inoculum of aggressive prions, genetically susceptible individuals can develop the clinical signs of TSEs. Their name reflects the finding *post mortem* of brain and central nervous tissue riddled with holes like a sponge.

The prion theory suggests that the responsible agent affects protease-sensitive protein production, so that, after a spontaneous or acquired genetic modification, the protein (a normal constituent of cell walls) changes conformation to become protease resistant. This change triggers a chain reaction: the rate of protein conformation change becomes exponential so that there is a rapid laying down of the mutated form of protein (designated PrPsc – the sc for scrapie, the oldest known prion disease).

The physical symptoms of the disease spectrum caused by prion agents arise from the alteration of cell-wall proteins into insoluble forms after exposure to and incorporation of prion proteins. The process then becomes a self-sustaining chain reaction, which produces sheets of insoluble protein in neural tissue and particularly in the central nervous system, with inevitably fatal results following segmentation and gradual, progressive destruction.

Animal TSEs and BSE

The best-known animal TSEs are bovine spongiform encephalopathy (BSE) affecting cattle, chronic wasting disease (CWD), which affects elk in Northern America, scrapie affecting sheep worldwide with the exception of the Antipodes, and transmissible mink encephalopathy (TME) which affects mink, polecats and ferrets. There are also related feline/canine diseases and certain rodent diseases. It is difficult to substantiate some of these diseases in other species because they tend to appear slowly and are usually seen in the mature animal. For some species, attaining sufficient age to display the disease may not be achievable, as death from other causes intervenes before clinical signs are seen, and postmortem examination will not be possible or routine.

The two most significant TSEs in the UK at present are BSE and scrapie, which have an associated link to vCJD in humans. Prion strain typing has shown scrapie to be closely related to the prion responsible for BSE in cattle, and that the causative agent of vCJD in humans is very close to BSE in its characteristics. In the USA, CWD is significant in deer and elk and, although as yet there is no definitive link to human illness, monitoring is ongoing.

BSE is a fatal neurological disease of cattle that was first identified in the UK in November 1986. The feeding of meat and bone meal (MBM) to cattle and changes to the method of rendering animal carcasses before incorporating them into MBM appears to have enabled the prion agent to survive and led to the outbreak. Feeding as little as 1 g infected material from the brain or spinal cord of a sheep has been shown to be sufficient to cause BSE in 70% of those animals genetically susceptible to the disease. After clinical onset is observed the disease is rapidly fatal, within either weeks or months. A ban was put in place in July 1988 by the UK to prevent the inclusion of ruminant-derived protein in cattle feed. In November 1989 a voluntary ban

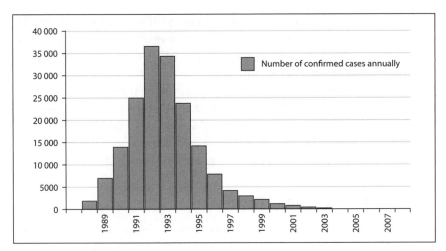

Figure 5.1 Confirmed cases of BSE.

supported by animal feed manufacturers stopped the inclusion of MBM in ruminant feeds. Since then various legislational measures have been taken to prevent a reoccurrence.[2]

By October 1996, BSE had been reported from 10 countries outside the UK, some arising from the importation of contaminated feed, and others linked to the importation of livestock from the UK for breed improvement or other purposes. As it is now known, once in the cattle herd, BSE can spread by maternal transfer; other cases arose in herds by this method.

After the first appearance and identification of BSE in cattle, a dramatic rise in incidence was seen, some of which could have been solely attributable to better surveillance. All cattle identified as suffering from the disease are slaughtered. The numbers have declined dramatically from a peak in the 12 months 1992–3 of 36 680 cases to 104 confirmed cases in 2006–7 (Figure 5.1).[3]

Measures at slaughter include a rigid adherence to non-invasive stunning, and the removal of all specified bovine material (SBM) from cattle carcasses, along with stringent inspection of meat at abattoirs, prevents contaminated material from entering the food chain. SBM includes the head, spinal cord, tonsils, spleen, intestines and thymus gland. All SBM must be rendered (temperature treated by boiling or steam heating), and then destroyed. The material must not under any circumstances be included in material for human consumption.

The significance of scrapie

Scrapie infection is important in our understanding of TSEs and is seen as the original source of BSE, and thus vCJD in humans. Research undertaken on scrapie has shown that susceptible animals need to be genetically predisposed to develop the disease, and for the infective agent to be present. It is now known from research carried out in the 1950s that, in sheep, inoculation stems from grazing on pasture contaminated with placental matter or other bodily material. Once in a susceptible animal population, further spread can occur by maternal transfer, so that it becomes a genetic inherited disorder in future generations. An infected animal can remain asymptomatic for a variable period of time. There is no evidence of the prion responsible for scrapie being able to cross the species barrier directly into humans.

Variant CJD and human TSEs

HG Creutzfeldt first described the disease now known as sporadic or classic Creutzfeldt–Jakob disease (CJD) in 1920. In 1921 another German neurologist, Jakob, described four more cases. CJD appears to occur as a sporadic disorder in 90% of known cases. Most of the remaining 10% show a strong relationship to a dominant inherited genetic trait. This was unexplained until the mapping of the human genome discovered that a mutation of chromosome 20 could lead to the damage necessary to initiate CJD. It appears that the genetic mutation, in association with ageing, produces a disease clinically indistinguishable from prion-mediated disease.

Several cases of CJD were related to the use of either brain tissue grafts originating from sufferers, or human growth hormone originating from the pituitary glands of cadavers. A case arose in 1974 after a corneal graft, and contaminated neurosurgical instruments have been implicated in several other cases. Following these cases a policy on destruction of surgical instruments and the use of synthetic hormones has prevented recurrence.[4]

The disease is invariably fatal and patients usually display a rapidly progressive state of dementia, with muscle spasm and tremor and a characteristic electroencephalogram (EEG) pattern. On postmortem examination, spongiform changes are found in the central nervous system.

The affliction occurs worldwide at a rate of about one case per million per year. There are higher rates in Slovakia and in a discrete group of Israelis who are all Libyan born. In these groups one case per year per 10 000 is seen. A blanket study of cell samples from postmortem examination of large cohorts of cadavers has shown that as many as 1 in 10 000 show signs of the mutation that can lead to CJD. It has also been suggested that, due to the limitations of the technique and the survey, this could be a substantial underestimate of the true incidence. Epidemiological surveillance of CJD was reinstated in the UK in 1990 to identify any changes in the occurrence of this disease after the epidemic of BSE in cattle.

There are three other human conditions that appear to be caused by similar but different modification of chromosome 20, each of which have slightly different clinical signs: Gerstmann–Sträussler–Schenker (GSS) syndrome (first described in 1928–36), fatal familial insomnia (FFI) (first described in 1986) and kuru. GSS and FFI are both related to an inherited genetic modification. Kuru may also be similar, but it exists solely in a single tribe from Papua New Guinea, the Fore Highlanders. A degenerative neural disorder, it was first described in 1957 by an Australian anthropologist. The disease was linked to the cannibalistic practice of eating deceased relatives' brains as part of an animistic religious rite. Since this practice has been discontinued the disease has virtually disappeared. Yet again the disease was characterised by gradual loss of neural capability. Postmortem findings of spongiform changes in the brain were also characteristic. Our knowledge of kuru and scrapie, the identification of their method of spread and how the disease progresses have been extremely important in gaining some understanding of the mechanism of spread of BSE and vCJD.

Variant Creutzfeldt–Jakob disease

Dr Robert Will first described vCJD in a 1996 paper in *The Lancet*. He stated:

> In the past few weeks we believe we may have identified a new clinico-pathological phenotype of CJD which may be unique to the UK. This raises the possibility of a causative link between BSE and CJD. The identification of a form of CJD that might be causally linked to BSE will result in widespread anxiety and concern.

This was an amazingly studied understatement.[5]

Initially known as new variant CJD, the 'new' designation for the disease was dropped by the Spongiform Encephalopathy Advisory Committee (SEAC) in March 1999, leaving the disease to be designated variant CJD. The identification of this variant arose from a series of deaths and postmortem findings which, although having many of the characteristics of classic CJD, did not fit the accepted case profiles. When compared with classic CJD cases, they were found to have an earlier age of onset, with a much longer period from clinical manifestation to death. The patients also did not have the characteristic EEG findings of sporadic CJD. At the time of the article in *The Lancet*, no similar cases had been seen in any other European country, thus triggering the possible link with BSE.

Patients suffering from vCJD have an average duration of illness of 2 years rather than the classic CJD pattern where it was unusual for a patient to survive for longer than 12 months. Classic (or sporadic) CJD affected patients aged 50–75, whereas vCJD affects a much younger group, with victims so far aged between 18 and 41 years.

Initially the hypothesis that vCJD and BSE were linked emerged from the association of two diseases of similar aetiology and clinical progress occupying the same location and time frame. It is now widely accepted that this disease is linked to BSE and that consumption of infected meat or other bovine material provides the inoculum (Figure 5.2). The evidence from studies in mice and monkeys supports the hypothesis.

It is still unclear how the prion invades the body after ingestion of infected material; however, a theory relating to Peyer's patches in the gastrointestinal tract of children and young adults is currently under development. Peyer's patches allow pathogens to be presented to the immune system in a controlled manner so that immunity can be developed. They recede in size and number as the child matures into adulthood. The theory proposes that the prion is absorbed from the gut, ingested by mobile lymphoid cells and then travels to other parts of the lymph node system, where it is subsequently able to develop in susceptible individuals. Neural pathways from the nodes can lead directly to the central nervous system, so the prion gains access by this route.[6]

The cumulative number of definite and probable cases to January 2008 totalled 166, including 46 where no diagnostic confirmation will ever be possible because the bodies were cremated, or the relatives refused permission for exhumation and postmortem examination (Figure 5.3). A particular genetic variation has been found in all of the cases tested to date with a modification of gene 20. This has been found to occur in approximately

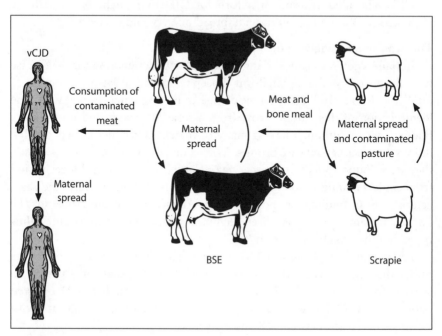

Figure 5.2 Diagrammatic representation of the most likely scenario for the emergence of variant Creutzfeldt–Jakob disease (vCJD). BSE, bovine spongiform encephalopathy.

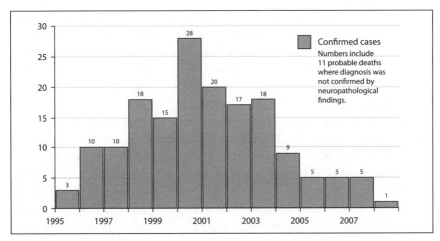

Figure 5.3 Number of deaths from variant Creutzfeldt–Jakob disease (vCJD) reported by year. (Figures courtesy of vCJD Surveillance Unit.)

40% of the population of the UK. This does not exclude the possibility of people without this genotype becoming victims of the disease.

In September 2000, the first report of possible maternal transmission of vCJD appeared. A baby born to a mother who subsequently died of vCJD was suspected of having the disease. The baby showed signs of brain damage with fits and convulsions, and was not developing normally. Confirmation of the diagnosis was not possible; however, the possibility of such an event is consistent with the findings in both BSE and scrapie.

Disease symptoms

Victims initially present with non-specific psychiatric symptoms. The clinical disease presentation shows progression from anxiety, depression, to gradually worsening changes in behaviour. Altered perception and painful sensory distortion are also seen in approximately 50% of patients.[7] There is a gradual loss of neuron density and function. After weeks, or months, the disease affects coordination and patients may have difficulty walking and picking things up; involuntary movements and convulsions occur. Memory problems develop and patients have reality perception difficulties, loss of motor control, dementia, paralysis and wasting. Patients deteriorate rapidly and require intensive nursing, as in the final phase of the disease total immobility occurs and the patient becomes mute. Death following overwhelming pneumonia is not uncommon.[8]

Diagnosis

Diagnosis in the initial stages of clinical onset is made difficult by the resemblance between this and other neurological and psychiatric disorders.

Differential diagnosis relies on the use of magnetic resonance imaging (MRI), computerised tomography (CT) and EEG. MRI has shown abnormal features in areas at the base of the brain in some vCJD patients, but the significance of these findings is not yet known. CT excludes other conditions, but does not definitively support the diagnosis. The use of lumbar puncture has proved of no benefit.[9]

The EEG findings in vCJD are consistently abnormal and do not show the distinctive changes associated with classic CJD. A mild elevation of hepatic enzyme levels has been seen, but is believed to be transient.

Confirmation of diagnosis is usually obtained only *post mortem*, where the characteristic spongiform changes with microscopic findings of abnormal protein clusters encircled by holes are seen, resulting in a daisy-like appearance described as 'florid plaques'. A biopsy specimen has been obtained in some cases before death, which can confirm the diagnosis, but the process may distress both the patient and relatives so it is unlikely to be used routinely in the future. There are some indications that testing tissue from the tonsils may allow definitive diagnosis to be made without the need for invasive techniques.

Treatment for vCJD patients and the BSE enquiry

As has been previously stated, many patients with vCJD are never properly diagnosed until after their demise. The disease is invariably fatal, and it is likely that, by the time signs and symptoms are seen, and a presumptive diagnosis made, the disease will be well advanced and death will follow swiftly. As the disease presents in a dramatic way, with mental illness, anorexia and loss of motor function, there is considerable distress for both patient and relatives.

In the interests of scientific research and public health, all patients suspected of suffering from a TSE are reported to the national Creutzfeldt–Jakob Disease Surveillance Unit (CJDSU), based in Edinburgh. Doctors from the unit visit all people with the disease and attempts are made to take a detailed history from the patient and relatives. The diagnosis of the case will also be reviewed at the same time. The CJDSU has produced a set of diagnostic guidelines that help place patients within classification groups of TSEs. Patients may be reclassified as their clinical symptoms and test results develop. Case notes are closed only after the death of the patient and when no further data is likely to be forthcoming.[2]

The task of the CJDSU is to identify and investigate all cases of CJD and other TSEs in humans occurring in the UK. The unit is also responsible for a comprehensive national surveillance programme. The programme aims to track case trends over time, and to detect case clusters. Research is also being undertaken to detect risk factors and mechanisms of transmission. This work is aimed at determining the magnitude of the public health problem, and to produce informed prevention strategies and valid diagnostic tests.

The annual report of the CJDSU and its database of cases have identified two clusters; these are examined later in this chapter.

Treatment

There have been a number of experimental drug therapies tried in an effort to slow the progression of the disease. Amantadine and amphotericin, although effective at slowing or arresting the condition in vitro, have little or no effect on the disease in sufferers. Aciclovir, interferon, antibiotics, steroids and other antiviral agents have also been tried and have failed to alter the outcome significantly.

Current trials centre on a number of agents. The first, pentosan polysulphate (PPS), which has been used with some limited success in several cases, is currently not licensed for human use, and each case has to be evaluated on an individual case basis before legal permission is given for it to be used.[10] It has to be directly infused into the brain. The second moiety is quinacrine, an antimalarial; a trial in CJD patients had been undertaken in the USA.[11] In the USA, three phenothiazines – chlorpromazine, promazine and acepromazine – are also under consideration, because they have displayed the ability in vitro to inhabit prion formation. In Germany, flupirtine has been undergoing trials in classic CJD patients.[12]

A decision is awaited on a clinical trial agreement for these drugs, but due to the nature of the disease there will be no placebo-controlled trials.

As patients deteriorate, rehydration and liquid feeds need to be used. Pain control may also be necessary. Clonazepam or sodium valproate can be given to control spasm and spasticity at normal doses, with titration to response.

Future hopes for therapies centre around protein stabilisers to prevent conversion of normal protein into prion protein. Anti-gene therapies are also proposed: such agents would destroy the gene responsible for producing the prion protein; however, it is unclear if this modification would carry with it a risk that the responsible gene has other metabolic functions, which may be currently unknown, within normal healthy body systems. Even these therapies may only slow progression, and are not seen as effecting a cure.

As the average age of the victims so far has been low in comparison to classic CJD, specialist strategies were not previously in place for dealing with young victims of degenerative disorders. Beds are now available in hospices or other facilities for the terminal care of these patients. Much of the health-care professional input in the care of victims of vCJD is palliative and relies heavily on good nursing practice. The Department of Health now provides a key coordinating worker to be appointed as soon as possible after diagnosis for every patient. The key worker ensures that there is an adequate care package in place, not only for the sufferer but also for relatives.

The BSE inquiry

A government-led enquiry into BSE commenced in December 1997 with it finally making its report in October 2000. The enquiry found that standards of care and support for families varied widely and suggested that improvements were needed, including speedy diagnosis with informed, sympathetic advice to relatives about the future course of the disease and the needs of the patient. It is now recognised that there is a requirement for rapid assistance for families to allow victims to be cared for in their own homes and access to hospice or similar care settings in the final phases of the disease's progress. The necessary measures include many of the items of care normally seen in association with care for elderly or disabled people, or those with cancer. They include home adaptations, respite care and, especially if the victim is the main breadwinner, financial support.

Epidemiological clusters

Clusters of cases form a very important part of the tools available to epidemiologists to identify not only past exposure and infection pathways, but also future trends. Through the work of the CJDSU, two clusters of cases have been identified. A cluster of cases of vCJD was first identified in the Leicestershire village of Queniborough in November 1998. In July 2000, when the investigation began, the number of possibly linked cases had risen to five. Between August 1996 and January 1999 five people developed the disease and subsequently died. All the victims lived in the area between 1980 and 1991, and this was the only time that a common exposure could have occurred.

An investigation was also undertaken into three deaths, in Armthorpe, near Doncaster. Two of the victims came from the same street, and the third visited the area frequently.

The expert findings into these two clusters excluded a number of factors that linked the victims including surgery and blood transfusions, dental surgery, occupational exposure, immunisations, injections, body piercing, cuts and animal bites, baby foods, school meals, drinking water and high manganese levels. All of these factors had been postulated as causing or contributing to the development of vCJD, but the links were unproven.

In each cluster the source appears to have been contaminated beef from cattle with BSE derived from animals that were Friesian–Hereford crosses born of dairy cattle and fattened on for slaughter. Such animals are slow to fatten and were therefore slaughtered at 30–36 months of age, rather than at the younger age normally associated with beef breeds. Being older, and given their feeding pattern, it was more likely that these animals could have had subclinical BSE at slaughter. This was compounded by slaughtering practice in local abattoirs. Cattle were slaughtered using a captive bolt as usual; however, in some local abattoirs and butchers, a pithing rod was also used to prevent the beast kicking after slaughter. The use of a pithing rod ruptures the brain structure and is more likely to release infective material into the work area, or onto the carcass, especially as the prion is most concentrated in brain material. Some local butchers also removed the brain from the head of the beast for further processing, increasing the chance of contaminating the meat.

Small abattoirs also often used a cloth to wipe down the beast after slaughter to remove any unwanted tissue, rather than hosing the carcass down as was usual practice in larger slaughterhouses. This practice increased the likelihood of contaminating the meat with infective material. At the time there was no legislation to define best practice.

The initial work of the enquiry team found that there was an association between the vCJD cases and the consumption of beef purchased from butchers where meat could have been contaminated with bovine brain. All the possible sources of meat were investigated to try to identify the butchery and slaughter methods used. The result showed that the victims were 15 times more likely to have purchased and consumed beef from a butcher who removed the brain from a beast compared with control groups who purchased meat from outlets where cross-contamination with brain material was not a risk.

The careful and exhaustive investigation of these clusters identified the likely timeframe for infection and has allowed the incubation period in humans of vCJD to be estimated as within the range of 10–16 years from infection.

Prevention of vCJD and BSE

The BSE enquiry[2] stated that government policy was 'All pathways by which vCJD may be transmitted between humans must be identified and all reasonably practicable measures taken to block them'.

The prevention of the passage of vCJD from sufferers to other humans is addressed in several ways: the World Health Organization (WHO) became involved soon after it became apparent that there might be a link between BSE and the emergence of vCJD. A series of consultations was undertaken with a variety of governmental bodies and eminent scientists. As a result, the WHO made a series of recommendations relating to foodstuffs and products derived from cattle. Milk was considered to be safe; however, tallow and gelatin were considered to be safe only if, during manufacturing, the process involved could inactivate or destroy any prion present. They also recommended that it is important that the pharmaceutical industry obtain bovine materials for use in parenteral, oral or other products from countries that have a surveillance system for BSE in place and that report either no or only sporadic cases of BSE. In addition, they encouraged the development of diagnostic methods and surveillance to ascertain the spread of vCJD.

In the UK regulations have been introduced covering the use of bovine materials in medicines and vaccines. The law came into effect on 1 March 2001 for human medicines, and from 1 June 2001 for veterinary medicines. All manufacturers of licensed medicinal products are affected and the Medicines Control Agency (MCA) and Veterinary Medicines Directorate (VMD) ensure compliance.[13]

All gelatin, collagen, tallow derivatives, amino acids and peptides made from bovine material and used in the pharmaceutical industry are derived from material obtained from animals slaughtered outside the UK.

Classic CJD has occurred by the transplantation of brain tissue or the use of brain-derived extracts. As a result, surgeons, especially neurosurgeons who treat CJD patients, are advised to destroy all surgical instruments after use. Disposable single-use instruments for tonsillectomies were introduced in 2001, although delays in their introduction led to a backlog of cases awaiting surgery.

Blood and blood products have been identified as carrying a particular risk of transmitting vCJD, with four cases being reported by the Health Protection Agency (HPA) to date. Measures have been taken to treat blood used in the UK by leukodepletion to reduce any transmission risk. Fresh frozen human plasma has been imported to produce certain blood products from countries where BSE/vCJD is unknown.[14]

The UK blood transfusion services are informed every 6 months of all definite and probable cases of sporadic and familial CJD who were reported as blood donors and blood product recipients. Whenever a suspected case of vCJD is confirmed as a 'probable' case, comprehensive information is passed to the transfusion service so that any donated blood can be withdrawn, and any blood donors whose blood has been given to the patient traced. Canada and the USA have banned blood donations from people who have spent long periods in the UK, and other countries are considering introducing similar measures.

Prevention strategies

Prevention of a recurrence of the BSE/vCJD outbreak is of paramount importance to the government of the UK, and its subordinate departments. As a result there are a series of measures in place to reduce the risks of BSE-infected meat entering the human food chain.[13]

Primary prevention focuses on preventing a resurgence of BSE in the UK cattle herd, and the presence of the disease in cattle at slaughter. Additional precautions are aimed at implementing and ensuring good butchery practice.

Any cattle suspected of having BSE are compulsorily slaughtered and their bodies destroyed. Milk produced by cows that are suspected of having BSE may not be used for any purpose other than feeding the cow's own calf. In addition to this very obvious measure there are several other measures in place to protect animal and, by implication, human health.

All cattle reared for beef destined for human consumption are ideally to be slaughtered at an age of less than 30 months. The requirement for removing the bones from meat before retail sale has now been lifted.

The Over Thirty Months Slaughter (OTMS) scheme banned the sale of meat derived from cattle aged over 30 months at the point of slaughter for human consumption and was introduced by the Spongiform Encephalopathy Advisory Committee (SEAC) in 1996. On 7 November 2005, following extensive consultation and risk assessments, a system of BSE testing was introduced for slaughtered cattle aged over 30 months (OTM) intended for human consumption. This system replaced the OTMS rule prohibiting the sale of beef for human consumption from OTM cattle. This scheme deals with dairy cattle that have reached the end of their productive lactations, old bulls, herd casualties and any other beasts.

Cattle identification and tracing

All cattle born or imported into the UK after September 1998 are registered on a national cattle tracing system managed and operated by the Department for Environment, Food and Rural Affairs (DEFRA). All movements of any particular beast are documented from birth until death. Each individual beast has a full passport on which the data are entered. All cattle are also numerically ear tagged to comply with European Commission regulations, making tracing easier.

Feed controls

Mammalian-derived meat and bone meal (MMBM) is outlawed from inclusion in ruminant feeds, and all feed mills and farms have had to be cleaned to remove any previous contamination from feed in which MMBM might have been present. A continuing inspection programme is coordinated by DEFRA. Feed is regularly inspected and sampled to ensure compliance.

Bull semen

The use of semen from infected bulls was identified as a possible method for introducing BSE into a country or herd of cattle previously certified as disease free. Following measures instituted by DEFRA to ensure that only disease-free semen was available, the export ban of this material was lifted to the European Union in 1996, and to other countries as bilateral agreements were reached based on guarantees of disease-free status. These are now in place in the USA, Canada, South Africa, Australia and New Zealand. The continuance of all these agreements hinges on no cases arising in cattle sired by exported semen.

Exported and imported meat

Regulations are now in place that prohibit the export or import of beef, or beef products, which are not certified free of BSE. The penalties and fines applicable to persons or organisations that break the rules are heavy, including fines of up to £5000 and up to 2 years' imprisonment. Any products detected as breaching the regulations are destroyed. Secondary prosecutions in the EU and other states are also possible. Meat for export must be accompanied by a valid Export Health Certificate, issued in accordance with the provisions of the Products of Animal Origin (Import and Export) Regulations 1992. Heavy fines are imposed for breaches of the regulations in conjunction with destruction of the produce. All exports of beef are deboned before dispatch under the provisions of the Date Based Export Scheme (DBES). The EU ban on exports of cattle and bovine products from the UK was lifted on 2 May 2006 and the UK BSE controls are now identical to those in other EU member states.

Offspring cull

To arrest the arrival in the adult cattle herd of calves born from cattle diagnosed with BSE, all suspect offspring have to be slaughtered. This eradication and slaughter programme was a prerequisite for the resumption of beef exports from the UK.

Specified risk material

Specified risk material (SRM) is controlled both by law in the UK and under a decision of the European Commission in Europe. Pithing is also to be outlawed both within the European Community and by import control in all countries wishing to export to the European Community. The measures aim to prevent material entering not only the human food chain but also animal feed, fertiliser or other cattle-derived materials. SRM may not be fed to any animal, nor may MMBM be incorporated in agricultural fertiliser. Controls on SRM prohibit the use of certain specified animal products that are known to harbour, or might theoretically harbour, the causative prion.

The future for vCJD

It is still uncertain what the future will hold in terms of case numbers; however, it is now seen as unlikely that there will be mass fatalities, although a few confirmed cases are expected annually.[15]

Situation in the USA

In December 2003, a single cow was diagnosed with BSE in Washington State. Precautions were taken to prevent meat derived from the carcass entering the food chain. The cow was traced back to a Canadian herd. Following this case, the US Department of Agriculture (USDA) announced a number of measures to further minimise the possibility of contaminated meat entering the food chain, including banning the use of 'downer' cattle (i.e. cattle found that are unable to rise) from being slaughtered for meat. In addition the Food Safety and Inspection Service (FSIS) requires SRM to be removed from all cattle aged over 30 months at slaughter.[16]

BSE surveillance was initiated in the USA in 1990, but this was the first case identified in the USA. The feeding of rendered cattle products to other cattle has been prohibited since 1997, and the importation of cattle and cattle products from countries with BSE or considered to be at high risk for BSE has been prohibited since 1989; these measures have minimised the potential exposure of animals and humans to the BSE agent.

In June 2005, the USDA confirmed BSE in an approximately 12-year-old cow born and raised in Texas. This was the first indigenous BSE case in the USA.

Imported human case

In October 2002, a clinical case of vCJD was seen in a Florida resident, who had been born and lived in the UK before emigrating to the USA; she died in 2004. It is assessed that the patient had been infected while in the UK. As the patient had not donated blood in the USA, or had any major surgery, it was considered that there were no medical risks that others had been infected from this case. This case and the proven blood-borne transmission of vCJD reinforces the necessity for continued surveillance.[17]

Monitoring

Since 1996, the Centers for Disease Control and Prevention (CDC) have used several mechanisms to conduct surveillance for classic CJD and vCJD in the USA. The CDC reviews data relating to cause of death to monitor the epidemiology of CJD in the USA. The CDC, in collaboration with state and local health departments, investigates CJD cases in persons aged <55 years to identify cases of possible vCJD. It routinely provides assistance in the investigation of suspected cases of vCJD spontaneously reported by health-care providers. The CDC, in collaboration with the American Association of Neuropathologists, established the National Prion Disease Pathology Surveillance Center (NPDPSC). These surveillance efforts have not detected any cases of indigenous vCJD in the USA.[18]

In the USA, the risk of blood-borne transmission of vCJD is low because of the absence of indigenous vCJD and a donor policy instituted by the FDA in 1999. This policy excludes from donating blood in the USA people who resided in or had extended visits to the UK or other European countries during periods of greatest concern for BSE exposure. In 2001, this policy was expanded to exclude donors who have travelled to other European countries for an extended period of time since 1980.

Suspected vCJD cases should be reported to local and state health departments. As the clinical manifestations and age distribution of vCJD patients can overlap with those of classic CJD patients, a brain postmortem examination should be conducted in all such cases to distinguish suspected or diagnosed vCJD from classic CJD.

Chronic wasting disease

CWD was first described in the USA in the 1960s and classified as a TSE in 1978. Previously localised to a contiguous endemic area in north-eastern Colorado and south-east Wyoming, since 2000, CWD has been found in free-ranging deer or elk in Illinois, Nebraska, New Mexico, South Dakota, Wisconsin, and outside the previously known endemic areas of Colorado and Wyoming. CWD has also been identified in captive deer or elk in Colorado, Kansas, Minnesota, Montana, Nebraska, Oklahoma, South Dakota and Wisconsin. Concern has been raised about the possibility that the prion associated with CWD might be transmitted to humans in a similar way.[19]

In February 2003, a retrospective study identified that there was a possibility that three individuals who had died of degenerative neurological disease had also participated in wild game feasts. Although two of the patients were found to have died of CJD, no evidence was found that this was associated with the consumption of meat contaminated with CWD. A previous investigation of unusually young CJD patients in whom the transmission of CWD was suspected also did not provide convincing evidence for a causal relationship between CWD and CJD. Subsequent investigations have not identified links between other cases of CJD-type illness and the consumption of venison; however, there is a need for continued surveillance. It is recommended that venison derived from animals with evidence of CWD is not consumed by humans, or animals.[20]

Useful addresses

There are a large number of organisations that now monitor CJD and vCJD across the world. The addresses given in Appendix 2 are solely as examples.

References

1. Zerr I, Brandel JP, Masullo C et al. European surveillance on Creutzfeldt–Jakob disease: a case–control study for medical risk factors. *J Clin Epidemiol* 2000; 53: 747–54.
2. Anonymous. *Report of the BSE Inquiry*. London: The Stationery Office, 2000.
3. Andrew NJ. Incidence of vCJD disease diagnoses and deaths in the UK January 1994–December 2007. Statistics Unit, Centre for Infections, HPA January 2008
4. Garske T, Ward HJT, Clarke P, Will RG, Ghani AC. Factors determining the potential for onward transmission of variant Creutzfeldt–Jakob disease via surgical instruments. *J R Soc Interface* 2006; 3: 757–66.
5. Will RG, Ironside JW, Zeidler M et al. A new variant of Creutzfeldt–Jakob disease in the UK. *Lancet* 1996; 347: 921–5.

6. St Rose SG, Hunter N, Matthews L *et al.* Comparative evidence for a link between Peyer's patch development and susceptibility to transmissible spongiform encephalopathies. *BMC Infect Dis* 2006; **6**: 5.

7. MacLeod MA, Knight R, Stewart G, *et al.* Sensory features of variant Creutzfeldt–Jakob disease. *J Neurol Neurosurg Psychiatry* 2000; **69**: 413–14.

8. Collins SJ, Lawson VA, Masters CL. Transmissible spongiform encephalopathies. *Lancet* 2004; **363**: 51–61.

9. Will RG, Zeidler M, Stewart GE *et al.* Diagnosis of new variant Creutzfeldt–Jakob disease. *Ann Neurol* 2000; **47**: 575–82.

10. Todd NV, Morrow J, Doh-ura K *et al.* Cerebroventricular infusion of pentosan polysulphate in human variant Creutzfeldt–Jakob disease. *J Infect* 2005; **50**: 394–6.

11. Barret A, Tagliavini F, Forloni G *et al.* Evaluation of quinacrine treatment for prion diseases. *J Virol* 2003; **77**: 8462–9.

12. Otto M, Cepek L, Ratzka P *et al.* Efficacy of flupirtine on cognitive function in patients with CJD: a double-blind study. *Neurology* 2004; **62**: 714–18.

13. Minor PD, Will RG, Salisbury D. Vaccines and variant CJD. *Vaccine* 2000; **19**: 409–10.

14. Llewelyn CA, Hewitt PE, Knight RS *et al.* Possible transmission of variant Creutzfeldt–Jakob disease by blood transfusion. *Lancet* 2004; **363**: 417–21.

15. Ghani AC, Donnelly CA, Ferguson NM, Anderson RM. Updated projections of future vCJD deaths in the UK. *BMC Infect Dis* 2003; **3**: 4.

16. Centers for Disease Control and Prevention. Bovine spongiform encephalopathy in a dairy cow – Washington state, 2003. *MMWR* 2003; **52**: 1280–5.

17. Belay ED, Sejvar JJ, Shieh W-J *et al.* Variant Creutzfeldt–Jakob disease death, United States. *Emerg Infect Dis* 2005; **11**; 1351–4.

18. Belay ED, Maddox RA, Gambetti P, Schonberger LB. Monitoring the occurrence of emerging forms of Creutzfeldt–Jakob disease in the United States. *Neurology* 2003; **60**: 176–81.

19. Belay ED, Maddox RA, Williams ES, Miller MW, Gambetti P, Schonberger LB. Chronic wasting disease and potential transmission to humans. *Emerg Infect Dis* 2004; **10**: 977–84.

20. MacWhinney S, Pape WJ, Forster JE, Anderson CA, Bosque P, Miller MW. Human prion disease and relative risk associated with chronic wasting disease. *Emerg Infect Dis* 2006; **12**: 1527–35.

6

Pandora's box

Pandora was the first woman to be created, fashioned from clay by Hephaestus at the request of Zeus. She was given every advantage by the gods that they were able to grant. Zeus then gave her a box to present to the man who married her. He planned to destroy man, who had been created by Prometheus, by giving a man Pandora as a wife. Knowing that Prometheus would be too wise to accept the gift, Zeus persuaded his less cautious brother Epimetheus to marry her. Later Pandora, against the instructions of the gods, opened the box and let loose upon the world all evils and diseases. In the bottom of the box only Hope remained.

Ancient Greek myth

Introduction

Most of the zoonoses already discussed in this volume lead to death only in an infected human after a prolonged untreated infection. The zoonoses discussed in this chapter are less benign. Their very names – anthrax, Ebola, plague and rabies – carry an echo of evil. This may be only a fantasy or a folk memory, yet the facts speak for themselves. Once infected, and they tend to be highly infective and pathogenic, the levels of associated mortality are higher than with other zoonoses, especially if treatment is delayed once symptoms appear.

Their impact having been dramatised in a variety of media, this chapter aims to realistically answer some of the questions relating to how dangerous these infections are, what their mortality statistics are and what treatments are available.

Although not endemic in the UK, all of these diseases could appear here carried by fomites, animals or humans, depending on their mechanism of spread. If robust measures were not put in place rapidly on the appearance of an initial case, a pestilence of biblical proportions could ensue. It is not for nothing that one of the horsemen of the apocalypse is named as pestilence or plague.

In the USA, rabies, although rare in humans, is widespread, and plague is found in natural reservoirs in some states. Anthrax is endemic in both the UK and the USA, although, due to industrial and domestic precautions, few clinical cases occur.

The UK is afforded some degree of protection by its temperate climate, geographical isolation and quarantine system. The system of quarantine has afforded comprehensive protection against rabies for many years, and the advent of a well-regulated system of pet passports has not compromised that system. The system cannot, however, quarantine human beings except in rare and exceptional circumstances, nor do all arrivals to our country – be they animal or human – stop at the immigration office on the way in, nor is it possible to tell if they are infected if they do. Migrating birds are believed to have been responsible for the outbreak of West Nile virus in New York, which killed eight people between September 2000 and September 2001, and has now spread across virtually the whole of the North American continent. Similarly, the current pathogenic strain of avian influenza – H5N1 – which has already killed millions of birds and some humans, and could under suitable circumstances cause a human pandemic, may be triggered by similar events. The case of the swan that died in March 2006 in Scotland emphasises well that wild birds do not stop at borders for a health check.

In the past, bubonic plague was introduced into the UK by rats from ships, and the outbreak known as the Black Death began with the first cases being seen at Melcombe in Dorset. The likelihood of a recurrence of plague from such a source is reduced by inspections and mandatory fumigation of vessels as well as the system of public health measures aimed at controlling rodent populations. Nevertheless there still remains a risk, and the price of safety is constant vigilance. Part of any system of vigilance has to be the education of healthcare professionals in the signs and symptoms associated with these diseases and this chapter aims to forward that objective.

It is not only animals and humans that travel today; goods are transported from far and near to fuel the appetite of our domestic market. Fomites transfer or objects contaminated with spores are particularly important in the transmission of anthrax. Recently the importation by both tourists and commercial companies of items made from goatskins in Haiti and the Dominican Republic has been banned because these items have been shown to be contaminated with anthrax spores. It is believed that the illegal import of infected skins, which he later turned into drum skins, led to serious illness in a drummer, Vado Diomande, in New York in February 2006, and may have been related to the death of another man who was also a drum maker in Scotland in a separate incident in October 2006.

There is another dimension to several of the diseases examined in this section. Biological warfare and bioterrorism have been the subject of a wide debate in modern society. The use of infectious disease in warfare, in either conventional or asymmetrical conflicts, has a long and less than glorious history, ranging from the catapulting of dead animals and humans into besieged strongholds by our ancestors, to the possibility of missiles loaded with anthrax being fired in recent, or future, conflicts. Biological warfare is banned by international treaty, and enforced by United Nation's inspection. However, as the anthrax attacks of 2001 in the USA have shown, this is not sufficient to prevent individuals or states pursuing this route in the hope of causing casualties to their adversaries. Some of the organisms discussed in this chapter have the potential to be biological agents for weapons of mass destruction and also to be used by terrorists. The aim of this chapter is to be realistic in the assessment of their potential, to dispel some of the wilder journalistic assertions and to give some understanding of the healthcare implications.[1]

Anthrax

Malignant pustule, woolsorter's disease, charbon, malignant oedema, splenic fever

Anthrax is an acute bacterial disease of animals and humans which can cause rapid fatality (hence the old English name of 'struck' for the disease in cattle). It is caused by *Bacillus anthracis*, a Gram-positive, encapsulated, spore-forming bacterium that spores rapidly on contact with oxygen. When cultured it produces dense colonies on agar with long chains of bacteria forming so-called 'medusa-head colonies' from their shape and appearance. This disease occurs worldwide and is an occupational hazard for those involved in processing the wool, hide, hair or bones of animals, such as farmers, slaughterers, skinners, hideworkers, tanners and woolworkers. Most mammals are susceptible to the disease. It is most commonly seen in cattle; goats, sheep, horses and pigs can also contract the disease.

Anthrax is a notifiable disease in the UK and the USA. Notification also applies to animals suspected of having died of the disease. Carcasses must be disposed of by burning or by liming followed by deep burial. Definitive diagnosis is not always possible because opening or moving suspect carcasses is also prohibited.

In the UK, the disease is rare. The last case before that of an amateur drum maker in Scotland in July 2006 (see case studies) occurred in November 2001 after a man involved in the animal hide trade was diagnosed as having the cutaneous form. After treatment he survived. There were a total of 14 cases of cutaneous anthrax confirmed in the UK between 1981 and 2000. Many of those affected were involved in the handling of dead animals, such as abattoir workers, or those whose work involved handling animal hides, bonemeal or wool.[2]

In the USA, before the cluster of cases associated with malicious contamination of mail in 2001 (see below), industrial processing of animal hair or hides was associated with 153 (65%) of 236 anthrax cases reported to the Centers for Disease Control and Prevention (CDC) in the period between 1955 and 1999. Of the remainder, products made from animal hair or hides accounted for an additional five (2%) cases. Of the total of 158 cases, the majority presented with the cutaneous form of the disease, with only 10 being inhalational anthrax. Many of the non-fatal cases in the USA associated with the handling of contaminated mail have also been of the cutaneous form (see Case history below).

An outbreak in 1979 at Sverdlosk, Russia, was later admitted by the Russian Government in November 2001 to have been related to an accidental release from a biological weapons research facility. Sixty-eight people died, although the authorities claimed at the time that the cases resulted from the ingestion of poorly cooked infected meat.[3]

A large outbreak in Zimbabwe from October 1979 to March 1980 caused more than 6000 (mostly cutaneous) cases. In Paraguay, 25 cutaneous cases were seen in 1987 after the slaughter of an infected cow. Currently the Department of Health (DH) considers South and Central America, southern and eastern Europe, Asia, Africa, the Caribbean and the Middle East as areas where the disease may occur in significant amounts.

There are sporadic occasional cases, in isolation or in clusters across eastern Europe, the Balkans and Turkey, usually associated with consumption of meat harvested from infected carcasses.

Disease in animals

Anthrax in animals often follows the grazing of pasture infected with viable spores. Symptoms in animals are usually acute, with high fever of sudden onset, localised swellings and profuse bleeding from orifices. Death usually occurs 24–72 hours after onset. Animals may be found dead or moribund.

In the USA, anthrax is endemic, with cases being reported on a regular basis, e.g. in September 2005, the *Journal of the American Veterinary Medical Association* reported that anthrax had been found in the states of South and North Dakota and Texas in the preceding months.[4] In South Dakota Animal Industry Board a group of almost 300 unvaccinated buffalo and rodeo bulls were believed to have been exposed to anthrax after grazing on contaminated pasture, with approximately 40 of the animals being found dead. The remainder of the herd were treated with antimicrobials, vaccinated and the carcasses safely disposed of.

Concurrently in the south-east of North Dakota, anthrax was detected at in excess of 20 locations, with confirmed cases in cattle, horses, bison and farmed elk. All surviving animals in the herds containing infected animals were quarantined and vaccinated.

The spores are resistant to a wide range of climatic conditions and can remain in contaminated ground for many years. In one reported incident from Hawaii, a cow died after grazing a pasture where the carcass of a cow suspected of having died of the disease 20 years previously was buried. Animals may also demonstrate in-species spread from infected meat or by close contact with an infected beast.

In April 2006, two cattle were confirmed as having died of anthrax on a farm in Rhonda Cynon Taff, South Wales, where there had been a previous outbreak 35 years before. Five cattle had also died in the previous month; however, the last two carcasses were the first to test positive for anthrax. No cattle from the farm had been sent for slaughter into the food chain for the previous 12 months. The source was identified as a pool on the farm, which is believed to have become contaminated.

Transmission

The spores present in the animal's blood or secretions, infected pastures, hides and bone or meat. Transmission to humans follows contact with these spores.

Disease in humans

The disease presents in distinct forms in humans depending on the route of infection. These are:

- Cutaneous, following physical contact with spores and their subsequent inoculation into wounds or abrasions
- Pulmonary, following inhalation of spores from infected hides
- Intestinal, following ingestion of spores or organism in undercooked meat from infected carcasses.

Infected individuals display the disease after a variable incubation period depending on route of infection. The cutaneous form develops after 2–10 days, the pulmonary after 1–5 days and the intestinal after 2–5 days.

The cutaneous form, once known as malignant pustule, is responsible for 98% of cases worldwide. After the incubation period, a papular spot develops on the skin. This papule becomes vesicular and turns black in the centre. This forms an eschar (a plug of dead tissue, skin and blood) which causes necrosis of the underlying tissue and then sloughs off. There is very little pain or tenderness associated with the condition, although local lymph nodes usually swell. Extensive oedema affecting the whole limb or upper body is often seen and is important in differentiating the disease from tick-borne disease where an eschar may also be present. Some patients will display fever, lethargy, sickness and severe headache. The skin lesion will often heal without treatment, but there is a 5–20% risk of untreated cases progressing to septicaemia or meningitis with fatal consequences after the eschar sloughs. Cutaneous spread to other people is possible.

In December 2004, a 31-year-old female Belgian traveller developed a cutaneous anthrax lesion on one finger following contact with dead antelope and a hippopotamus while touring South Africa.[5]

Pulmonary anthrax, known as woolsorter's disease, follows inhalation of spores from infected hides or wool. It presents as a flu-like illness after the incubation period, followed by cough and severe shortness of breath. This develops into respiratory failure and can be fatal within 24 hours, usually following septicaemic spread.

All of the fatal cases seen in the US terrorist attacks during 2001 were from the pulmonary form. Before the extensive number of cases seen in this incident, this form of the disease was believed to be fatal in all cases regardless of the rapidity with which treatment was commenced. This has proved erroneous, with death occurring in only 40% of cases.[6] There are still no known cases stemming from pulmonary spread from existing patients to other individuals, although precautions have been taken to prevent such an eventuality.

Intestinal anthrax follows ingestion of infected meat. The rarity of the condition is related to the low incidence of the disease in meat in developed countries, and the unlikely nature of ingesting enough viable spores or organisms to cause disease.

Severe copious diarrhoea occurs after the incubation period. Half of untreated cases will die.

Diagnosis

Identifying the causative organism in blood smears is diagnostic. Growing samples on standard culture media leads to the development of characteristic colonies, with the bacterium showing centrally placed spores. Immunofluorescent and enzyme-linked immunosorbent assay (ELISA) techniques can also be used.

Treatment

In the UK, the Health Protection Agency (HPA) makes the following recommendations for the treatment of anthrax. The antibiotics of choice are ciprofloxacin and doxycycline. Later therapy may be switched to amoxicillin if the infective strain is susceptible. Cephalosporins must **not** be used because they are ineffective.

As with any other therapy, the latest recommendations from the DH or HPA should be checked before initiating therapy. It should be noted that ciprofloxacin is not licensed for use in children or pregnant women, but may be indicated in life-threatening illness, and also that doxycycline is not recommended in childhood or pregnancy; however, its use would be considered in a serious infection such as anthrax.

Where a diagnosis of infection by anthrax is suspected due to clinical signs or patient history, an early initiation of therapy before laboratory confirmation may be required to reduce fatalities. Usually a short course (3 days) of ciprofloxacin is used until blood culture results become available. It should be noted that, in this case, other likely causes of acute respiratory illness need to be investigated and treated concurrently.

In cases of inhalational and ingestional anthrax, ideally drug therapy should be administered intravenously initially. As the patient improves and once the drug sensitivity of the bacterium is identified, treatment can be continued using oral antibiotics.[7]

In addition to ciprofloxacin, there is some evidence that additional antibiotics or vaccination may be incorporated into a multidrug antibiotic regimen and that this can reduce mortality in inhalational anthrax.[8] In anthrax meningitis, moieties with good central nervous system (CNS) penetration are essential additions, with penicillin, ampicillin, meropenem, vancomycin and rifampin being proposed as suitable. Corticosteroids have been used concomitantly to reduce cerebral oedema in some cases.[9]

The detailed HPA recommendations as of December 2008 are as follows.

Inhalational/ingestional anthrax
- Adults (including pregnant women):
  - ciprofloxacin 750 mg i.v. every 12 h (750 mg twice daily by mouth when appropriate)
  - or doxycycline 100 mg i.v. every 12 h (100 mg twice daily by mouth when appropriate)
  - plus one or two additional antibiotics (agents with in vitro activity include rifampicin, vancomycin, gentamicin, chloramphenicol, penicillin, amoxicillin, imipenem, meropenem and clindomycin).
- Children:
  - ciprofloxacin 10 mg/kg i.v. every 12 h, with the total dose not to exceed the adult dose of 1500 mg/day (when changing to oral therapy if appropriate, dosage is to be altered to 15 mg/kg by mouth, not to exceed the adult dosage of 1500 mg/day)
  - or doxycycline initiated intravenously and then changed to oral therapy when appropriate dosages are

orally – older than 8 years and weighing more than 45 kg: 100 mg every 12 h

intravenously – older than 8 years: 2.2 mg/kg every 12 h

 – plus one or two additional antibiotics (agents with in vitro activity include rifampicin, vancomycin, gentamicin, chloramphenicol, penicillin, amoxicillin, imipenem, meropenem and clindamycin).

• In all cases, both adults and children, therapy should be continued for 60 days.

Cutaneous anthrax

Treatment as in inhalational anthrax is normally using ciprofloxacin or doxycycline as first-line therapy. Unlike inhalational anthrax, treatment can be initiated in adults with oral ciprofloxacin 750 mg or doxycycline 100 mg twice daily for 7 days. If later the organism is found to be susceptible, or the patient cannot tolerate fluoroquinolones or tetracyclines, this can be changed to oral amoxicillin 500 mg three times a day.

For children, the doses of ciprofloxacin or doxycycline follow the same oral regimen as that already detailed for inhalational anthrax. If using amoxicillin, a total daily dose of 80 mg/kg divided into three equal portions and given every 8 hours is an option for completion of therapy after clinical improvement. The oral amoxicillin dose needs to be sufficient to achieve minimum inhibitory concentration levels.

Where cases of cutaneous anthrax show signs of systemic disease, with extensive oedema, or lesions on the head or neck, intravenous therapy may be required, with multidrug therapy being recommended.

If a deliberate release is suspected, treatment may need to be continued for up to 60 days, so as to provide cover for inhalational anthrax, which may have been acquired concurrently.

Prophylaxis

In people known to have been exposed to anthrax, and where no clinical disease is currently present, prophylaxis using antibiotics must be initiated as soon as possible.

Ciprofloxacin is the current drug of choice for all patients. Ciprofloxacin is also the drug of choice in prophylaxis against two other biological agents that could be deliberately released, plague and tularaemia, so its use covers the risk in advance of laboratory testing and identification. The risk of adverse effects associated with administration of antibiotic prophylaxis has to be weighed against the risk of developing a life-threatening infection. The prophylaxis should continue for 60 days to cover the prolonged latency period possible before germination of inhaled spores.

In the UK, usually only 5 days' supply of ciprofloxacin is initially made to individuals, especially in an incident believed to be a deliberate release, in accordance with DH guidelines, and the emergency drug 'pods' deployed by the HPA. After the initial treatment with ciprofloxacin, doxycycline may be substituted to complete the 60-day prophylaxis, this needs to be supplied through local prescribing or dispensing systems. There are patient group directions (PGDs) in place for the initial and further supply of ciprofloxacin and the further supply of doxycycline in the event of exposure to a suspect biological agent (details may be found on the DH/HPA websites).

Made under Article 7 of the Prescription Only Medicines (Human Use) Order 1997 (the POM Order) PGDs make it legal for medicines to be given to groups of patients, e.g. in a mass casualty situation, without individual prescriptions having to be written for each patient. This empowers staff other than doctors (e.g. paramedics, pharmacists and nurses) to legally give the medicine, but only in accordance with the detailed provisions of the PGD.

If anthrax exposure is confirmed, and the organism is identified as being susceptible to penicillin, prophylaxis may be continued using oral amoxicillin as an alternative to ciprofloxacin or doxycycline.

The detailed HPA recommendations as of December 2008 are:

- Adults (including pregnant women), initial (5-day) therapy:
  - ciprofloxacin 500 mg orally twice a day followed by a further (55-day) therapy of either ciprofloxacin 500 mg or doxycycline 100 mg orally twice daily
  - if the strain is found to be susceptible, amoxicillin 500 mg orally three times a day may be substituted.
- Children, initial (5-day) therapy:
  - the dose of ciprofloxacin is age and weight dependent, with the recommendation being that newborn babies up to the age of 6 months receive 100 mg/day in divided doses, and older children receive 15 mg/kg orally twice a day (dose not to exceed 1 g/day, i.e. adult dosage) followed by a further (55-day) therapy of either ciprofloxacin at the same dosage or doxycycline
  - only if older than 8 years and weighing more than 45 kg, at a dose of 100 mg orally every 12 h
  - if the strain is susceptible, amoxicillin may be substituted at a rate of 80 mg/kg per day, in three divided doses (not to exceed 500 mg/ dose).

In the USA, ciprofloxacin was the primary antibiotic used during the outbreak in 2001 in the USA, with doxycycline and amoxicillin being used only if a contraindication to fluoroquinolones existed. Combination therapy was also used.

The current CDC recommendations are similar to those of the HPA, with in addition, levofloxacin now being approved by the US Food and Drug Administration (FDA) for prophylactic therapy for *B. anthracis* exposure.[10,11]

In Europe, BICHAT (Task Force on Biological and Chemical Agent Threats) have made similar recommendations.[12]

Prevention

A vaccine derived from a cell-free filtrate of killed bacteria is available and licensed for human use in the UK. Supplies are kept by the HPA and usually issued for use in workers considered to be at a high occupational risk. The vaccination regimen consists of three doses given over a period of 6 weeks with a booster dose given after 6 months. An annual booster is necessary to maintain immunity. A vaccine is also available for animals, but it is only for emergency use and is obtained through the Department for Environment, Food and Rural Affairs (DEFRA).

Physical prevention methods are based on preventing or limiting contact with infected animals or their hides, hair or meat. All surface wounds should be disinfected and covered. Physical disinfection of hides and hair is considered to be good practice in the tanning and wool industry. The use of formaldehyde as a disinfectant is carried out by specialist companies for imports of hide, bones and bonemeal (much reduced in volume since the advent of bovine spongiform encephalopathy (BSE)) and wool. Heat treatment is also used. Animals suspected of having died of the disease are to be handled in accordance with biohazard procedures. Suitable protective clothing and filtered ventilation helmets should be worn.

Spores may be killed by heat with autoclaving or boiling infected materials or instruments where appropriate. In areas where anthrax is endemic, meat should be thoroughly cooked or avoided.

Formaldehyde and glutaraldehyde are effective disinfectants for dealing with local contamination and spillages, although it is recommended that clothing and other articles of victims should be incinerated carefully.

Cases associated with drum makers

Vado Diomande, a dancer and drum maker, domiciled in New York, but originally from the Ivory Coast, was hospitalised and then diagnosed with inhalational anthrax in February 2006. He appears to have become infected from spores present on hides that he had imported into the USA from West Africa to make his own drumskins. Diomande may have inhaled the spores when, after soaking and stretching them, he scraped the hair off the hides. He was also working untreated hides purchased from US suppliers at the same time, so the source cannot be accurately determined. After extensive antibiotic therapy he survived. Most of the contents of his workshop and apartment were removed and destroyed by public health officials in the ensuing decontamination operation. Close associates were tested for the disease and given antibiotic prophylaxis.[13]

In July 2006, a Scottish artist who lived in Hawick, Scottish Borders, died of anthrax. This was the first fatal case of anthrax in the UK for 30 years, with the previous fatality occurring in 1971. The victim, Christopher 'Pascal' Norris, apparently became infected after he used infected, imported, untreated animal hides to make drum skins. The hides were scraped and worked in a manner that could produce aerosols of infected matter. He developed a rapidly progressive septicaemia and subsequently died. He had previously been treated for cancer, and it is possible that the progress of the disease was increased due to his impaired immune system. It was only retrospective testing of postmortem samples that identified the causative agent as anthrax, and by then his body had been cremated.

His house was quarantined, and had to be systematically decontaminated. Most of his close friends and relatives had to be screened for infection, as a wake was held in the house after the funeral, with guests being encouraged to take away items as keepsakes.

Another case in late 2008 led to the death of another drum maker/drummer in the East End of London.

These were not the first cases associated with the conversion of untreated animal hides into drum skins, with a similar case being recorded in Florida in 1974.

In 2001, a woman was hospitalised in Vancouver, British Columbia, Canada, with cutaneous anthrax on the palm of her hand, which she contracted while handling animal hides during a drum-making class.

Potential as a biological warfare agent

Anthrax can be cultured successfully and its spores harvested. The spores can then be turned into a dry powder. During World War I, the Germans produced sugar lumps inoculated with anthrax for feeding to allied draught horses. There were also incidents of bags of powder containing anthrax spores being dropped from German aircraft. In 1942–3, the British conducted trials on Gruignard Island off the north-west coast of Scotland to investigate the feasibility of biological warfare using anthrax. (The island was finally declared safe in 1990.) In an associated programme, Britain developed cattle cakes inoculated with anthrax for retaliatory strikes against Germany. These were to have been dropped from bomber aircraft in the event of a German strike. In Germany warheads containing anthrax were developed for attachment to V1 and V2 weapons. The escalation of hostilities that such weapons would have caused led to neither side employing them offensively.

In Japan, during the 1990s, the Aum Shinrikyo cult released anthrax spores in Tokyo. Luckily there were no fatalities. Following the Iran–Iraq war and the Gulf War, Iraq was shown to have produced shells and missile warheads packed with spores.

Many authorities view anthrax as the greatest threat for use in biological warfare or terrorism. With the cases caused by contaminated mail in the USA in the aftermath of the events of 11 September, it has become apparent that as a terrorist weapon it has a tremendous potential to cause widespread concern with some fatalities, even when the potency has not been enhanced by finely grinding the powder containing the spores.

Amerithrax: the 2001 cases in the USA

In September and October 2001, there were a cluster of cases of cutaneous and inhalational anthrax, after maliciously contaminated mail was sent through the US Postal Service to addressees in the US Congress, US government departments, prominent journalists and other media figures across the USA (Florida, New York, Washington, New Jersey).[14]

Initial diagnosis of patients was slow; however, once it was recognised that a bioterrorism attack using anthrax spores had occurred, tracing and screening were initiated.[15] There were 22 cases, of whom 19 were confirmed and 3 classed as probable, with 5 being fatal. Cases were seen in people directly exposed to the contaminated letters, and indirectly by secondary spread from sorting machines, or other post that was passing through the mail facilities at the same time as the contaminated letters.

All the contaminated mail contained powder containing anthrax spores The four letters that were recovered during the investigation also contained notes, purporting to be from Islamic extremists, although this was later dismissed as misdirection by the perpetrator. It is believed that seven letters were sent in total; however, the other three have never been found.

Following detection of cases, work places where the letters had been handled were screened for contamination, and then decontaminated. All workers were tested for exposure, and given antibiotics (ciprofloxacin, doxycycline or amoxicillin) as either treatment or prophylaxis; however, in the cases of some postal workers and other victims this was not initiated rapidly enough to prevent fatalities. Some suspected cases were never confirmed as the bacterium could not be isolated from initial samples and, as antibiotics were given on a precautionary basis, re-testing was negative.

Some of the fatal cases were sporadic (i.e. not linked to direct exposure to the contaminated letters), with one in a healthcare worker apparently after secondary exposure to infected clothing in a hospital emergency room, and another (an elderly woman in Connecticut) being notionally linked to mail contaminated by passing through a sorting machine at the same time as one of the deliberately contaminated letters.[16]

A criminal investigation was launched by the FBI; however, it was initially hampered by the need to focus on the events following the 9/11 attack on the World Trade Centre and the Pentagon. With the strain identified as one normally associated with scientific establishments, the FBI focused on using profiling to try to identify suspects. To date nobody has been charged in relation to the attack.

Facilities contaminated included mail offices, sorting offices and other premises. The clean-up to date has cost many millions of dollars, and it has been difficult to agree the level of decontamination required by workers' unions to allow premises to re-open.

Before and since the Amerithrax incident, there have been a number of hoax letters containing powder across the world, notably in Canberra in 2005 and again in 2008, against the Church of Scientology in the USA in 2006 and 2008, and by anti-abortionists in the USA and Canada, a campaign that pre-dated the Amerithrax incident; there has been a total of 655 letters to date, including 554 mailed by one US activist in November 2001. The aim in all these incidents, none of which to date has contained anthrax, seems to be to cause the maximum amount of disruption while making a political or ethical point. The costs of dealing with such incidents are high, requiring specialist staff and equipment to contain, identify and control possible contamination.

Ebola
African haemorrhagic fever; Ebola haemorrhagic fever

Ebola is probably one of the most dramatic zoonotic infections. It is caused by a virus similar in form to Marburg virus but distinguished by differences in antigen testing profile. The virus is named after a river in The Democratic Republic of the Congo (DRC; formerly Zaire). Classified as an RNA filovirus, it shows strange branching and filamentous forms displayed by no other viral group. There are four subtypes of the virus. The three demonstrated to be pathogenic in humans are Ebola–Ivory Coast, Ebola–Sudan and Ebola–Zaire. The fourth, Ebola–Reston, has been shown to be pathogenic in apes but not for infected humans. This last type was identified in monkeys imported from the Philippines into Italy and North America for laboratory use. Several research workers became infected with the virus, although none became ill.[17]

Ebola haemorrhagic fever was first recognised in 1976, when large outbreaks occurred in southern Sudan and neighbouring northern Zaire. Since then it has appeared sporadically in these and other areas of Africa. There has been only one case recorded outside Africa with a single non-fatal case in a laboratory in the UK after a needlestick injury. The pathogenic forms of the virus are not known to be native to other continents.

Transmission

The natural reservoir of Ebola virus is not proven fully; however, it has been detected in three species of fruit bats. Scientists from the Institut Pasteur, Paris, have also detected it in small rodents in the Central African Republic. There is still work to be done to discover how the virus is transmitted to apes and monkeys, which have previously been identified as the link to human infection. The handling of ill or dead infected chimpanzees was shown to be the source of human infection in outbreaks in the Ivory Coast, Gabon and the DRC.[18,19]

The main concern for countries outside Africa stems from the latent period of the infection. In theory it would be possible for an infected individual to carry the disease into a city or country where, unrecognised, the disease could rapidly spread. Mortality rates have been as high as 90% in some outbreaks so the fear is not unfounded.

Disease in humans

The virus has an incubation period of between 2 and 21 days after exposure and infection in humans before clinical signs are seen. Weakness and lethargy follow a sudden onset of fever with a temperature as high as 39°C. Muscle and joint pain are seen in most cases, with sore throat, headache and occasionally hiccups. More severe symptoms follow with anorexia, nausea, vomiting and diarrhoea. The development of a severe skin rash and mental confusion is concurrent with the progression of the illness. Kidney and liver damage occurs and catastrophic internal and external haemorrhage leads to death towards the beginning of the second week. The virus is present in high concentrations in the blood, tissue fluids and most organs of the body. Patients lucky enough to survive require extended periods of care.

Human-to-human transmission occurs after direct contact with the blood, secretions or semen of infected patients. Following the first confirmed or index case, transmission occurs to those in closest contact with the victim. These can be friends, family or healthcare workers. Nosocomial spread or spread from a clinic or hospital to staff or other patients has occurred several times in major outbreaks, leading to high mortality rates. In Africa limitations on availability of disposable equipment and protective clothing have also led to transmission. The disease can also be sexually transmitted through semen up to 7 weeks after clinical recovery. All Ebola virus subtypes have displayed the ability to be spread through aerosols under research conditions, although aerosol spread has not been demonstrated during outbreaks.

Outbreak statistics

In the first recorded outbreak, between June and November 1976, the Ebola virus infected 284 people in Sudan, with 117 deaths. During the outbreaks 76 of the 230 staff at Maridi Hospital contracted Ebola fever, with 41 subsequently dying. In Zaire (now the DRC) there were 318 cases and 280 deaths in September and October 1976.

There was an isolated case in the DRC in 1977 and a second outbreak in Sudan in 1979. One human case of Ebola haemorrhagic fever and several cases in chimpanzees were confirmed in the Ivory Coast in 1994 when a scientist contracted the disease after conducting a postmortem examination on a wild chimpanzee found dead with signs of haemorrhagic disease. Fortune favours the foolish and the brave and he spontaneously recovered.

A large epidemic occurred in Kikwit, DRC in 1995 with 315 cases, 244 of whom died. This outbreak was thought to have occurred after the index case handled a monkey and smoked its flesh.

Ebola virus infections were not reported again until the autumn of 2000 when an outbreak occurred in the Gulu district of northern Uganda. This was the first outbreak ever documented in Uganda and, by the time that it was declared over in February 2001, there had been 425 cases, including 224 deaths. Spread had been dramatic both in the community and in hospitals, with healthcare workers among the dead.

In Gabon, Ebola haemorrhagic fever was first documented in 1994 and two outbreaks occurred in February 1996 and July 1996, with 37 cases and 21 deaths in Mayibout related to cooking a chimpanzee, and 61 cases and 45 deaths in Booue. Another outbreak occurred in Gabon, and the neighbouring area of the DRC, between October 2001 and March 2002 with 122 cases, of whom 96 died.

Since then there have been series of outbreaks in the DRC, between December 2002 and April 2003, November and December 2003, and May and June 2005. All of these outbreaks were in the Cuvette Ouest Region of the DRC. In the 2005 outbreak, only one case was laboratory confirmed and 11 others epidemiologically linked; of these 12, 9 subsequently died. Other contacts were monitored for 21 days after the last reported death, but none was infected.

In 2004, a small outbreak occurred in Sudan with a concurrent measles epidemic. This confused the differential diagnosis, with the final number of cases actually attributable to Ebola being revised to 17 cases and 7 deaths.

The latest outbreaks were in 2007 and 2008, in the DRC and Uganda. The 2007 outbreak in the DRC started in August, and finished in October with 249 suspected cases and 183 deaths; another outbreak began in December 2008. The last outbreak in Uganda was between November 2007 and February 2008. There were 149 cases with 37 deaths. Characterisation of the virus in the Uganda outbreak has led to the conclusion that this may be a new species of Ebola virus, which as yet remains unnamed.

Treatment

There is no therapeutic treatment for the disease. Supportive measures, such as rehydration by intravenous fluids, blood transfusion, use of nutritional supplements (again by intravenous route) and management of kidney failure, can improve the outcome of the disease. Rapid treatment of secondary infections is also very important, especially in the convalescent patient. During the Kikwit outbreak in 1995, eight patients were given blood donated by survivors. Seven of the eight patients recovered, probably as a result of the conferred immunity, although this treatment has not been properly clinically evaluated.[20] Research continues to try to develop a vaccine, and some progress has been made with experimental protection using a live-attenuated, recombinant, vesicular, stomatitis virus vector expressing the Ebola virus glycoprotein.[21] This product has been experimentally shown to completely protect rodents and non-human primates from lethal Ebola virus challenge.[22]

Prevention

Since 1989, there have been a number of cases of Ebola–Reston, fatal to monkeys, but so far harmless in humans in quarantine facilities in the USA, Philippines and Italy, all linked to primates sourced from the facility in the Philippines where fresh-caught and captive-bred apes were mixed. The recommendations from the CDC and other responsible bodies are that any imported apes that have not been bred in captivity must be strictly quarantined. For best practice this should be extended to all primates. Strict hygiene measures should be employed. Appropriate protective clothing should be worn at all times.

Suspected Ebola haemorrhagic fever is a notifiable disease in the UK and the USA, both domestically and to the World Health Organization (WHO). For healthcare workers strict barrier nursing and the use and careful disposal of gloves, syringes, needles and dressings are essential. All clinical specimens have to be handled according to guidelines for extremely hazardous substances. Immediate disposal of bodies in secure body bags with prompt burial or cremation is necessary during an outbreak.

Case contacts or individuals exposed in laboratories must be placed under health surveillance for 3 weeks after their last possible exposure to infection. If there is the onset of febrile symptoms they must be placed in strict isolation until diagnostic test results have been obtained.

In Africa, as the infection route is still incompletely understood, prevention of Ebola poses a major problem. Educating healthcare workers and others to identify a suspected case early and be able to isolate the patient with appropriate barrier nursing techniques is seen as the main thrust of current limitation strategies. The main obstacle to the success of such a strategy is the availability of sterile materials, protective clothing and appropriate facilities. Usually once a case has been confirmed by diagnostic tests an outbreak is already under way.

Plague
The Black Death, Bubonic and Pneumonic plague

Any book about zoonoses would not be complete without a section on plague, and any section on plague must detail the historical importance of the ravages associated with the disease. Even today, it is not unusual to see children in the playground singing and acting out 'Ring-a-ring o'roses, a pocket full of posies, a-tishoo, a-tishoo, we all fall down'. This anonymous nursery rhyme, originating in the middle of the seventeenth century, is a graphic and simple representation of the effects of an outbreak of pneumonic plague. The importance of rat control is emphasised in the same way, with the telling of the tale of the Pied Piper of Hamelin.

Historians differ in their view of the worst results of epidemic plague, and the numbers of casualties quoted for pandemics are probably in legal terms 'unsafe'. The widest geographical epidemics are usually known as pandemics and the consensus of opinion is that in recorded history there have been three outbreaks that could be thus classified.

The first to spread across Europe started in the sixth century, and was known as the Plague of Justinian. There were widespread fatalities. This outbreak was seen as a visitation by God on a sinful people; however, the religiosity that it engendered was no protection against flea bites and disease.

The outbreak now termed the Second Pandemic, or the Black Death, started from a natural focus somewhere in Mesopotamia in western Turkey during the eleventh century. Plague-infected rats and their associated fleas, carried aboard trading ships, spread the Black Death from Tana in the Crimea, Ukraine, to Messina in Sicily in 1347. In the ensuing European plague, which endured up to the end of the seventeenth century, it is variously estimated that a quarter to a half of the population died as a result of this disease alone. At the height of the epidemic in the fourteenth century, the effect upon all aspects of social and international development was profound: large swathes of land in Europe became uninhabited. The epidemic in the UK in the 1660s, which caused the Plague of London and other local outbreaks, stemmed from this pandemic. Although important in British history, it was insignificant in world terms, with only 70 000 fatalities.

The third and last pandemic occurred during the late nineteenth century. It owed its rapid spread to commercial shipping, with infected rats becoming stowaways on fast steam packets leaving Hong Kong and Canton in 1894 for many other ports the world over. Within a decade it had spread to over 70 ports on 5 continents. Coming as it did at a time when scientific endeavour and disciplines were developing, the bacterium, its association with rats and the rat flea as a vector were soon identified, allowing prevention strategies to be put in place.

The disease

The pathogen responsible for plague is *Yersinia pestis*, a Gram-negative coccobacillus. A facultative anaerobe, the bacterium is capable of forming an encapsulated spore swiftly when exposed to the air. The risk of infection from the spores, which are able to survive under suitable conditions for prolonged periods of time, is considered to be significant in archaeological excavations of burial sites.

During World War II, part of the Blitz upon London was aimed at disturbing the plague pits used for burials during the Plague of London three centuries previously, in the hope of releasing viable spores into the environment. Had this succeeded, the death toll from this disease, let loose in a city with increasing rodent numbers, poor sanitation and a displaced human population, would arguably have been high.

This was not the first use of the disease as a weapon of war. Corpses of humans and animals that had died of this and other diseases have in the past been hurled into besieged cities using catapults. This stratagem was used in the hope and certainty of infecting the garrison from the earliest recorded incidents of siege warfare until modern times. In 1346 a Tartar army besieging the city of Kaffa, in what is now Turkey, suffered from plague. They threw their dead into the city over the walls, and the resulting epidemic forced the defenders to surrender.

Plague has been identified as a pathogen at the centre of several countries' programmes of biological warfare development. Russia is known to have designed for use a genetically manipulated strain. Both North Korea and Israel are known to have studied the use of this pathogen extensively in an offensive military role. If employed, the pathogen would be delivered using an air-borne route, so giving pneumonic plague to victims.

Wild foci

Wild plague foci, where suitable rodent populations and habitat conditions exist, are found in the western USA, some countries in South America, extensive areas of north-central, eastern and southern Africa, Madagascar, Iran, and also along the frontier between Yemen and Saudi Arabia, central and south-east Asia, and portions of the former Soviet Union[23] (Figure 6.1).

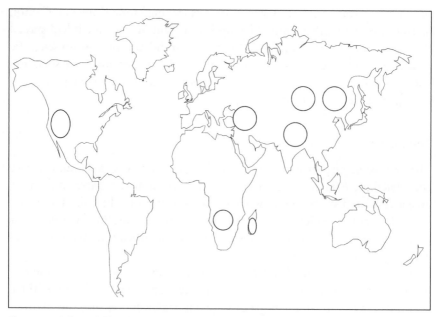

Figure 6.1 Sylvatic (wild) plague foci across the world.

These foci are associated with dry areas, usually where desert or prairie-type landscapes form. Foci are normally away from urban areas because of their inaccessibility, or their inhospitable nature. It is therefore unusual to find human cases emanating from wild foci sources; however, in the USA where there has been rapid expansion of urban areas and isolated condominium building, an increasing number of human cases come from this source.

Rodents in a natural plague focus become immune to the disease. However, if they spread from the focus into another distinct rodent population, especially one linked to an urbanised site, infection of a susceptible population of rodents may produce massive fatalities. This can lead to the phenomenon known as rat-fall, where a large number of rodent corpses are seen in open areas. Associated with this event are usually reports of fleas biting humans: the rat fleas leave the corpses in search of new hosts, and this results in disease transfer.

The world picture

The WHO and the CDC have formed the World Health Organization Colloborating Center or WHOCC for Plague at the CDC, Fort Collins, Colorado, USA. The centre provides epidemiological assistance, with advice on prevention strategies, diagnostic support (including a reference collection of strains), and in-country training. It also supports research into all aspects of plague. Plague is one of only three infectious diseases subject to international health regulations. All confirmed cases should be reported to the WHO.[23]

The last worldwide study of plague was completed by the WHO in 1997, and the overall world picture remains consistent with that study; however, this may change in the future as alterations in climate may alter the epidemiology (see below).

In 2003, when the CDC conducted a survey, there were 2118 recorded cases of plague worldwide with 1882 fatalities. Over 98% of the cases and 98% of the fatalities occurred in various plague foci in Africa.

In Africa, Madagascar reports the highest number of cases in most years, probably due to the large numbers of rodents in its unique ecosystem. The disease has also been reported in Algeria, the DRC, Malawi, Tanzania and Uganda.[24]

In the USA, there are two main regions where natural plague foci are found: northern New Mexico, northern Arizona, southern Colorado and California, southern Oregon and far western Nevada.

Plague also occurs across South America with cases being reported recently from Bolivia, Brazil, Ecuador and Peru.

In Asia, cases have been recorded in China, India, Indonesia, Kazakhstan, Mongolia, Myanmar and Vietnam. Although cases are reported it is possible that reporting may be incomplete.

Epidemiology

In terms of the development of an epidemic, the re-emergence of plague in India in 1994 after a gap of reported cases of almost 30 years was dramatic. In 1993 a severe earthquake hit areas previously identified as having wild plague foci. The resulting devastation allowed the rat population to increase dramatically, with a corresponding increase in the population of their associated fleas. In August 1994 a village in the Beed district reported rat-fall and subsequent flea nuisance. An outbreak of bubonic plague followed, with 596 cases but no fatalities.

A separate outbreak in Gujarat followed flooding associated with a record monsoon rainfall. During the clean-up operation, workers came into contact with infected animal corpses. The initial cases turned into secondary pneumonic plague, and subsequently, during an influx of people into Surat City for a religious festival, an outbreak of pneumonic plague ensued. Of 151 cases, 52 died.

Only sporadic cases were seen in India from 1994 until 2002, when a cluster of cases was seen in Himachal Pradesh. The index case had killed a sick wild cat, and then skinned it; he subsequently developed pneumonic plague, infecting 13 of his relatives (probably due to close contact and poorly ventilated living accommodation) and 2 other people who acquired the disease while in the same hospital as other victims.

In the USA, there were 107 cases and 11 deaths from human plague between 1990 and 2005; of these cases 81 were bubonic, 19 septicaemic, 5 pneumonic and 2 unclassified. In 2006 there were thirteen cases, of which two were fatal, in four US states: seven in New Mexico, three in Colorado, two in California and one in Texas; five were septicaemic and eight bubonic.

The most dramatic cases in the USA, and the ones that caused a major public health response, were a married couple from Santa Fe, New Mexico who travelled to New York City in November 2002. After arriving in New York they both became ill, and were diagnosed with plague. An alert emergency doctor who carried out the initial case assessment became aware that the couple might have the disease, and a comprehensive health response led to a number of healthcare workers and other contacts receiving antibiotic prophylaxis. No further cases resulted. This case highlighted the risk that infected people might travel to different areas, where the disease might not be recognised during the pre-patent period.

There have been a number of outbreaks in Africa: Malawi (2002), Uganda (2004) and the DRC (2005). The DRC outbreak in Oriental province was unusual in that there were 130 suspected cases of pneumonic plague, of whom 57 died. Thousands of people fled the region to avoid the infection.[25]

An outbreak in Oran, Algeria in 2003 was not linked to a previously identified focus; however, it may have been triggered by the building of a new flour mill with subsequent rodent colonisation. Oran had historically had a number of outbreaks, notably in the last two pandemics.[26]

In Tanzania, a natural focus has been identified in Lushoto province. This focus is believed to have led to 7600 cases of plague in the period 1980–2004.

The area of most concern in plague infection in Africa is currently Madagascar. A strain of *Y. pestis* showing multiple antibiotic resistance has emerged there.[24] The island has an unusual animal population: rodent species are widespread, leading to an atypical pattern of foci with a higher risk to the human population. The majority of cases are bubonic, due to the virtually universal source of infection being primary contact with rodent fleas.

Climate change

The current changes in world climate with warmer springs and wetter summers might increase the incidence of plague. This could stem from a number of factors, such as increases in the numbers of rodents and more fleas (which because of the higher temperatures are more active and breed faster). A 1°C increase in temperature in Kazakhstan over spring and summer has led to a 59% increase in the number of reported cases of plague. Increased temperatures were also associated historically with the previous pandemics.

A similar pattern has been seen in the USA around foci, with high rainfall in spring, and cool summers increase the numbers of rodents and fleas, leading to pressure on rodents to move outward from the foci, thus contacting susceptible rodents or humans.

Disease in animals

The primary wildlife reservoirs of plague are rodent species. The rat, either the domestic black rat (*Rattus rattus*) or the urban brown rat (*R. norvegicus*), was the most important reservoir and rodent vector in terms of previous pandemics. Other species may be involved depending on the site and situation of the natural foci involved. In the USA, ground squirrels, rabbits and chipmunks have been identified as important maintenance hosts. Under the normal circumstances in a natural wild focus, the disease cycles within the rodent population and is transferred by fleas, which are often specific to the rodent species involved[27] (Figure 6.2).

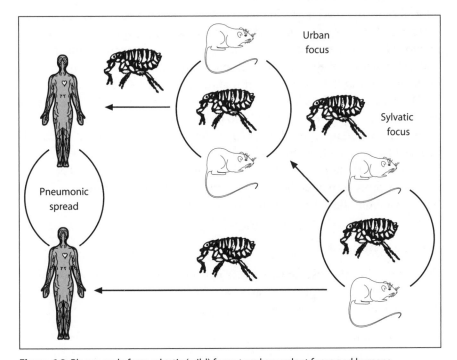

Figure 6.2 Plague cycle from sylvatic (wild) focus to urban rodent focus and humans.

Other animal species capable of carrying, amplifying or transmitting plague include goats, dogs, cats, squirrels, camels and rabbits. Dogs usually have a brief illness and often recover; cats are not so fortunate. They will often have severe fatal infection with high fever, swollen lymph nodes, pneumonic symptoms and encephalitis. Cats have caused human infection, usually after bites or scratches or inhalation by the human of aerosolised cat secretions. Other non-rodent species are also theoretically able to infect humans via similar routes.

Transmission

The infection of the first, and sometimes only, victim in an outbreak can almost be classed as accidental, following bites from rodent fleas, either in a natural focus or after a rat-fall. The infection may also follow direct contact with rodents or other infected animals, especially if they are butchered or skinned. The route of infection under these circumstances can be by direct transfer of blood, ingestion of infected tissue, or inhalation of infected aerosols of blood or mucus. There is some evidence that fomite spread by knives or other instruments used to slaughter or butcher rodents is also possible.

Once an infected host has been bitten, the bacterium is ingested and multiplies in the flea's gut. The bacterium secretes a coagulase, causing an occlusive clot to form in the mid-gut of the flea. This causes blood from a previous bite to be regurgitated during the next bite, due to the obstruction and the structure of the flea's mouth parts. Inevitably this leads to transfer of the bacteria in the most efficient manner possible.

Once infected, fleas can remain infective for a period of weeks or months. The coagulated mass can also ultimately kill the flea. The inoculum necessary to initiate clinical disease, if delivered by the bite of a flea, is believed to be a single viable organism.

The usual route of infection for humans is by rat flea bite. There have also been cases of plague being transmitted from human to human via the bite of a human flea. This is believed to be extremely rare.

Disease in humans

The course that the disease then takes depends upon the route of infection and the symptoms displayed. Cases are classified as bubonic, septicaemic, meningeal, pharyngeal or pneumonic plague.

Bubonic plague

This is the classic pattern of infection following the bites of infected fleas or inoculation of a wound with contaminated material. After infection, an incubation period of 2–6 days is normally seen. As with many other diseases, the initial signs and symptoms after inoculation can be very generalised and non-specific, but with an acute onset. A fever with headache, chills, fatigue, sickness, joint pain and sore throat are the first clinical signs, indistinguishable from infection with other pathogens.

Following these initial symptoms, and the development of a persistent fever that may increase, there is a progressive swelling of the lymph nodes. This usually commences with the node nearest the site of inoculation. The nodes become tender and are known as buboes, hence the condition's name. Vomiting and muscle pain with delirium usually follow. The swollen nodes fill with pus and the disease spreads, through both the lymphatic system and the bloodstream. The skin over the node becomes reddened, shiny and swollen.

On treatment the reddening starts to resolve. However, the buboes, especially the first, subside only over a period of time. The initial site can remain swollen for weeks and may require surgical removal for full recovery to take place. In untreated cases, more than half of patients will die.

Septicaemic plague

Primary septicaemic plague does not present with a bubo. There is a high fever, with gastrointestinal disturbance. Symptoms may be confused with urinary tract or chest infections, appendicitis or a viral infection. Pneumonic plague may develop. The disease is progressive, and mediated by an endotoxin secreted by the pathogen. There is an overwhelming immunological response, resulting in a syndrome similar to anaphylactic shock. Intravascular coagulation may occur with multiple-organ failure and respiratory distress, thrombosis and subdermal haemorrhage leading to the blackening and focal necrosis (the symptom from which the soubriquet 'Black Death' comes) of the skin. Meningeal plague can be present, as can ophthalmic involvement and hepatic or splenic abscesses.

Meningeal plague

Usually seen as a complication of bubonic or septicaemic plague, it can also be a primary infection. Fever, headache and stiffness of the neck, with increasing delirium and confusion followed by coma, are normally seen. The pathogen can be isolated from the cerebrospinal fluid. Most cases follow delayed, inappropriate or bacteriostatic antibiotic therapy. The use of any antibiotic incapable of crossing the blood–brain barrier carries with it the risk of developing this form of disease.

Pharyngeal plague

Pharyngeal plague follows inhalation and deposition in the nose, mouth or throat of large droplets of infected pulmonary exudate or ingestion of infected raw or undercooked meat. Clinical signs mimic bacterial or viral pharyngitis, with severe lymph node swellings. The only way of characterising the infection and the responsible pathogen is by identification from a throat swab and subsequent culture. The course of the disease is variable; however, it normally progresses to a bubonic infection if the patient survives that long.

In 1994 (finally reported in 2005), there was a cluster of cases of pharyngeal plague associated with eating raw camel liver from an infected animal. The index case slaughtered the camel, and presented with the bubonic form, although he also did not eat any meat from the animal. People who ate raw liver contracted pharyngeal plague, and a large number of other people who ate the cooked meat or liver remained disease free.[28]

Pneumonic plague

Patients suffering from bubonic or septicaemic plague may have a dissemination of infection to form a focus in the lungs, known as secondary pneumonic infection. Although their infection remains mainly bubonic, and the clinical course is relatively unaltered, they can develop cough with production of aerosolised infected pulmonary exudate. This can transfer infections to other individuals who then develop a primary pneumonic form of the disease. Once individuals display pneumonic symptoms, they are extremely contagious and the spread of the disease within human outbreaks is usually by this rapid route, without the further involvement of rodents or fleas. For the infection to spread, other individuals need to usually be within 2 m of an actively coughing patient. Humid overcrowded living areas encourage and promote human-to-human spread by this transmission route.[29]

Pneumonic plague is the form of the disease associated with the highest rate of fatality. The pre-patent period is very short: 24–72 hours after exposure. The initial symptoms are similar to other forms of the disease but there is marked physical weakness and respiratory difficulty. A productive cough with copious thin sputum, gradually increasing chest pain, breathing difficulties and the coughing of blood are progressive signs as the condition worsens. Deterioration is very rapid and death occurs within 3 days in almost all untreated patients.

To avert this outcome, antibiotic therapy must be commenced within 18–24 hours of clinical onset. Development of concurrent septicaemic plague and associated complications make supportive therapy and nursing difficult.

Diagnosis

The WHOCC recommends that, immediately a diagnosis of human plague is suspected on clinical and epidemiological grounds, appropriate specimens for diagnosis should be obtained and the patient should be started on specific antimicrobial therapy without waiting for laboratory results. Victims suspected of having the pneumonic form should be placed in isolation wards and barrier nursed.

Confirmation of the diagnosis follows isolation, culture and identification of *Y. pestis* from specimens. Staining with Wayson or Giemsa stain leaves the pathogen showing a distinctive bipolar appearance. On microscopic examination they have a distinctive 'safety-pin' shape. Serological testing, ELISA and antibody testing can also be used if available. In some cases, diagnosis is only confirmed retrospectively *post mortem.*

Treatment

The first response to plague infection is antibiotics. The following notes come from the WHO, CDC and HPA; however, not all drugs are licensed in every country for use in plague. Any cases seen in the UK or the USA would be treated by specialists.

Streptomycin, tetracyclines and chloramphenicol have been traditionally used to treat plague, with streptomycin being the treatment of choice, especially in severe infections, in particular the pneumonic form. However, the HPA now recommends gentamicin instead. Two pieces of research suggest that gentamicin (either alone or in combination with a tetracycline – doxycycline) was as effective as streptomycin and that doxycycline can be used on its own as a monotherapy.[30,31]

Chloramphenicol

Chloramphenicol is a suitable alternative to aminoglycosides in the treatment of bubonic or septicaemic plague and is the drug of choice for treatment of patients with meningeal, ophthalmic or pleural complications. Chloramphenicol may be used together with either streptomycin or gentamicin.

Tetracyclines

The tetracyclines are bacteriostatic, and their use can lead to the development of complications. However, they are deemed suitable for use in uncomplicated cases. Tetracyclines can be used in addition to other agents.[32]

Other antibiotics

Fluoroquinolones such as ciprofloxacin and levofloxacin have been shown to be effective against *Y. pestis* in laboratory and animal studies.[33] Penicillins, cephalosporins and macrolides have been shown to be ineffective or of variable effect in the treatment of plague and they should not be used for this purpose.

In the UK the current HPA recommendations are:

- Adults:
  - gentamicin (first choice in pregnancy) 5 mg/kg i.m. or i.v. once a day or 2 mg/kg loading dose followed by 1.7 mg/kg i.m. or i.v. three times daily (renal function should be monitored and blood taken for gentamicin or streptomycin levels)
  - if aminoglycosides are unsuitable ciprofloxacin 400 mg i.v. twice daily may be used (in milder cases only, 500 mg orally twice daily may be used), or doxycycline 100 mg orally twice daily (for ciprofloxacin, other fluoroquinolones with proven activity, e.g. ofloxacin, levofloxacin, may be substituted, at equivalent doses)
  - if plague meningitis is suspected chloramphenicol 25 mg/kg i.v. four times daily may be given.
- Children:
  - ciprofloxacin 10 mg/kg i.v. twice daily (max. 400 mg) not to exceed 800 mg/day (in milder cases only, 15 mg/kg orally twice daily may be given with total dose not to exceed 1 g/day)
  - or doxycycline 100 mg orally twice daily in children > 8 years and who weigh > 45 kg; in children > 8 years but weighing < 45 kg the dosage of doxycycline should be 2.2 mg/kg every 12 h
  - in cases of suspected meningeal plague, chloramphenicol 25 mg/kg (max. 500 mg) orally or i.v. four times daily can be used.
- In both adults and children therapy should be continued for 14 days.

Prophylaxis

Healthcare workers or others who come into close contact with infected patients should receive prophylactic treatment. It may also be suitable for scientific fieldworkers investigating plague foci. Tetracycline, doxycycline or co-trimoxazole is currently used. Chloramphenicol has fallen from favour, due to the incidence of severe side effects.

In the event of exposure to a deliberate release, or contact with a case of pneumonic disease, prophylactic antibiotic therapy should be initiated immediately. Contacts of cases of bubonic plague should be assessed for the need for prophylaxis. For adults, children and pregnant women, ciprofloxacin is the drug of choice.

The risk of adverse effects from antibiotic prophylaxis must be weighed against the risk of developing clinical disease in both adults and children. Other antibiotics, such as chloramphenicol or co-trimoxazole, could be used in individuals who cannot tolerate the antibiotic, or where the risk is considered to be too great.

After initial treatment with ciprofloxacin, doxycycline may be substituted to complete the 7-day prophylaxis. People who come into contact (< 2 m) with patients with pneumonic plague should receive antibiotic prophylaxis for 7 days. In healthcare and laboratory staff with continuing exposure, prophylaxis should be extended to 7 days after the last contact with a patient or sample considered to be infectious. Prophylaxis should continue until exposure has been excluded.

As with anthrax, in the UK, the duration of initial course of antibiotic treatment is currently 5 days from the HPA emergency system, and a PGD has been developed to provide the necessary continuation course. Details may be found on the DH website. In the UK the current HPA recommendations are:

- Adults (including pregnant women), initial (5-day) therapy:
  - ciprofloxacin 500 mg orally twice a day followed by a further (2-day) therapy of either ciprofloxacin 500 mg or doxycycline 100 mg orally twice daily.
- Children, initial (5-day) therapy:
  - the dose of ciprofloxacin is age and weight dependent, with the recommendation being that newborn babies up to the age of 6 months receive 100 mg/day in divided doses, and older children receive 15 mg/kg orally twice a day (dose not to exceed 1 g/day, i.e. adult dosage) with a further (2-day) treatment of ciprofloxacin at the same dose
  - doxycycline may also be used at the following dosages: if the child is > 8 years and weighs > 45 kg at a dose of 100 mg orally every 12 h; in children > 8 years but weighing < 45 kg the dosage of doxycycline should be 2.2 mg/kg every 12 h.

Prevention

Vaccination is available; however, the likelihood of travellers contracting plague is very low. People going to work or live in areas where there is a known wild focus may be vaccinated. Laboratory workers who could be exposed to plague through clinical samples should be vaccinated in endemic areas, especially if investigating the focus. Development of immunity takes at least 1 month after immunisation. Immunisation with the vaccine does not protect against developing primary pneumonic plague, so workers in risk areas, especially if geographically isolated, should be educated about signs and symptoms and encouraged to carry suitable antibiotics for immediate use if required. The vaccine is available in the UK through specialised centres, such as the Hospital for Tropical Diseases and the DH, and in the USA through the CDC. It is unlicensed in the UK, although if needed this is probably not significant. The vaccine does not offer immediate protection and should be used only for prophylaxis.

Avoiding exposure to rodents and their fleas, and controlling rodents and their fleas, remain the best methods of prevention. Domestic and companion animals in endemic areas should be treated for fleas, and bites and scratches avoided wherever possible.[21]

Rabies (hydrophobia)

Classic rabies is caused by a genus *Lyssavirus*, family *Rhabdoviridae* virus, sometimes known as genotype 1 virus, to distinguish it from other closely related viruses that have been identified as causing similar illnesses (see below). It is a continual challenge to public health systems worldwide, especially in developing countries, with an estimated 55 000 deaths, and approximately 10 million people receiving post-exposure prophylaxis (PEP) annually worldwide, mainly in Africa and Asia.[34]

The expense of vaccine as PEP for patients exposed to animals suffering from the disease or potentially rabid animals is a significant cost for the public health purse in countries or areas where the disease is endemic.

The UK and Europe

The UK benefits from a geographical advantage when it comes to rabies. As an island it has been possible to eradicate the disease in the past and prevent its re-introduction. The last indigenous case of rabies was in 1902, and after a nationwide campaign and enforcement of a system of strict quarantine the country was declared disease free. The continued enforcement of these regulations and the strict rules relating to the issuing of pet passports has maintained the UK in this status; however, this is not true of continental Europe.

Rabies is believed to have crossed the Polish border into Europe in the late 1930s. At this point, the virus transferred from dogs (its previous reservoir) into its main reservoir species in western Europe, the red fox (*Vulpes vulpes*); however, it is now believed that it also spread into the raccoon dog (*Nycterentes procyonides*). This has led to the current pattern of dog-mediated rabies in eastern Europe, fox-mediated rabies in east and central Europe, and raccoon dog rabies in north-eastern Europe. Currently, only Turkey has 'dog-mediated rabies', where wild and feral dogs form the main disease reservoir. The southern portion of the former Soviet Union is unique in having a mixed pattern of dog- and fox-mediated infection.[35]

The area where the disease was considered to be endemic advanced towards the English Channel at approximately 20–60 km (12–36 miles) each year, and had engulfed Paris by the late 1970s. A concerted effort by European governments over a number of years to vaccinate domesticated animals and wildlife (by using baits loaded with an oral vaccine) has led to many states being declared 'rabies free'. The effectiveness of such schemes can be gauged from the reduction seen in Germany, from 10 000 animal cases per year in the late 1970s, to 56 cases in 1999, to 6 bat-linked cases in 2007.

During 2007, the WHO European rabies monitoring centre reported a total of 9563 cases. Of these, 54% occurred in wild animals and 45% in domestic animals. There were only nine human cases, with six in the Russian Federation, two in the Ukraine and one in Romania.

Cases in domestic animals totalled 4329, of which cats and dogs were the most significant species. Cattle, horses, sheep and other farm animals can also contract the disease, but onward transmission is unlikely. Rodents and other small mammals may also carry and suffer from the disease. The WHO programme also records and includes the detection of bats with lyssavirus; however, although in 2007 26 bats were found with the disease, reporting is probably incomplete.

Many European countries are now considered to be rabies free, but this status can be lost due to unforeseen circumstances, e.g. in September 2004, France notified the WHO of a recent case of rabies in a dog illegally imported from Morocco into France, which could have transmitted rabies to humans and other dogs during August 2004; 187 people were given PEP, no secondary cases were detected in animals during this period and the area was declared rabies free again in March 2005.

In March 2008, France lost its rabies-free status after the illegal importation of an infected dog, which subsequently infected two other dogs. A low but increased risk of rabies was declared in three areas of France (Gers, Grandpuits and Calvados). If no cases had been detected following this case, the 'rabies-free' status should have been reinstated later in 2008.[36] However, after another case of rabies in an infected dog in October 2008, France is still not considered to be rabies free. Similar incidents have occurred elsewhere in Europe, notably in Switzerland in 2003.

Rabies in North America

Historically, rabies was endemic across the USA. The pattern of rabies infection in the USA has altered dramatically since the early twentieth century when canine rabies predominated. Following extensive vaccination programmes and a culling policy from the 1850s, domesticated animals, and particularly dogs, as a source of rabies declined from 82.6% of reported cases in 1950 to 7.9% in 2006. The total number of rabies cases in animals – both wild and domesticated – across the USA in 2006 was 6490, of which 318 (4.6%) were in cats. Cases of canine rabies have been seen stemming from imported animals posing the risk of accidental reintroduction.[37]

New reservoirs of infection have now been identified in wild animal populations, with raccoons, skunks, ferrets, beavers and bats forming disease reservoirs. Raccoon rabies has spread across the eastern USA since 1981, and has also spread into skunks. It is possible that, in a similar manner to the change seen in western Europe in the 1940s, a new genotype will emerge. This would have implications for control measures which centre around oral inoculation using baits, as the vaccine used is efficient in raccoons, but less so in skunks. The first known human death occurred in Virginia in 2003 with a man aged 25 becoming ill after being bitten by a rabid animal.[38]

In Canada, efforts have been made to eliminate the disease. A comprehensive vaccination by bait programme in Toronto, Canada has virtually eliminated fox-mediated Arctic variant rabies with over 300 000 baits being distributed between 1989 and 1999. Only 5 cases of rabid foxes were seen between 1990 and 2006 compared with 19 cases between 1972 and 1989, with the last rabid fox in the greater Toronto area being reported in 1996.

Rabid bats have been detected in every US state except Hawaii since the 1950s, and have also been detected in Canada. Approximately three-quarters of rabies deaths in the USA are now associated with bat rabies. Between 1990 and 2000, of 32 human cases of rabies, 24 were linked to bats, and only 2 cases reported being bitten. Bats are difficult to control; they are nocturnal, capable of living in large colonies in urban areas and often protected by wildlife preservation statutes.

Bat bites can be unrecognisable, or easily overlooked, and transmission may have followed inoculation of wounds, mucous membranes or abrasions with infected saliva. In many cases victims could not identify having been bitten or exposed to contact with a bat, although they or their families recalled bats being present in the patient's work place or home. This has led the CDC to issue guidance to clinicians that aggressive use of post-exposure vaccination in individuals suspected of possible exposures to bats should be considered.

Rabies elsewhere in the world

In Asia and Africa, canine rabies predominates and is considered to be the most significant animal reservoir worldwide, and control of rabies in canids is seen as a high priority for preventing human infection. Rabies control measures have improved in many South American countries, and the pattern of infection has changed with canine rabies becoming less prevalent; however there is another transmission path that has become more important – transmission of the disease by vampire or haematophagous bats. Outbreaks of bat-transmitted rabies have occurred in several remote areas in Brazil, Peru and Venezuela, with sporadic cases occurring in Mexico, Chile and Colombia.

The increase in vampire bat attacks and the transmission of rabies appear to be linked to deforestation, and the change of roost from forest to caves and disused mines.

During 2006, there were two rabies outbreaks in Portel and Viseu municipalities in Para State, northern Brazil associated with vampire bats. A total of 21 human deaths occurred. There had also been a outbreak in Turiacu, northern Brazil in October 2005 which killed 12 people, and another outbreak in Para in 2004.[39]

Disease in animals

The causative rhabdovirus is shed in large numbers into the saliva of infected mammals. Transmission follows inoculation of a bite wound or abrasion with infected saliva. Any animal suffering from rabies will display symptoms of CNS disturbance. After the incubation period and before the 'mad' or excitative phase, the animal may display certain prodromal symptoms. Behaviour will start to change: animals may display antisocial behaviour, becoming solitary and sexually aroused, and having increased urinary frequency.

The animal shows a lack of appetite for food and will not drink. After a few days the animal may become very excitable and vicious, biting or attacking anything or anybody in close proximity. This phase may be prolonged or short, and in some species is totally absent. The third or paralytic stage of the disease follows. As paralysis sets in, the animal becomes progressively more docile and death follows rapidly, usually within 10 days of the start of clinical signs.

Transmission

Humans contract the disease from bites of rabid animals, or by inoculation of wounds with virus-containing saliva. The possibility of air-borne droplet transmission has been demonstrated in caves where there are large populations of bats. The possibility of contracting the disease by organ or corneal transplantation from patients dying of undiagnosed disease has also been documented (see below). There is a theoretical risk of transmission of rabies from the consumption of milk or meat from an infected animal, although pasteurisation or thorough cooking is known to inactivate the virus.

Disease in humans

The virus is localised for a period post-exposure in the immediate vicinity of the wound. The area around the site of entry may be painful or itch. Localised numbness, especially of the limb nearest the site, may be reported.

There is a pre-patent period following infection: this period seems to vary according to where the wound is in relation to the CNS – the closer the wound, the shorter the period. However, it is usually between 3 and 12 weeks, with variations linked to amount of inoculum and age of the patient; higher inocula and younger patients show more rapid onset of disease. Incubation periods of more than a year have occasionally been reported, with the longest being 19 years and the shortest 4 days. Of infected people 93% show symptoms earlier than 12 months after exposure.

The virus migrates from the point of inoculation during this period, and enters the CNS. Early symptoms are very generalised, consisting of fever, headache and lassitude. As the CNS involvement begins, more serious clinical signs occur, often with acute onset. Symptoms progress as the neurological involvement increases. These can include insomnia, confusional states, anxiety, paralysis, hypersalivation, with swallowing difficulties caused by spasm of the oesophageal and laryngeal muscles (leading to the classic symptom of foaming at the mouth), altered perception and aggression. The patient may be extremely excited and often has convulsions. Disturbances of normal breathing and cardiac function are also seen. In the final stages of the disease, most victims pass through phases of delirium, convulsions to the almost invariable outcome of death.

The synonym hydrophobia for the disease relates to the physical difficulties of drinking experienced by humans and animals, which are probably exacerbated by the abnormal mental state that occurs. The duration of the disease is short: death follows within a few days of the start of clinical signs.

Person-to-person transmission is extremely rare; however, precautions should be taken to prevent exposure to the saliva of the diseased person.

Diagnosis

Diagnosis is often presumptive from the patient's history or presence of bite wounds. The virus can be isolated from bodily fluids or tissue samples and identified by microscopy, after treatment with fluorescent antibody-staining techniques. Rabies nucleic acid can also be detected using polymerase chain reaction tests. Isolating and identifying the virus from brain tissue or saliva *post mortem* often confirms diagnosis.

Treatment

Vigorous cleansing of bites or wounds with copious amounts of surfactant disinfectants or soap and water is a vital measure to reduce the risk of infection. This must be carried out immediately or as soon after the event as is practicable. In children, any bites are usually on the limbs, head, face or neck, and they must be cleaned very thoroughly. Rapid use of post-exposure vaccination is recommended. Suturing should not take place because this can spread the virus more rapidly.

Post-exposure treatment also uses human rabies immunoglobulin (HRIG) (also known as antirabies immunoglobulin) locally infiltrated around the wound site with concurrent administration intramuscularly. The dose used is calculated on a weight basis at a rate of 20 units/kg; if all of the dose cannot be infiltrated locally, or the wound has healed or is not visible, the remainder may be given intramuscularly in the thigh, but not the buttocks. HRIG is manufactured by Bio Products Laboratory and is available in the UK from HPA laboratories and regional blood transfusion centres in England and Wales. It is also available to the Scottish National Blood Transfusion Service (see Appendix 2).

In patients with overt clinical signs intensive care is required to maintain respiration. If convulsions and seizures are controlled using anticonvulsants, there is a small chance of survival.

In 2004, a 15-year-old girl who had contracted rabies after a bat bite in Wisconsin, USA, was placed in a drug-induced coma and treated with intravenous ribarvin. She was kept in the coma for 7 days, and her antirabies IgG titre rose steadily. On day 33 of her illness she was taken off a ventilator and 3 days later transferred to a rehabilitation unit.[40]

This case was the sixth known human recovery from rabies; however, the case was unique because the patient received no rabies prophylaxis either before or after symptoms were seen. Previously no unvaccinated patients had survived. All other survivors were either previously vaccinated or received some PEP before symptom onset.

The treatment method has been used in several cases since, with some clinical variations; however, no other patient has survived.

Prophylaxis

Vaccination programmes in domestic animals, with rigid guidelines on the control of stray or feral dogs, cats and other mammals, are important in reducing risks and exposure in countries where the disease is present. The vaccination of wild animal populations using inoculated baits has become very important in reducing levels of disease in the wild animal reservoir within endemic areas. Rigid control of animal imports, and the use of pet passport schemes or quarantine facilities, allow risks to be reduced and disease-free status to be maintained.

Travellers to rabies-endemic countries should be warned about the risk of acquiring rabies, although rabies vaccination is not a requirement for entry into any country. The avoidance of bites and scratches from stray dogs or companion animals in countries where rabies is endemic is the most important part of any prevention strategy.

Pre-exposure rabies vaccination should be considered for patients who will be staying a month or more in countries where dog rabies is endemic. The necessity of post-exposure rabies prophylaxis after an animal bite should be discussed with patients planning to travel to a non-industrialised country. They should be made aware that vaccination within a few days after a bite is capable of preventing the disease developing. Prophylaxis is recommended for travellers going to countries where there is a risk that post-exposure therapy may be unavailable, or available only using products of dubious quality.

All travellers to such countries may wish to ensure that they carry sterile packs containing needles and syringes. In the event of the need for vaccination, clean equipment is then available. Travellers should be encouraged to avoid handling, feeding or caressing wild and feral animals unless wearing appropriate protective clothing.

Individuals at risk of occupational exposure, such as workers in laboratories, quarantine facilities, port officials, customs officers, animal and bat handlers, and veterinary surgeons, whose employment is likely to carry a higher risk of exposure, should be considered for routine immunisation. Healthcare workers likely to be exposed to patients with the disease must be immunised wherever possible.

Vaccination regimens

There are wide regional variations in the types of rabies vaccines available. In the UK a human diploid cell rabies vaccine (HDCV: Pasteur Mérieux) is available, as is a purified chick embryo cell (PCEC) vaccine (Rabipur: Novartis, MASTA); both are inactivated, containing no live virus, and may be used interchangeably in the event of supply disruption.

In other countries, especially developing nations, other products may be in use. These include neural tissue vaccines prepared from sheep or mouse tissue. These vaccines have a high incidence of associated neurological complications; however, they may be the only product available. Some countries also use more modern vaccines prepared on different substrates to those in common use in western Europe or the USA. These include purified Vero cell rabies vaccine (PVRV) and purified duck embryo vaccine (PDEV).

The UK DH recommends that for prophylactic use HDCV vaccine should be given in a three-dose schedule on days 0, 7 and 28, with booster doses every 2–3 years if the individual is at continued risk. The last dose may be given from day 21 if insufficient time is available before the individual travels to an endemic area. A booster dose should be given 12 months after the first dose for those at regular or continuous risk, with further doses at 3- to 5-year intervals thereafter. For people at intermittent risk, or where they are returning to risk areas, and where no ready access to safe medical care is available, a subsequent dose after every 2 years is required.

Although pre-exposure vaccination does not eliminate the need for additional therapy after an incident, it does simplify post-exposure treatment by removing the need for rabies immunoglobulin and by decreasing the number of doses of vaccine required.

Where it is not known what regimen (if any) a patient has been given as prophylaxis, a full post-exposure regimen must be adopted unless there is serological evidence of antibody response following a risk assessment.

Recommended post-exposure regimens differ according to the previous vaccinations given. Fully immunised patients exposed to whatever level of risk should be given two booster doses on days 0 and 3. Individuals who have not been previously immunised, or who may have inadequate or out-of-date prophylaxis, should receive a course of injections starting as soon as practicable after exposure on days 0, 3, 7, 14 and 30, with a dose of HRIG on day 0 if considered to be at high risk.

Concomitant treatment with antimalarials, such as chloroquine and mefloquine, interferes with the antibody response to HDCV. For patients taking these medicines, intradermal vaccination is not recommended. The intramuscular route must always be used.

As with other immunisations, there may be a reaction to the injection. Pain can occur at the injection site, with reddening, swelling or itching. Headaches, nausea, gastrointestinal disturbance, generalised aching and dizziness have been reported. Due to the serious nature of the disease, post-exposure programmes must be continued despite mild localised or systemic symptoms, or other factors such as pregnancy. The gluteal muscle must not be used as an administration site, because past experience has shown that there is a poor response to vaccine administered here.

WHO recommendations

The WHO endorses the use of the Essen or five-dose regimen in post-exposure vaccination. This consists of five injections of one dose of vaccine intramuscularly on days 0, 3, 7, 14 and 28. Day 0 is considered to be either the day of the injury or the date at which treatment begins. In theory both should coincide; however, in practice this may not always be the case.[41]

There is also a four-dose regimen with two doses of vaccine being given on day 0, one in each deltoid/thigh, followed by one dose on days 7 and 21. In addition to these vaccination schemes, there are other regimens that have been developed to reduce the cost but not the effectiveness of post-exposure treatment.

Both of the following regimens use intradermal inoculation, reducing the amount of vaccine required to produce a sufficient immune response. The eight-site scheme requires injection of 0.1 mL at eight sites (one in each upper arm, one in each lateral thigh, one on each side of the suprascapular region, and one on each side of the lower quadrant of the abdomen) on day 0, one injection in each upper arm and each lateral thigh on day 7, and one dose in each upper arm on days 30 and 90.

The two-site scheme requires one injection of 0.1 mL at two sites on days 0, 3, 7 and 28.

Other related viruses

There are a number of related lyssaviruses often referred to by genotype that can cause a disease which in general terms is clinically similar to rabies. They are closely related to the classic virus (genotype 1), and rabies vaccine cross-reacts with these viruses, giving prophylaxis and treatment in human cases. There are a number of other lyssaviruses identified in Russia that have not yet been fully genotyped but are also capable of causing rabies-like disease. These are known as Aravan, Khajard, Yuli, Irkut and West Caucasian bat virus (Table 6.1).[42]

Lagos bat virus is carried by bats and has never been associated with known human disease to date; it has recently been detected in bats in South Africa, and appears to be sporadic, possibly reflecting bat migrational patterns.[43]

Mokala virus is unusual in that it is carried by shrews, rodents, cats and dogs. Mokala virus is believed to have caused disease in humans in Nigeria during the 1970s shortly after its discovery, but no recent human cases have been identified, although it has been identified in cats and dogs in South Africa.

Duvenhage virus is also carried by bats, with the last recorded clinical human case being recorded in 2006, when after a bat scratch a 77-year-old South African man died; this was only the second human case ever attributed

Table 6.1 Other lyssaviruses capable of causing rabies-like disease	
Genotype	**Name**
2	Lagos bat virus
3	Mokala virus
4	Duvenhage virus
5	European bat lyssavirus 1
6	European bat lyssavirus 2
7	Australian bat lyssavirus

to the virus, with the previous case occurring in 1970, when the virus was first identified.[44]

European bat lyssavirus (bat rabies)

The risk of European bat lyssavirus (EBLV) is thought to be low; however, much emphasis is placed on it in British public health circles. Since 1977 there have been five human deaths in Europe (three confirmed, two possible) from EBLVs, all in cases where the human had been bitten or scratched by bats and had not received rabies vaccination either before or after the incident. Many other people have been bitten or scratched by bats; however, they all received PEP.[45]

EBLV is split into two distinct genotypes: EBLV-1 is the predominant genotype across Europe, but has been identified only in one (of 273 examined) serotine bat (*Eptesicus serotinus*) in southern England. EBLV-2 has been detected in the UK with seven Daubenton's bats (*Myotis daubentonii*) testing positive: a pregnant female in 1996 in Sussex, a juvenile female in 2002 and an adult male in 2002 in Lancashire, a juvenile female in 2004 in Surrey, an adult female in Oxfordshire in 2006, an adult female in Shropshire in 2007 and another in Shropshire in 2008. In November 2002 in Scotland, a bat handler became the first victim of EBLV-2 in the UK, after a bite from an infected bat. Healthy bats often show lyssavirus antigens, although they are not clinically ill, and are therefore believed to be capable of surviving rabies-like disease.

All bats in Britain are protected species and should not be handled, particularly if sick or injured, except by professional bat handlers. In the USA the situation is similar, and bats should not be handled by the general public, if at all possible.

Australian bat lyssavirus

In 1996 a rhabdovirus related to rabies, now known as Australian bat lyssavirus, was found in a sick bat. A bat handler died after being infected with this pathogen in 1996, and in a separate incident in 1998 a further human fatality occurred. It has been found sporadically since in bats, but no other human cases have been seen.

Case histories

Classic rabies

A rabid kitten that had been handled by members of 60 female softball teams at an interstate competition in July 2007 held in Spartanburg, South Carolina, led to a multistate health alert. The kitten was taken home by one of the team coaches, where it became ill and later died. On investigation it was found to have been rabid. Following tracking and investigation of people exposed to the kitten, 27 were given prophylaxis: 1 from South Carolina, 15 from Georgia and 11 from North Carolina. No clinical cases of rabies followed.

Bat rabies (non-EBLV)

There have been a number of incidents of human rabies after exposure to infected bats since 2000 in the USA. In March 2002, a 28-year-old man from Glenn County, California died of rabies after exposure to a Mexican free-tailed bat, probably from a colony in his home. A previous case in Amador County, California in September 2000 was associated with the same species. Also in 2002, a 20-year-old man in Iowa died after exposure to either infected silver-haired or pipistrelle bats. This was the first case of rabies in Iowa since 1951. A boy from Tennessee, aged 13, died in the same year in a case also associated with silver-haired or pipistrelle bats.

Since 2002, there have been on average one or two cases each year in the USA across a number of states.

In Alberta, Canada, a 73-year-old man died of rabies in April 2007 after a bite from a silver-haired bat.

Imported cases

There have been a number of cases of imported rabies in Europe, the UK and the USA in the last decade.

In 2003, a 3-year-old child died in France after returning from Gabon having been bitten by an infected dog. The following year there were three separate incidents, with an Austrian tourist dying after being bitten in Morocco, a young German girl died in Germany after holidaying in India (see below), and a 41-year-old man died in Florida of canine rabies after visiting Haiti on holiday.[46,47]

The latest case of imported rabies in a human in the UK was in 2005, and followed a bite from a dog in Goa, India, while the patient was on holiday. Vaccination was not sought post-exposure and the patient subsequently died after returning to the UK. There had been three previous cases of imported rabies: the first in 1996 after a bite from a stray dog in Nigeria, the second from a dog bite in the Philippines in 2001 and the third also from a bite in Nigeria.[48]

In November 2006, an 11-year-old boy in California died of rabies, from a virus type associated with canine-borne rabies in the Philippines. His family had immigrated from the Philippines 2 years earlier, with the child being bitten just before their departure for the USA.

In 2007, another German national died after being bitten by a stray dog in Morocco.

All of the victims were unvaccinated and all cases were fatal. These cases highlight the need for travellers to be educated about this disease, and to realise that a bite from an animal requires medical attention as soon after it occurs as possible.

Organ transplantation

In June 2004, an organ donor from Arkansas died (of undiagnosed rabies); his liver and two kidneys were used in three subsequent transplantations in Alabama, Oklahoma and Texas, with all the recipients dying of rabies. Rabies has also followed corneal transplantations in eight people across five countries.[49]

In similar circumstances, in February 2005, German officials reported that three of six patients who received organs transplanted from a single donor who died in December 2004 were infected with rabies. The donor appears to have been infected while on holiday in India (see above), but was symptom free when she died from cardiac arrest. Two of the three infected died; the other was in a critical condition but later survived; the other three who had received corneal and liver transplantations remained disease free, but received PEP.[50]

UK guidelines state that individuals must not donate blood or tissue for 12 months (and until fully cleared by a clinician) after a known exposure to an infectious disease. Although rapid diagnosis tests are available, accurate travel and clinical history as well as exact identification of causes of death remain essential to reduce the risk of disease transmission.

Prevention

As mentioned previously, part of the protection and prevention measures in place in the UK and the USA is a strict quarantine system. Recently this has undergone a slight modification in the UK to allow a pet passport scheme to undergo trials (see below). The effectiveness of the quarantine system in the UK was demonstrated in April 2008, when a social worker involved in bringing Sri Lankan street dogs into the UK was bitten by a puppy that later died of rabies while in quarantine. She and two kennel workers were given PEP. No further cases occurred.

In the USA, it is recommended by the CDC that all cats be vaccinated against rabies because they are more frequently seen with clinical disease than dogs (269 cases in cats in 2005 compared with 76 in dogs in the same year). Imported dogs must be immunised in accordance with CDC vaccination requirements.

The CDC also recommends that livestock that are particularly valuable, especially breeding stock, should be vaccinated, as should animals used in petting zoos, agricultural fairs and horses that move from state to state. All wild animals caught for use in zoos should be quarantined for 6 months and employees of exhibitions or zoos with animals should be immunised on a precautionary basis.

In healthcare settings, adherence to standard infection-control precautions minimises the risk for healthcare workers' exposure to rabies; however, PEP should be provided to healthcare workers who care for patients with rabies where their mucous membranes or open wounds may have been exposed to infectious body fluids or tissue (e.g. saliva, tears, cerebrospinal fluid or neurological tissue) from infected patients.

Children should be taught to be cautious in their interactions with animals, especially those that are unfamiliar, to avoid potential exposures to rabies and other infectious diseases. An apparently healthy dog, cat or ferret that bites a person should be confined and observed daily for 10 days. If the animal becomes ill or dies during this observation period, its brain should be examined for evidence of rabies virus infection. If rabies is detected, prompt administration of PEP is indicated. If the animal is unavailable for testing, public health officials should be consulted.

In the UK, the advice on the provision of PEP has changed since the detection of EBLV in UK bats. As classic rabies vaccine offers complete protection to this virus, the latest guidance stresses that clinicians need to be aware of the risk of rabies after significant exposure to bats. If a person is bitten or scratched, or there is direct contact with a bat to mucosa or broken skin, the area should be cleaned thoroughly with water and soap and medical advice sought urgently and expert assessment performed. PEP (vaccination and possibly administration of immunoglobulins) is recommended. Any member of the public finding a bat behaving abnormally, found in an unusual place, or under unusual circumstances, should not attempt to handle or move the animal, but contact their local bat conservation group or the Bat Conservation Trust. All bat handlers and other people likely to be at risk of exposure through the close handling of bats should be vaccinated against rabies and this is provided free of charge by the HPA through the NHS.

Awareness in the general public and healthcare professionals of this small risk needs to be addressed without creating unnecessary fear of these endangered and protected animals.

Anyone who is bitten or scratched by a bat should contact a doctor immediately, who should, in turn, seek expert advice. This is available 24 hours from relevant centres: in England, the HPA Virus Reference Department (tel: +44 (0)20 8200 4400) or Communicable Disease Surveillance Centre (tel: +44 (0)20 8200 6868); in Wales, the National Public Health Service for Wales (tel: +44 (0)29 20742178, out of hours (tel: +44 (0)29 20747747. In Scotland the Scottish Centre for Infection and Environmental Health (tel: +44 (0)141 300 1100); and in Northern Ireland, the Consultant in Communicable Disease Control in the relevant health board or the Communicable Disease Surveillance Centre (Northern Ireland) (tel: +44 (0)28 9026 3765).

In the USA, medical services should contact local county and state health officials and the CDC.

Pet Travel Scheme (PETS)

This scheme was introduced in the UK in April 2000. The regulations, made under SI 1999 no. 3443 The Pet Travel Scheme (Pilot Arrangements) (England) Order 1999, form the basis of the scheme. European Union (EU) Regulation 998/2003, which has applied since July 2004, has updated the scheme and sets the requirements for the movement of dogs, cats and ferrets travelling within the EU, and into the EU from third countries. The rules of entry to the UK remain largely unchanged by the Regulation. The scheme aims not only to prevent rabies entering the UK, but also to prevent establishment of *Echinococcus multilocularis* and certain tick-borne diseases endemic elsewhere in Europe and the rest of the world. It does not replace the quarantine system; however, it does allow cats, ferrets and dogs, especially hearing dogs for the deaf, or guide dogs for the blind, to accompany their owners abroad. The scheme allows owners and their animals to travel to a number of EU and non-EU destinations and return without needing formal quarantine.

To enter an animal into the scheme, it must have a microchip inserted to identify it permanently, and be verifiably and effectively vaccinated against rabies. A certificate is then issued under the scheme. This allows the animal to enter or leave the UK by specified routes and carriers. Details can be found on the DEFRA website (http://maff.gov.uk/defra). Booster injections have to be given as recommended by the rabies vaccine manufacturer to maintain immunity and validity of the certificate.

In addition to this certificate, there is a requirement for the animal to be treated for ticks and tapeworms between 24 and 48 hours before it enters or re-enters the UK. Again a certificate is issued by a vet to verify that the treatment has taken place with approved products on each occasion. These certificates must be obtained before travelling, otherwise the animal may not be accepted by the travel company or may be turned back at the border.

During 2006, 8375 cats, 74 285 dogs and 31 ferrets successfully entered the UK under the Scheme. In total, 362 602 pet animals have entered the UK under the PETS since 2000 (ferrets have only been able to enter under the Scheme since July 2004). There have been no cases of imported rabies in the UK in animals that have used PETS.

Deliberate release – bioterrorism

Initial definitions

- Biological terrorism: use of biological agents or toxins (e.g. pathogenic organisms that affect humans, animals, or plants) for terrorist purposes.
- Deliberate release: the spreading of a pathogen or toxin deliberately to cause casualties, fear or disruption.
- Threat: the capability of an adversary, coupled with intentions, to undertake malevolent actions.

Background

Following almost immediately after the attacks on the World Trade Centre in September 2001, the anthrax letters in the USA prompted the WHO, CDC, HPA and other healthcare bodies to explore for the first time, in the public domain, the issue of bioterrorism.[51]

Biological warfare is not new, but it was not until the twentieth century that state-sponsored programmes to develop biological weapons began to be established, reaching their zenith in the latter years of the Cold War. By then many nations had either established or sought to establish biological weapon programmes, often known as the 'poor man's atom bomb' (a reflection of the likely level of fatalities and casualties that such attacks might cause).

Estimates vary as to the level of casualties a deliberate release would cause; however, a study at Stanford University in California in 2003, using a computer model, estimated that a kilogram of anthrax spores released efficiently in a city of 10 million people could cause as many as 123 000 victims if antibiotic treatment was not administered within 48 hours. This was almost identical with UK estimates made in the 1970s.

As the threat increased a Biological and Toxin Weapons Convention (BTWC) was proposed, being initially signed in 1972, and ratified by more than 100 nations in 1975, in an attempt to control the spread of such weapons.

Many nations have since chosen to destroy their stockpiles of these weapons and scale down or cease their offensive programmes in accordance with the BTWC, retaining only a defensive or protective programme. Since then the UN has sought to prevent proliferation of the technology, materials and information that would allow other nations or organisations to develop such programmes and destroy bioweapon programmes and stockpiles.

The Australia Group

The Australia Group grew out of the BTWC in 1985, being an informal arrangement aimed at reducing the proliferation and export or transhipment of biological warfare materials or production techniques. It currently has 40 members plus the EU. It develops and updates lists of organisms and toxins that it considers to be of concern. Although not all the organisms that are listed under the Australia Group, or covered by the legislation such as the UK Anti-terrorism, Crime and Security Act (ATCSA) 2001 and the associated orders, or the Public Health Security and Bioterrorism Preparedness and Response Act of 2002 and the Uniting and Strengthening America by Providing Appropriate Tools Required to Intercept and Obstruct Terrorism (USA PATRIOT) Act of 2001 in the USA, are zoonotic pathogens, many are. Many of the moieties known to have been developed within state programmes were also zoonoses, because they had the essential attributes necessary for warfare agents, being easily transmissible to humans, aggressive in terms of pathogenicity, and capable of both causing massive fatalities or severely ill casualties and fear or panic among the 'worried well'.

The Global Health Security Initiative

Since 2001, although there are still concerns over state programmes, such as those of Iran and North Korea, the main emphasis has shifted to an act of bioterrorism or a deliberate release resulting from malicious activity by a terrorist or terrorist-related organisation.

Part of the international response to this threat has been the establishment of the Global Health Security Initiative (GHSI), an informal, international partnership focused on strengthening health preparedness and coordinating the global response to threats of biological, chemical or radionuclear terrorism (CBRN) initially. Its remit has since been widened to include in addition planning and response to pandemic influenza.

Launched in November 2001 by Canada, the EU, France, Germany, Italy, Japan, Mexico, the UK and the USA, the GHSI has appointed the WHO as an expert adviser on health and has started a series of initiatives, including exploring and encouraging joint projects to procure and develop vaccines and antibiotics to counter biological agents, share emergency response plans, collaborate on risk assessment and management, and agree frameworks for countries to share expertise and laboratory linkages.

Surveillance of data and epidemiological information are seen as key indicators in detecting a deliberate release or bioterrorism incident, so the GHSI also seeks to ensure that such data is rapidly shared so that a speedy response can be mounted.

Likely agents

The literature on state-sponsored biological warfare is now extensive and identifies anthrax, Ebola virus and other haemorrhagic fevers (Marburg, Crimean–Congo haemorrhagic fever or CCHF), botulinum toxin, plague, tularemia, Q fever, brucellosis, Lassa fever and associated arenaviruses as organisms that have been investigated and in some cases fully developed into bioweapons.

Luckily obtaining and developing the majority of these organisms is currently believed to be beyond the capability of terrorist groups according to the CDC; however, the main fear is that a terrorist group might attempt to use a bioweapon.

Historically, terrorists or other extreme groups have attempted to use deliberate releases. In 1984, followers of the Bagwan Shree Rajneesh, in Oregon, attempted to influence the outcome of a local election by contaminating salad bars with pathogenic *Salmonella* spp.[52] In a similar incident at a medical centre in Dallas, Texas in 1996, 12 people were severely ill after a disgruntled colleague deliberately contaminated cakes with a *Shigella* spp.

Anthrax in particular has attracted the attention of terrorists, with Al Qaeda allegedly attempting to develop the bacterium into a viable weapon at a number of sites in Afghanistan before the invasion in 2002. After the invasion of the country and the destruction of a number of sites, it is unclear whether they are currently attempting to reconstitute this programme.[53]

Slightly more unusual were the attempts by the Aum Shinrikyo cult in Japan to use botulinum toxin on a number of occasions in the early 1990s. They also cultured anthrax, which they attempted to disseminate. There is no evidence that there were any casualties from their efforts, unlike their successful attack with sarin nerve gas in 1995 on the Tokyo underground, where 12 people died and thousands required medical or hospital treatment.[54]

In the USA, the CDC has classified likely agents into three categories: A, B and C (see list below – zoonotic diseases in bold). In essence those agents in category A are considered to pose the highest risk in terms of ease of dissemination and should be treated as the highest priority in terms of both risk to human health and secondary spread, category B are the second highest priority and category C the third priority, and include pathogens that are emerging and might be engineered in the future to become capable of mass spread.[55]

Category A

Anthrax (*Bacillus anthracis*)
Botulism (*Clostridium botulinum* toxin)
Plague (*Yersinia pestis*)
Smallpox (variola major)
Tularemia (*Francisella tularensis*)
Viral haemorrhagic fevers (filoviruses, e.g. Ebola, Marburg and arenaviruses, e.g. Lassa, Machupo).

Category B

Brucellosis (*Brucella* spp.)

Epsilon toxin of *Clostridium perfringens*

Food safety threats (e.g. *Salmonella* spp., *Escherichia coli* O157:H7, *Shigella* spp.)

Glanders (*Burkholderia mallei*)

Melioidosis (*Burkholderia pseudomallei*)

Psittacosis (*Chlamydia psittaci*)

Q fever (*Coxiella burnetii*)

Ricin toxin from *Ricinus communis* (castor beans)

Staphylococcal enterotoxin B

Typhus fever (*Rickettsia prowazekii*).

Viral encephalitis (alphaviruses, e.g. **Venezuelan equine encephalitis, eastern equine encephalitis, western equine encephalitis**)

Water safety threats (e.g. *Vibrio cholerae*, *Cryptosporidium parvum*)

Category C

Emerging infectious diseases such as Nipah virus and hantavirus.

Public health dimension

A deliberate or accidental release of a biological pathogen poses a threat to the public, and therefore it is unsurprising that in the UK, the USA and the EU there have been measures taken to try to put plans in place to tackle any incident. It is also complex, because it requires, subsequent to the realisation that an incident has occurred, a coordinated approach from health services (primary and secondary care, government, public health authorities and voluntary organisations such as the Red Cross), police and emergency services, and also the media.

In the UK and the USA, the police will always have the lead in such situations, because it is likely to stem from a criminal act; however, emergency preparedness, and the mitigation of such an attack, is a civil authority responsibility within national guidelines, so health authorities and administrations should have a plan in place to deal with any incident quickly and appropriately.[56]

The HPA is pivotal to the response to any such incident in the UK, and has issued guidance (which can be found on its website) for health professionals and public bodies, including the recent update of the HPA's *CBRN Incidents – Clinical Management and Health Protection* manual in September 2008.[57] Importantly the response in the UK relies on health workers recognising new or unusual clusters of infections, where a number of people becoming ill, at or around the same time, especially where associated with unusually high morbidity or mortality, or where a single case is seen that demonstrates unusual or particularly severe symptoms, where there is no associated history to suggest an explanation of the illness. Where such cases are seen contact should be made immediately with the medical micro-biologist or infectious disease consultant at the local hospital. Failing this, contact the Director of Infection Prevention and Control, the local health protection unit or the HPA direct on +44 (0)20 8200 4400. Full details may be found on the HPA website at www.hpa.org.uk.

In the USA, the county and then state and federal health authorities should be contacted along with the CDC. More information can be found on the CDC website – bioterrorism links (see Appendix 1).

Preparedness

In both the USA and the UK, emergency preparedness plans are exercised regularly, sometimes using simulated casualties. Stockpiles of antibiotics, protective clothing and decontamination materials are also maintained. As healthcare professionals, the main role is to initially identify that an event has occurred and be prepared to support the response to such an event with the knowledge of treatment, prevention and infection control.

References

1. Pearson GS. The threat of deliberate disease in the 21st century. In: Stimson Centre report no. 24. *Biological Proliferation: Reasons for concern, courses of action.* Bradford: Stimson Centre for Peace Studies, Bradford University, 1998.
2. Metcalfe N. The history of woolsorter's disease: a Yorkshire beginning with an international future? *Occup Med (Lond)* 2004; **54**: 489–93.
3. Meselson M, Guillemin J, Hugh-Jones M *et al.* The Sverdlovsk anthrax outbreak of 1979. *Science* 1994; **266**: 1202–7.
4. JAVMA News Alert. Anthrax found in three states, 1 September 2005.
5. Van den Enden E, Van Gompel A, Van Esbroeck M. Cutaneous anthrax, Belgian traveller. *Emerg Infect Dis* 2006; **12**; 3.
6. Jernigan JA, Stephens DS, Ashford DA *et al.* Bioterrorism-related inhalational anthrax: the first 10 cases reported in the United States. *Emerg Infect Dis* 2001; **7**: 1–26.
7. Holty J-EC, Bravata DM, Liu H, Olshen RA, McDonald KM, Owens DK. Systematic review: A century of inhalational anthrax cases from 1900 to 2005. *Ann Intern Med* 2006; **144**: 270–80.
8. Vietri NJ, Purcell BK, Lawler JV *et al.* Short-course postexposure antibiotic prophylaxis combined with vaccination protects against experimental inhalational anthrax. *Proc Natl Aacd Sci USA* 2006; **103**: 7813–16.
9. Sejvar JJ, Tenover FC, Stephens DS. Management of anthrax meningitis. *Lancet Infect Dis* 2005; **5**: 287–95.
10. CDC. Evaluation of postexposure antibiotic prophylaxis to prevent anthrax, January 25, 2002. *MMWR* 2002; **51**: 49–72.
11. CDC. Update: Investigation of bioterrorism-related anthrax and interim guidelines for exposure management and antimicrobial therapy, October 2001. *MMWR* 2001; **50**: 909–19.

12. Bossi P, Tegnell A, Baka A *et al*. BICHAT guidelines for the clinical management of anthrax and bioterrorism-related anthrax. *Eurosurveillance* 2004; **9**(12): 1–7. Available at: http://www.eurosurveillance.org.

13. CDC. Inhalation anthrax associated with dried animal hides – Pennsylvania and New York City, 2006. *MMWR* 2006; **55**: 280–2.

14. Doolan DL, Freilich DA, Brice GT *et al*. The US Capitol bioterrorism anthrax exposures: clinical epidemiological and immunological characteristics. *J Infect Dis* 2007; **195**: 174–84.

15. Cinti SK, Saravolatz L, Nafziger D, Sunstrum J, Blackburn G. Differentiating inhalational anthrax from other influenza-like illnesses in the setting of a national or regional anthrax outbreak. *Arch Intern Med* 2004; **164**: 674–6.

16. Griffith KS, Mead P, Armstrong GL *et al*. Bioterrorism-related inhalational anthrax in an elderly woman, Connecticut, 2001. *Emerg Infect Dis* 2003; **9**: 681–8.

17. World Health Organization. *Ebola Haemorrhagic Fever*. WHO fact sheet no. 103. Geneva: WHO, 2000.

18. Leroy EM, Kumulungui B, Pourrut X *et al*. Fruit bats as reservoirs of Ebola virus. *Nature* 2005; **438**: 575–6.

19. Morvan J, Colyn M, Deubel V, Gounon P. *Ebola: Virus marks detected in terrestrial small mammals*. Paris: Institut Pasteur, 2000.

20. Mupapa K, Massamba M, Kibadi K *et al*. Treatment of Ebola hemorrhagic fever with blood transfusions from convalescent patients. *J Infect Dis* 1999; **179**(suppl 1): S18–23.

21. Ströher U, Feldmann H. Progress towards the treatment of Ebola haemorrhagic fever. *Expert Opin Investig Drugs* 2006; **15**: 1523–35.

22. Feldmann H, Jones SM, Daddario-DiCaprio KM *et al*. Effective post-exposure treatment of Ebola infection. *PLoS Pathog* 2007; **3**(1): e2.

23. Dennis DT, Gage KL, Gratz N *et al*. WHO *Plague Manual: Epidemiology, distribution, surveillance and control*. Geneva: World Health Organization, 1999.

24. Ratsitorahina M, Chanteau S, Rahalison L, Ratsifasoamanana L, Boisier P. Epidemiological and diagnostic aspects of the outbreak of pneumonic plague in Madagascar. *Lancet* 2000; **355**: 111–13.

25. Nebehay S, World Health Organization. Thousands flee as plague kills 61 in Congo. *Reuters Health* 18 Feb 2005.

26. Bitam I, Baziz B, Rolain JM, Belkaid M, Raoult D. Zoonotic focus of plague, Algeria. *Emerg Infect Dis* 2006; **12**: 1975–7.

27. Lowell JL, Wagner DM, Atshabar B *et al*. Identifying sources of human plague exposure. *J Clin Microbiol* 2005; **43**: 650–6.

28. Bin Saeed AA, Al-Hamdan NA, Fontaine RE. Plague from eating raw camel liver. *Emerg Infect Dis* 2005; **11**: 1456–7.

29. Kool JL. Risk of person-to-person transmission of pneumonic plague. *Clin Infect Dis* 2005; **40**: 1166–72.

30. Boulanger LL, Ettestad P, Fogarty JD, Dennis DT, Romig D, Mertz G. Gentamicin and tetracyclines for the treatment of human plague: review of 75 cases in New Mexico, 1985–1999. *Clin Infect Dis* 2004; **38**: 663–9.

31. Mwengee W, Butler T, Mgema S *et al*. Treatment of plague with gentamicin or doxycycline in a randomized clinical trial in Tanzania. *Clin Infect Dis* 2006; **42**: 614–21.

32. Russell P, Eley SM, Green M *et al*. Efficacy of doxycycline and ciprofloxacin against experimental *Yersinia pestis* infection. *J Antimicrob Chemother* 1998; **41**: 301–5.

33. Steward J, Lever MS, Russell P *et al*. Efficacy of the latest fluoroquinolones against experimental *Yersinia pestis*. *Int J Antimicrob Agent* 2004; **24**: 609–12.

34. CDC Recommendations and Reports – April 6 2007/56(RR03); 1–8. *Compendium of Animal Rabies Prevention and Control*. Washington DC: National Association of State Public Health Veterinarians, Inc. (NASPHV), 2007.

35. Bourhy H, Kissi B, Audry L *et al*. Ecology and evolution of rabies virus in Europe. *J Gen Virol* 1999; **80**: 2545–57.

36. Servas V, Mailles A, Neau D *et al*. An imported case of canine rabies in Aquitaine: Investigation and management of the contacts at risk, August 2004–March 2005. *Eurosurveillance* 2005; **10**(10–12): 222–5.

37. Blanton JD, Krebs JW, Hanlon CA, Rupprecht CE. Rabies surveillance in the United States during 2005. *JAVMA* 2006; **209**: 1897–911.

38. Guerra MA, Curns AT, Rupprecht CE, Hanlon CA, Krebs JW, Childs JE. Skunk and raccoon rabies in the eastern United States: temporal and spatial analysis. *Emerg Infect Dis* 2003; **9**: 1143–50.

39. da Rosa EST, Kotait I, Barbosa TFS *et al*. Bat-transmitted human rabies outbreaks, Brazilian Amazon. *Emerg Infect Dis* 2006; **8**: 1197–20

40. Willoughby RE Jr, Tieves KS, Hoffman GM *et al*. Survival after treatment of rabies with induction of coma. *N Engl J Med* 2005; **352**: 2508–14.

41. WHO Geneva. Rabies vaccine – WHO position paper. *Weekly Epidemiological Record* 49/50 2007; **82**: 425–36.

42. Botvinkin AD, Poleschuk EM, Kuzmin IV *et al*. Novel lyssaviruses isolated from bats in Russia. *Emerg Infect Dis* 2003: E-pub.

43. Markotter W, Randles J, Rupprecht CE *et al*. Lagos bat virus, South Africa. *Emerg Infect Dis* 2006; **12**: 504–6.

44. Paweska JT, Blumberg LH, Liebenberg C *et al*. Fatal human infection with rabies-related Duvenhage virus, South Africa. *Emerg Infect Dis* 2006; **12**: 1965–7.

45. Fooks AR, McElhinney LM, Pounder DJ *et al*. Case report: isolation of a European bat lyssavirus type-2a from a fatal human case of rabies encephalitis. *J Med Virol* 2003; **71**: 281–9.

46. Anonymous. Human case of rabies in a child in France who had visited Gabon. *Eurosurveillance Weekly Release* 2003; 7(46): 1–5.

47. Strauss R, Gränz A, Wassermann-Neuhold M *et al*. A human case of travel-related rabies in Austria, September 2004. *Eurosurveillance* 2005; **10**(10–12): 225–6.

48. Solomon T, Marston D, Mallewa M *et al*. Paralytic rabies after a two week holiday in India. *BMJ* 2005; **331**: 501–3.

49. Srinivasan A, Burton EC, Kuehnert AJ *et al*. Transmission of rabies virus from an organ donor to four transplant recipients. *N Engl J Med* 2005; **352**: 1103–11.

50. Hellenbrand W, Meyer C, Rasch G, Steffens I, Ammon A. Cases of rabies in Germany following organ transplantation. *Eurosurveillance Weekly Release* 2005; **10**(8): 224–6.

51. Jernigan JA, Stephens DS, Ashford DA *et al*. Bioterrorism-related inhalation anthrax: the first 10 cases reported in the United States. *Emerg Infect Dis* 2001; **7**: 933–44.

52. Török TJ, Tauxe RV, Wise RP *et al*. Large community outbreak of salmonellosis caused by intentional contamination of restaurant salad bars. *JAMA* 1997; **278**: 389–95.

53. Inglesby TV, O'Toole T, Henderson DA *et al*. Anthrax as a biological weapon, 2002: updated recommendations for management. *JAMA* 2002; **287**: 2236–52.

54. Arnon SS, Schechter R, Inglesby TV *et al*. Botulinum toxin as a biological weapon: medical and public health management. *JAMA* 2001; **285**: 1059–70.

55. CDC. Biological and chemical terrorism: strategic plan for preparedness and response. *MMWR* 2000; **49**(RR-4): 1–14.

56. Butler JC, Cohen ML, Friedman CR, Scripp RM, Watz CG. Collaboration between public health and law enforcement: new paradigms and partnerships for bioterrorism planning and response. *Emerg Infect Dis* 2002; **8**: 1152–6.

57. Heptonstall J, Gent N. *CBRN Incidents: Clinical management and health protection*, version 4.0. London: Health Protection Agency, 2008.

7

Viral zoonotic diseases

This chapter describes viruses that have shown their zoonotic potential dramatically by causing human illness, usually with associated fatalities.

Notes on arrangements of monographs

A decision has been made to use viral classification to group the following conditions, as viral taxonomy has moved on dramatically since the first edition of this book. Readers should be aware that there are other classification methods.

One of these methods that may be seen in current literature is the overall grouping of viral pathogens into a heterogeneous generalised classification of arboviruses. An arbovirus is defined as any arthropod-borne virus transferred from its normal reservoir (either animal or human) to humans via biting insect vectors. The usual arthropods involved in transmission of the viral pathogen from one host to another are either mosquitoes or ticks, both soft and hard bodied.[1] Most arboviruses can be classified as either dengue fever like or encephalitides. They can be further subdivided into mosquito- and tick-borne groups.

Alphaviruses

Chikungunya

Caused by an alphavirus, Chikungunya fever is transmitted to humans by the bite of infected mosquitoes. It is found in west, central and southern Africa and many areas of Asia. The animal reservoir is considered to be monkeys. Following recent epidemics of the disease in Africa and Reunion, the disease has been seen in returning travellers. There have been clusters of cases in Italy, and there are fears that the disease has now adapted to indigenous European species of mosquito, which may lead to further outbreaks.

Initial non-specific symptoms are followed by a debilitating illness, with muscle pain, rash and extreme fever. Incapacitating joint pain and arthritis may continue after clinical recovery from the acute phase, but is not similar to that seen in dengue fever.

Treatment is symptomatic, but aspirin should be avoided because there are risks of haemorrhagic sequelae. Chloroquine phosphate has also been used, but opinion still remains divided as to its efficacy.[2]

Eastern equine encephalomyelitis

An alphavirus, eastern equine encephalomyelitis virus (EEEV) is mosquito borne, and usually infects wetland birds and horses. Western equine encephalomyelitis virus (WEEV) and Venezuelan equine encephalomyelitis virus (VEEV) are related but genetically distinct alphaviruses. EEEV and VEEV are lethal in up to 90% of horses showing clinical symptoms, whereas WEEV is least virulent in horses, which have a mortality rate of approximately 40%. EEEV is also capable of causing fatal encephalitis in humans with a case mortality rate between 50% and 75%.

In the USA, EEEV occurs mainly from New England to Florida and along the Gulf Coast, with rare reports of foci as far inland as Michigan and South Dakota. The virus is maintained in mosquito pools, and then amplifies in birds. Subsequent transmission to horses occurs, and human cases usually follow equine outbreaks. Human survivors are frequently left with persistent neurological damage, including epilepsy and focal damage in portions of the brain tissue. Initially starting with flu-like symptoms, patients rapidly pass into a coma and are often severely disabled if they survive.

Recent cases

The first case of eastern equine encephalitis in the UK occurred in early October 2007. A man who had been to New Hampshire in the USA on a fishing holiday developed symptoms after his return to the UK.

In late summer 2005, 11 laboratory-confirmed cases of EEEV disease were reported in New Hampshire and Massachusetts, of whom 4 subsequently died. All the patients worked or socialised in areas near swamps, cranberry bogs or other wetlands capable of supporting mosquito vectors, and had potential exposure at dawn or dusk in the fortnight before the onset of clinical disease. Investigations confirmed the presence of the virus in mosquito populations in the vicinity of the patients.[3]

The virus was also found in wild birds, horses, alpacas, two emus and a llama in New Hampshire, and in horses and an emu in Massachusetts. During 2005, 21 confirmed cases of EEEV were reported across the USA to the Centers for Disease Control and Prevention (CDC), a distinct rise over the annual average between 2000 and 2004 of 8.2 cases per year. The reason for the rapid rise in cases numbers remains unknown.

Mayaro virus

Mayaro virus is a zoonotic alphavirus found in Latin America, transmitted from its reservoirs of primates (monkeys and sloths), rodents and birds by mosquitoes. Little is known of its clinical course in humans, but it can cause an influenza-like disease and possibly encephalitis.[4]

Arenaviruses

Arenaviruses are normally associated with a range of rodent vectors, mostly species of rats and mice. The first arenavirus to be identified was lymphocytic choriomeningitis virus in 1933. Since then, approximately 20 other arenaviruses, some of which cause human disease, have been identified. They are split into two main groups: the Old World (Lassa), and New World (Tacaribe) complexes. The Lassa complex includes Ippy, Lassa, lymphocytic choriomeningitis, Mobala, Mopeia and Mozambique viruses. The Tacaribe complex consists of Allpahuayo, Amapari, Bear Canyon, Flexal, Guanarito, Junin, Latino, Machupo, Oliveros, Parana, Pichinde, Pirital, Sabia, Tacaribe, Tamiami and Whitewater Arroyo viruses.[5]

Infected rodents are asymptomatic, and may acquire the virus by maternal transfer, traumatic injury such as bites or scratches or faecal–oral transfer. Human infection follows inhalation or contamination of wounds/abrasions by rodent faeces, saliva or urine. Contaminated food may also cause infection.[6]

Once across the species barrier, some of the arenaviruses such as Lassa, may spread by human-to-human or fomite transfer.

Zoonotic arenaviruses

Guanarito virus

A zoonotic arenavirus, this virus has been found only in the Guanarito municipality of Barinas state, Venezuela. The reservoir is cane rats, with the disease being transmitted either via a vector or by direct contact with rats or their body fluids. In humans it can cause severe disease, characterised by fever, malaise and sore throat, followed by abdominal pain, diarrhoea, haemorrhagic manifestations, convulsions and death.

Diagnosis is confirmed only by viral isolation and treatment is purely symptomatic.[7]

Junin virus

Also known as Argentinian or South American haemorrhagic fever, cases of Junin virus are seen only in the Junin region, east of Buenos Aires. Disease outbreaks are normally seen between February and August during the agricultural growing season, when agricultural workers become exposed to infected rodents or their urine and faeces in soil or aerosols. Person-to-person transmission has also been reported. Symptoms are similar to Lassa fever and other arenavirus infections. There is no treatment, and fatality rates range from 3% to 30% depending on lethality of the strain prevalent in the outbreak.

Lassa virus

Lassa virus causes Lassa fever, an acute viral haemorrhagic fever first described in 1969 in the town of Lassa, Nigeria. It is endemic in west Africa with approximately 300 000 cases annually, of which up to 5000 are fatal. Cases have been seen elsewhere in the world due to the movement of infected patients during the incubation period via airlines.[8]

Following infection, by exposure to infected rodent faecal matter or urine, or by patient-to-patient spread often through contaminated blood, there is an incubation period of 6–21 days during which the virus initially colonises the mucosa, intestines, lungs and urinary tract, followed by spread into the vascular system.

Most infected patients are asymptomatic, but in about 20% of cases it can cause severe disease. Generalised symptoms include fever, facial swelling, fatigue, conjunctivitis and mucosal bleeding with bloody vomiting or diarrhoea. There may be involvement of the vascular system, with cardiac complications, respiratory difficulty, and encephalitis or meningitis with associated seizures. Clinical cases may not be easy to differentiate from those caused by Ebola or Marburg virus or malaria. Clinical cases in pregnant women usually require abortion, because the virus has a particular affinity for the placenta, and only 10% of infected fetuses survive.[9]

The overall mortality rate is approximately 1% of cases, although in some case clusters this can reach 50%, especially where early therapy or supportive measures are unavailable.

There is no vaccine currently available for Lassa fever; however, development is being undertaken, with the closely related, but less virulent, Mozambique virus being considered as a possible candidate because it shows cross-reactivity without the lethality.

Case of imported Lassa fever, New Jersey, 2004

In August 2004, a New Jersey resident died of Lassa fever following travel to west Africa. He had been in Liberia (where he had been born) and Sierra Leone, and had returned to the USA via England. Luckily none of the fellow travellers who were traced and tested was infected in either the USA or the UK. About 20 cases of imported Lassa fever have been reported worldwide.

Lymphocytic choriomeningitis virus

Lymphocytic choriomeningitis virus (LCMV) is endemic in house mice worldwide. Pet rodents such as hamsters, guinea-pigs or rats may acquire the infection by contact with infected mice. Normally LCMV in humans is asymptomatic, causes a mild, self-limiting viral infection similar to influenza or in rare cases causes an aseptic meningitis that is occasionally fatal, following a pre-patent period of 7–14 days. However, in patients who are already immunocompromised, LCMV may result in serious infection leading to death. LCMV infection during pregnancy, although uncommon, can cause abortion or severe birth defects, and fetuses may be infected from birth by maternal transfer. A study undertaken in the USA indicated that 5% of the human population had immune system markers for LCMV, indicating widespread infection.[10]

Pregnant women and immunocompromised patients should reduce their exposure to rodents whenever possible. Children and the owners of pet rodents should adopt hygiene procedures such as hand washing, and not allowing faecal matter, saliva or urine to be inhaled, or come into contact with wounds or abrasions. Wild rodents should be controlled routinely in all domestic and industrial premises.

LCMV in transplant recipients

In April 2005, LCMV infection was passed to four transplant recipients from an infected donor who had acquired the infection from an infected hamster. Three of the four died. The investigation after the incident demonstrated that LCMV-infected pet rodents were extant across pet shop distribution chains.[11]

Machupo virus

Found in Bolivia and first identified in 1959, Bolivian hemorrhagic fever or black typhus is caused by Machupo virus, a group V arenavirus related to Junin virus of the Old World arenavirus group.[12]

Infection is caused by inhaling aerosols of rodent urine or droppings specifically from the vesper mouse. It may also follow contamination of open wounds with infected material. Infected rodents are asymptomatic.

The incubation period is between 7 and 16 days. The infection is of slow onset with fever, lethargy, headache and muscular pains. Facial flushing and reddening of the throat may follow, with bleeding from the nose and gums, vomiting of blood and blood blisters as the disease progresses into the haemorrhagic phase, usually within 7 days of onset. The mortality range is between 3% and 30% of cases. Person-to-person transmission has been reported especially in healthcare settings.

Reducing contact between infected rodents and humans has been effective, with few recent cases being reported. A vaccine developed for Junin virus has shown cross-immunisation potential and could be used in individuals at risk of infection.

Mobala virus

A novel arenavirus found only in the Central African Republic, and possibly Argentina, the natural reservoir is rodents, and in particular soft fur rats. The disease caused is similar to Lassa fever or Ippy virus. The transmission pathway is unclear, but it is possibly via aerosol or vector routes. Diagnosis follows isolation of viral particles and classification using antigen test methods.

Sabia virus (Brazilian haemorrhagic fever)

An arenavirus that has been found naturally in only one clinical case in Sabia, Sao Paulo, Brazil (1990). Only three clinical cases have ever been recorded: the index case, the physician who examined clinical samples from the index case and the third case after a laboratory accident at a reference collection. The animal reservoir is as yet unknown, but believed to be rodents. Transmission is believed to be by aerosolised infected body fluids.

In humans it presents with fever headache, myalgia, nausea, vomiting, conjunctivitis, acute hepatitis, diarrhoea and gastrointestinal haemorrhage.

Bunyaviruses

Crimean–Congo haemorrhagic fever

The causative agent of Crimean–Congo haemorrhagic fever (CCHF) is a bunyavirus carried by *Ixodes* ticks. It is found in eastern Europe, the Balkans, Greece, Turkey, central Asia, Africa, China, the Middle East, India and the former Soviet Union.[13]

In 1944, an outbreak occurred in the Crimea; this together with a further outbreak in 1969 in the Congo led to the naming of the disease. Infected ticks act as both a vector and a reservoir for the disease, with transovarial spread occurring. Wild and domestic animals such as cattle, goats, sheep, rabbits and hares act as both a reservoir and an amplifying host for the pathogen.

In humans, following a bite from an infected tick, there can be an acute onset of symptoms, with severe headache, rapidly elevating temperature, arthralgia, muscle pain and gastrointestinal disturbance. Eyes may become bloodshot, the throat inflamed and reddened, with focal blood blisters. As the disease progresses there may be altered mental states, jaundice, massive haematomas and bleeding from the nose and throat. This may continue for 14 days, if the patient survives, with fatalities ranging from 9% to 50% in some outbreaks. Agricultural workers in regular contact with animals in endemic areas are at risk. Person-to-person transmission is possible because infected blood or fluids can cause nosocomial spread.

Diagnosis is by polymerase chain reaction (PCR) or enzyme-linked immunosorbent assay (ELISA). There is no specific treatment and treatment is usually symptomatic; however, ribarvin has undergone trials as a treatment and, as a result of the severity of the side effects, a case-by-case assessment must be made before treatment. A vaccine has been developed but it is not licensed in the UK or the USA.[14]

Hantaviruses

The first occasion on which a hantavirus was recognised as a cause of human fatality occurred in Hantaan, Republic of Korea, in 1978. A bunyavirus, approximately 14 species of closely related viruses have since been identified within the genus *Hantavirus*, named for the locations in which they were first identified.

Rodents form the natural reservoir for these viruses, and different species of rodent are linked to specific geographical areas and viral species. Infected rodents do not generally show clinical symptoms of the disease. The virus has also been found in birds in Russia and cats in China.

There are approximately 150 000–200 000 cases of hantavirus-related disease reported annually, with about 50% occurring in the People's Republic of China. Classic hantavirus infection usually presents with renal involvement and haemorrhagic features. Hantaviruses cause haemorrhagic fever with renal syndrome (HFRS) in Eurasia and hantavirus pulmonary syndrome (HPS) in the Americas. In both Eurasia and the Americas, people with occupational exposure to rodents are considered to be at greater risk than the general population.

Human disease

After infection, clinical symptoms may appear between 7 and 28 days. Initial symptoms mirror those of many viral diseases, with fever, headache and non-specific gastrointestinal symptoms. Later, cough, breathing difficulties and circulatory collapse may follow, particularly in HPS. Kidney failure may occur in HFRS after renal inflammation or destruction. Patients who survive normally recover fully.

HFRS

HFRS is endemic in Eurasia. In Europe, three hantaviruses have been identified as causative: Puumala virus (PUUV), Dobrava virus (DOBV) and Saaremaa virus (SAAV).

The Balkan area has two forms of HFRS, with the less severe causing virtually no fatalities, and a severe form in which more than 10% of patients die. In Denmark, Estonia, Germany Latvia, Lithuania, Slovakia and other European countries, no fatal cases have been reported.[15]

There was a large outbreak in Serbia and Montenegro in 2002, with 128 confirmed cases; subsequently, in 2003, there were 34 cases in the same area and 31 in 2004. This may have been caused by climatic conditions, the increase in the rodent population and the years of armed conflict, which had led to drastic alterations in social and environmental conditions.

In 2005, there was a large increase in confirmed hantavirus infections in Germany, with 448 confirmed cases from both rural and urban areas. This was almost three times the number of patients recorded in previous years and appeared to be associated with an explosion in the population of bank voles, the rodent reservoir of PUUV.[16]

A similar marked increase of hantavirus infection was observed in Belgium and France in the same year, although patients living in densely populated urban areas were reported only from Germany.

HPS

HPS was first recognised in 1993 after an outbreak of severe respiratory disease in the Four Corners Region of the USA; of 42 confirmed cases, 26 died. The Sin Nombre virus (SNV) was identified as the hantavirus responsible. The hantavirus disease symptoms associated with Sin Nombre virus are atypical, with fever; headache, diarrhoea, muscle pain and respiratory symptoms gradually worsen into acute respiratory distress.[17]

Since then a clade (group of viruses with common genetic ancestry) of four other hantaviruses – Bayou virus, Black Creek Canal virus, New York virus and Monongahela virus – has been identified as responsible for HPS in the USA. HPS cases have also been reported in Argentina, Bolivia, Brazil, Canada, Chile, Panama, Paraguay and Uruguay.

North America

Between 1993 when the disease was recognised, and early 2006, the CDC has confirmed 438 cases of HPS across 30 US states, with a 35% fatality rate. In early 2006, nine cases of HPS occurred in Arizona, New Mexico, North Dakota, Texas and Washington.[17]

South America

In late 1996, there were 18 cases of HPS in El Bolson, Argentina. A new hantavirus, subsequently named Andes virus, was identified. All the patients were either local residents or had visited the area. Three doctors who had treated patients also became ill, probably from the first recorded instance of person-to-person transmission. Andes virus is responsible for most of the cases recorded in Argentina, Chile and Uruguay.

An outbreak of HPS occurred in Chile in 1997; of a total of 25 cases, there were a number of family clusters, in which nosocomial spread may have occurred.[18] In addition during mid-January 1999, an outbreak of HPS occurred in Panama. The causative hantavirus was designated Choclo virus.[19]

In 2000, a total of six male patients in Bolivia (aged 15–49 years) were serologically confirmed to have HPS; five died. Five of the six cases occurred between April and July, the sixth in November. All the patients lived and worked in rural areas in a 70-km radius around Bermejo. The hantavirus responsible is closely related to Andes virus and is now known as Bermejo virus.[20]

Transmission

Transmission is not by arthropod vector, but usually follows inhalation of infected aerosols of rodent saliva, urine or faecal material. Cases have been reported after rodent bites or wound inoculation with infected material.

Human-to-human transmission has been seen in HPS, and may be possible in patients with HFRS, where infected blood or body fluids could cause nosocomial transmission.

Diagnosis

Diagnosis follows PCR or ELISA testing of clinical samples.

Treatment

Supportive treatment is essential to maintain organ function. HPS cannot be effectively treated with antibiotics; however, in early disease patients should be placed on broad-spectrum antibiotics until the diagnosis of HPS is well established, because differential diagnosis between bacterial shock and hantaviral shock may be difficult. Ribarvin is effective in HFRS but it has shown no clinical effectiveness in HPS cases.[21]

Prevention

Prevention revolves around reducing exposure to infected rodents and their faeces or urine. For some areas in the USA, the problem is complicated by the range of infected rodents coinciding with natural plague foci, and the demise of rodents may lead to associated, possibly infected, fleas seeking alternative hosts and provoking a plague outbreak.

Cache Valley virus

Cache Valley virus (CVV) disease is caused by a mosquito-borne bunyavirus and is widespread in North America, where its animal reservoir consists of deer, sheep, cattle and horses.

Only two human cases have been seen, probably because it is seldom tested for; one of the patients died of acute encephalitis. The other case presented with severe headache, nausea, vomiting and generalised fatigue. The illness then progressed to an aseptic meningitis. Therapy was purely supportive and the patient made a full recovery. The route of infection is unknown.[22]

The closely related Ngeri virus caused an outbreak of haemorrhagic fever in Africa in 2004.

La Crosse virus

The bunyavirus that causes La Crosse (LAC) virus encephalitis, which mainly affects children, is widespread in the mid-western and south-eastern USA, and was first identified in La Crosse, Wisconsin. Approximately 75 cases are seen annually. It is transmitted by mosquito bite, and the virus can be transferred from mosquito to offspring via the transovarial route. The animal reservoir is squirrels and chipmunks, with transmission by mosquito bite.[23]

Symptoms are often non-specific and progress to coma, paralysis and permanent brain damage in severe cases. Treatment is purely symptomatic.

Oropouche virus

A bunyavirus, Oropouche virus causes a febrile illness known as Oropouche fever. Transmitted by mosquitoes to humans from sloths, it occurs in the Amazon region of South America, the Caribbean and Panama. First isolated in Trinidad and Tobago, it has since been responsible for several large epidemics in Brazil in the 1970s and 1980s.[24]

The illness presents with a fever of abrupt onset, with other generalised symptoms of chills, headache, anorexia, muscle and joint pain, and vomiting, which may progress to meningitis. Diagnosis follows detection of viral antibody in serum samples.

Treatment is non-specific with anti-inflammatory drugs or other symptomatic relief. Aspirin should be avoided because there is a summative risk of haemorrhagic complications. The illness is usually self-limiting with most patients making a full recovery.

Rift Valley fever

The causative is a bunyavirus, and the virus is passed to humans via the bites of infected arthropod vectors, which have previously fed upon infected animals, usually cattle, sheep, camels or goats. The virus may also be transferred by direct contact with infected animals, slaughtering or butchering beasts, or the consumption of infected meat or milk.

First recorded in Kenya in 1930, it is widespread in east Africa; epidemics are often associated with high rainfall, because this increases the mosquito population which is the prime vector for the spread of the disease. In animals the disease often causes abortion and death, especially in young animals.

In humans, the initial symptoms resemble influenza, but onset of severe disease (usually in only about 8% of cases) is manifested by the onset of acute fever, associated with severe headache, arthralgia and myalgia; there may also be unexplained bleeding, visual disturbance and alteration in mental state, with meningoencephalitis.

Survivors of severe disease may have permanent visual impairment and may never fully recover. Animals can be vaccinated against the disease, but there is no treatment and, although a vaccine for humans has been developed, it is not yet licensed.

Outbreaks

The largest recorded outbreak was in Kenya in 1997–8 with an estimated 89 000 cases and 478 deaths. In 2000, the disease appeared in Saudi Arabia and Yemen, possibly following the importation of infected livestock with 800 and 1000 cases, respectively.[25]

An outbreak of Rift Valley fever occurred in Kenya between November 2006 and January 2007. There were a total of 404 confirmed cases with 118 fatalities. The outbreak was controlled by banning the slaughter and movement of animals, with immunisation of apparently healthy animals in the areas unaffected but contiguous with the infected area, and a widespread spraying programme to reduce mosquito populations and breeding rates.[26]

In October 2007, an outbreak occurred in Sudan which, by November 2007, had 125 confirmed cases with 60 fatalities.

Coronaviruses

SARS

In November 2002, an outbreak of a pandemic of coronavirus that caused severe acute respiratory syndrome, or SARS, occurred. The outbreak was brought under control in July 2003, although sporadic outbreaks were reported from the People's Republic of China, where the original outbreak had occurred in late 2003 and early 2004. During the initial outbreak the virus spread to 33 countries in 5 continents and caused at least 8000 cases, of which more than 700 were fatal.

The causative coronavirus was later discovered to have a natural reservoir in several species of horseshoe bats, along with a number of other novel viruses from the same genus.[27]

The SARS virus is capable of infecting a number of animal species and humans, with virus being detected in live animal markets and in the wider environment in rats, palm civets, raccoon dogs and ferret badgers. It is unclear if bats transmitted the virus direct to the initial human cases, or whether the route was via other animals including the masked civet or other susceptible intermediary species; however, it would appear that the infective reservoir is species of bats, in a manner similar to Nipah and Hendra viruses.[28]

The transmission route for SARS is unknown and there is still debate as to whether this is from infected aerosols, blood, urine or faeces.

The discovery of SARS-like coronaviruses in bats highlights the increasingly recognised importance of bats as reservoirs of emerging viruses.

Filoviruses

Marburg virus

Marburg virus is caused by a filovirus closely related to but distinct from Ebola virus. It causes a haemorrhagic fever similar to Ebola fever, and has been isolated from fruit bats. The main range for the disease is Uganda and eastern Congo.[29]

The animal host is now believed to be bats, following the detection of antibodies/isolation of the virus from bats and fruit bats living in underground mines in The Democratic Republic of Congo (DRC). It still needs to be determined whether the bats are either infected by parasites or by consuming infected arthropods, or the primary reservoir.[30]

The bats are believed to shed the virus in their blood, saliva, faeces and urine, in a manner similar to many other bat-borne viruses. The initial outbreak among laboratory primates, which then spread to humans in Marburg, Germany in 1967, is believed to have arisen after the monkeys were held in a holding facility in Uganda where they were exposed to fruit bats that may have been infected.

Outbreaks

There were isolated cases of Marburg haemorrhagic fever in 1975 (South Africa), 1980 and 1987 (Kenya). There was a protracted outbreak of

Marburg virus in the village of Durba in the DRC between late 1998 and late 2000. There were 154 patients with a fatality rate of 83%. The primary cases were seen in young male miners; secondary spread occurred to families and healthcare workers.

In 2004–2005, there was a major outbreak in Angola, with an unrecorded number of cases, which led to more than 300 deaths.

Disease in humans

Human infection follows exposure to infected blood, saliva or faeces, probably from the animal host in primary infections, and then from primary patients in secondary cases. The incubation period is between 3 and 9 days, initial symptoms are non-specific and early differential diagnosis is almost impossible. Five days after the initial symptoms a maculopapular rash appears on the trunk, which may be followed by organ involvement, causing hepatitis, jaundice, pancreatitis, anorexia and altered mental states, with haemorrhage, fluid loss and organ failure. The clinical course lasts from 1 week to 3 weeks when the infection regresses or kills the patient. Full recovery in survivors may be prolonged.

Treatment is purely supportive, with administration of intravenous fluids to prevent hypotension and volaemic shock as a mainstay; however, patients with symptoms of haemorrhagic fever may respond poorly, and pulmonary oedema can occur. A vaccine is under development in both the USA and Canada.

Patients must be barrier nursed with strict controls on use of protective clothing at all times. In 2007, there were two cases in Uganda with the primary case being a male miner, who survived, and the second one of his co-workers who cared for him during his illness, and who subsequently died.

Paramyxoviruses – henipaviruses

Hendra virus

This pathogen was first identified after a respiratory tract illness was seen in 20 horses and 2 humans in Hendra (a suburb of Brisbane), Queensland, Australia, during September 1994. The resulting fatalities included 13 of the horses and their trainer. A stable hand who became infected survived. A second unconnected outbreak was identified as having occurred in Mackay, Queensland, in or about August 1994. The Mackay outbreak was much smaller – only two horses died and one human was infected, and later died. The outbreak was identified only retrospectively after the death of the man, 14 months after his exposure to infected horses. There have been four more outbreaks, each of which resulted in the death of one horse, the first in January 1999 in Cairns and the latest on the Sunshine Coast in June 2006.

The only human case seen was in a vet involved in the postmortem examination of the horse in 2004, who recovered.[31]

Initially the causative virus was named equine morbillivirus; this was later changed to Hendra, after the geographical site of the first-documented outbreak. A paramyxovirus, closely related to measles and rinderpest, it had not been identified previously as responsible for disease in either humans or horses.

Disease in animals

In horses, the disease causes respiratory distress, fever, pulmonary oedema, and nasal and oral discharge with blood present. As the disease progresses, there is central nervous system (CNS) involvement. Serologically positive fruit bats, which are usually asymptomatic, have been found in Australia and Papua New Guinea. Experimentally the virus can cause severe disease in cats, which can pass viable organisms in their urine, as can horses. Horses could be initially infected by consuming feed contaminated with the virus, but the route of infection is unknown.[32]

Transmission

The route of transmission from horse to human initially seemed to be by contact with infected blood or secretions. Investigations since have shown the presence of the causative pathogen in fruit bats, which seem to form the normal reservoir in which no clinical signs of disease are seen.

Close contact seems to be sufficient for horse-to-horse spread; however, the route of transmission from bat to horse is believed to be from aerosols of infected urine, amniotic fluid from pregnant bats or nasal discharge. There has been no evidence of bat-to-human spread, or human-to-human spread in this disease.

Disease in humans

The virus is not deemed to be highly contagious. Clinical presentation starts as a flu-like illness with fever and aching muscles. Sore throat, dizziness, drowsiness and confusion follow. Haemorrhage into or oedema of the lungs may follow, with meningitis. Death usually follows respiratory and renal failure.

Prevention

Good hygiene practice and quarantine of infected animals help control outbreaks.

Nipah virus

In the period between late 1998 and mid-1999, there were cumulative reports of a novel form of encephalitis causing fatalities and neurological damage in pig workers in Malaysia. Three major clusters of cases were seen. The first was near Ipoh in the state of Perak, the second in Sikamat in Negri Sembilan, and the third and largest in Bukit Pelandock, also in Negri Sembilan.[33]

At first the disease was considered to be Japanese encephalitis. However, the pattern of infection, the scale of the outbreak and the predominance of mature male Chinese pig farm workers led to the conclusion that a novel zoonotic agent was implicated.

Transmission

A novel paramyxovirus related to but not identical with Hendra virus was identified as the causative organism. Most victims were of Chinese ethnicity – an important factor in determining the animal origin of the virus. In Malaysia, where there is a diverse ethnic mix, ethnic Malays are predominantly Islamic and are therefore not involved in the pig industry. No cases were seen in this group. If a widespread environmental vector such as a mosquito had carried the pathogen responsible for the disease, this distinct identification of victims by ethnicity and employment would not have been seen.[34]

Of the patients identified as suffering from the disease, 93% were involved in pig farming or associated activities. When histories were taken from those patients who were able to respond to questioning, the majority reported contact with swine before developing symptoms, and a large proportion of these patients stated that they had contact with pigs that were already ill. This evidence strongly indicated that pigs were the source of the disease, particularly because, on farms where human cases were seen, the pigs were also dying of a disease characterised by symptoms of respiratory tract infection and airway insufficiency. This led to the conclusion that the route of infection could be the inhalation of infected aerosols.

Disease in humans

The period between exposure to swine and overt disease was estimated to be usually less than 14 days from the histories taken from patients or their relatives. The main symptoms seen at the onset of clinical disease were neurological, with drowsiness and lowered levels of consciousness, loss of muscle tone, sensory and cerebral dysfunction, progressive disorientation, seizures, muscle spasm and spasticity. Generalised symptoms such as headache, dizziness and sickness were also seen in some cases, before or associated with the onset of more serious symptoms.

The disease progressed to encephalitis, with 32% of patients dying, 53% recovering fully and 15% surviving but with persistent neural abnormalities and damage. In the Malaysian outbreak, of the 265 people affected 105 died.

No human-to-human transmission was documented, although familial clusters were seen. This probably relates to the pattern of employment on the pig farms, with whole families employed in the same enterprise. Healthcare workers who cared for patients suffering from Nipah virus or who were involved in their postmortem examinations were all monitored for disease: none showed any clinical signs of contracting the condition.

Soldiers employed in the culling of pigs, abattoir workers and veterinary surgeons involved in outbreak control were also screened for antibodies to the virus.

Diagnosis

Confirmation of diagnosis was obtained by isolation of viral particles from the blood and cerebrospinal fluid of victims, both swine and human. In humans there were demonstrable abnormalities in both fluids. The viral particles, later genetically sequenced, were found to be identical in both pigs and humans, confirming the theory that the agent was zoonotic and had arisen in humans from initial swine infection.

Treatment

The only treatment available was generalised supportive therapy using aspirin and theophyllines. Half of the cases admitted to hospital lost consciousness and half of these patients required intubation and respiratory support. No intervention appeared to show any influence on the eventual mortality rate. On postmortem examination, damage was found in the CNS, lungs and kidneys. Using staining techniques, the virus was found to be present in neural and endothelial cells in the brain.

Prevention

It was decided that the main method of preventing further cases should be a comprehensive cull of all pigs in the Malay states of Negri Sembilan, Perak and Selangor. Approximately 890 000 pigs were slaughtered. Measures were put in place to prevent pig movements, to implement a health education programme, and to provide protective clothing and equipment to pig farmers. A system for national surveillance to identify and destroy any other herds identified as being infected was established. Following the cull, no new cases of the disease were seen.[35]

In Singapore, by mid-March 1999, there were 11 cases of acute symptoms associated with the disease in abattoir workers reported to healthcare officials, of whom one subsequently died. All the infected individuals had handled imported pigs. A decision was swiftly taken to stop all imports of pigs from peninsular Malaysia and to close all abattoirs on 19 March 1999. Subsequent to these decisions no further cases were reported. Singapore also banned racehorses and other horses from entering or returning from any of the constituent states of Malaysia.

Retrospective analysis of the infective pattern associated with the outbreak led to the conclusion that the spread of the disease was related to the transportation of infected pigs, either from farm to farm or from farm to abattoir. A dead dog was found to have the virus *post mortem*; however, this was an isolated case. It is now believed that, in common with Hendra virus, the viral reservoir is fruit bats. Cats are susceptible to Nipah virus and can shed the virus in urine and nasal mucus, but research has shown that they are rarely exposed in nature by contact with fruit bats. The cats found to be infected in the Malaysian outbreak had probably been infected by contact with pigs that were dead or dying from the disease.

One of the less important but still publicly significant effects of this outbreak was the lack of pork available for Chinese cookery, reducing the variety of dishes available in restaurants across the Malay peninsula.

The Nipah virus outbreak prompted much research and investigation work to be undertaken into the normal host for the virus, and to map its geographical spread.

An outbreak of encephalitis in Faridpur, Bangladesh in April–May 2004 was identified as being caused by Nipah virus which appears now to be endemic in the region. Of 36 cases, 75% died. Analysis of the outbreak confirmed person-to-person transmission which was suspected following outbreaks of the same pathogen in Siliguri, India and Mehrepur, Bangladesh in 2001; further outbreaks followed in Naogoan, Bangladesh in January 2003 and in Rajbari and Faridpur, Bangladesh in January–February 2004. The lack of transmission during the Malaysian outbreak is probably linked to different healthcare and social practices. There are other paramyxoviruses that spread easily from person to person, and Nipah virus has now been isolated from respiratory mucus.[36]

There was another outbreak in Tangail, Bangladesh from late 2004 until early 2005; of 12 clinical cases, 11 died (92%). Two-thirds of the victims had drunk raw date palm sap, which fruit bats could have contaminated (as it was being collected) with saliva, faeces, urine or by drowning in the collection containers.

The latest outbreaks were between February and May 2007 in Nadia, India and Kushtia, Bangladesh. In both outbreaks there were approximately 50 cases with a 10–12% fatality rate.

Eleven isolated cases of Nipah virus encephalitis have also been documented in Bangladesh since 2001.

Other unusual paramyxoviruses in fruit bats

As a result of the emergence of Hendra virus, a research and investigation programme was set up to monitor diseases associated with fruit bats. Within the first 4 years two other viral diseases capable of zoonotic activity were identified in Australia.

Another paramyxovirus, now named Menangle virus after its first place of identification, caused an outbreak of disease at a piggery in New South Wales, Australia, in 1997. The pigs suffered illness, and sows spontaneously aborted. Human workers showed symptoms similar to influenza. Serological testing showed the virus to be the same in pigs and humans. The suspected reservoir is also fruit bats.

Tioman virus is another group V *Mononegavirales* paramyxovirus. It was first isolated from the urine of fruit bats on Tioman Island, Malaysia in 2000 while efforts were being made to identify the natural host of Nipah virus. Related to Menangle virus, there is no evidence that Tioman virus can cause human illness; however, as it is closely related to other zoonotic paramyxoviruses, continuing monitoring of any suspected cases is required.[37]

Range

Fruit bats across Malaysia, Thailand and Cambodia have tested positive for Nipah virus infection, although it is possible that the virus circulating in Cambodia may be another closely related henipavirus. Nipah, Hendra and Tioman viral antibodies have been found in fruit bats from Madagascar. It is possible that these viruses are prevalent in fruit bats across their whole geographical range including Africa. No human cases of henipavirus infection has been seen outside Malaysia, Australia or Bangladesh.[38,39]

Flaviviruses

Apart from the diseases listed in the following section, the flavivirus group also includes Ebola (see Chapter 6) and yellow fever (found in wild primates, transmitted by mosquito, but not considered to be zoonotic, although possibly reverse zoonotic, i.e. humans to animals, because the main reservoir is now believed to be humans).

West Nile virus/Kunjin virus

West Nile virus (WNV) was first identified in the West Nile province of Uganda in 1937. A flavivirus, closely related to the causative pathogens of Japanese encephalitis and St Louis encephalitis, historically it has been confined to Africa, the Middle East and the Mediterranean coast. In the biggest outbreak recorded in 1974 in the Cape Province of South Africa, almost 3000 people were infected. Kunjin virus, which is very closely related and is believed to be a subtype of WNV, is found in Australasia and south-east Asia.[40]

In Europe, WNV was first detected in Albania in 1958. The pathogen has since been detected in Portugal, France, Italy, the Czech Republic, Slovakia, Hungary, Romania, Moldavia, the Ukraine and Belarus. Most cases have coincided with periods of maximum activity for mosquitoes, usually July to September, when adjusted for the infectious pre-patent period. Work in the USA has now demonstrated that the virus can over-winter in adult mosquitoes. Reintroduction into previously disease-free or quiescent areas may follow an influx of infected migrating birds.

Disease in animals

The natural reservoir for the virus is wild birds, where its presence is especially significant in migratory species, because this forms a highly mobile infectious reservoir. Birds that become infected are believed to suffer from clinical symptoms of disease. As most are wild species, the course of infection is not easily determined, although it is believed that the outcome is either death or survival. Birds that survive can become carriers.

The introduction of a carrier into a susceptible population of birds at a time when there is high seasonal mosquito activity can produce widespread infection, with a resulting 'die-off' of birds similar to that associated with the introduction of plague (*Yersinia pestis*) in susceptible rodents. Once the virus enters the mosquito population, it is also spread into any other mammals, including humans, that the insect bites. Transfer vertically through a generation of mosquitoes occurs by transfer from female adults to eggs laid post-infection. The other mammals usually affected include horses, bats, rodents, cats and raccoons.

Transmission

The disease is spread from bird to bird, and from bird to human, by a variety of mosquito species, depending on the geographical area involved (Figure 7.1). The spread of the disease into either local bird or human populations is solely dependent on the presence or absence of suitable vectors if infected or carrier birds are present. Much work has been done to identify the main species involved; however, the spectrum is so diverse that it is best to assume that all migratory birds under suitable conditions can suffer from or carry the pathogen.

Incidence

There were a series of notable outbreaks in the late twentieth century, with Senegal in 1993, Romania in 1996 (of 500 reported cases approximately 10% were fatal), Israel and Kenya in 1998, and Volgograd, Russia, in 1999

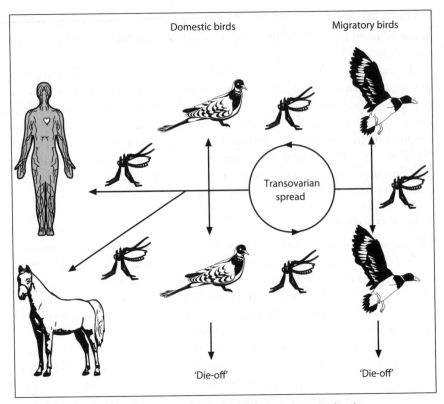

Figure 7.1 Cycle of infectivity and maintenance for West Nile virus in bird and vector populations.

with 826 cases, of which 84 progressed to meningitis, with approximately 40 fatalities. Cases have also been seen in the Camargue region of southern France, where an outbreak killed 20 partially feral horses in 2000, although no human cases were reported. Case distribution follows migratory bird patterns.

Although endemic in several regions of the globe, the disease did not receive any particular media attention until 1999, when an outbreak occurred affecting the eastern seaboard of the USA. Between August and October there were 62 human cases reported and confirmed, with 7 deaths. The centre of the outbreak was in Queens, New York City, where a large 'die-off' of birds, particularly crows, was seen shortly before the first human cases. Many birds across a wide variety of species in the Bronx Zoo also died. Once confirmed by serological testing, the outbreak was determined to be the first outbreak ever seen in the USA.

This outbreak seems to have arisen as a result of the coincidence of a number of environmental changes. The mosquito population had increased markedly, partially due to prevalent climatic conditions during the previous year, and also as a result of the cessation of insecticide treatments on areas of standing water in public parks. The cases in humans coincided with the active feeding phase of the mosquito life cycle.

Subsequent to this outbreak the virus seems to have managed to establish a presence in the mosquito population, with further outbreaks occurring on an annual basis. In 2000, 18 cases, including one fatality and one patient left in a permanent vegetative state, were seen in New York and New Jersey. The virus was detected in mosquitoes and birds before the cases occurred. In 2007, there were 3304 cases of WNV reported from 43 states across the USA, of which 93 were fatal; 286 viral positive blood donors were identified, of whom 2 later progressed to neuroinvasive disease and 59 to clinical fever.

Since 2000 the WNV Surveillance System, set up in response to the 1999 outbreak in the USA, has demonstrated an increase in the geographical range of WNV activity. Surveillance included monitoring mosquitoes, sentinel chicken flocks, wild birds and potentially susceptible mammals (e.g. horses and humans). In 1999, WNV activity was detected in only four areas: Connecticut, Maryland, New Jersey and New York.

In 2007, across 34 states, nearly 1600 dead crows and 500 other birds were reported as testing positive for the virus. Horses across 33 states tested positive for WNV, along with dogs in 3 states and squirrels in 2 states. Seroconversion to WNV was reported in 764 sentinel chicken flocks in 11 states. A total of 7772 WNV-positive mosquito pools have been reported from 36 states, the District of Columbia and New York City.[41]

Since the arrival of WNV in the USA, monitoring in the Caribbean and Central and South America has shown the presence of the virus across a wide geographical area. Surveillance in sub-Saharan and west Africa has shown that the virus is endemic.

Disease in humans

After an infective bite there is a short pre-patent period of about 3–14 days, followed by generalised symptoms similar to influenza. There may also be a widespread rash, conjunctivitis, diarrhoea, localised lymph node swelling and respiratory difficulty; this seems to be related to the particular strain of WNV responsible. The acute phase of the disease follows swiftly, with stiffness of the neck, high fever, vomiting and headache. There may be onset of either meningitis or encephalitis, with fatalities in more than 40% in cases where symptoms are most severe and where onset is swiftest. Neurological symptoms of confusion, altered states of consciousness, tremor, convulsions and coma may be seen related to the onset and progression of CNS infection. The highest mortality is associated with cases in elderly patients. Loss of coordination, tremor and neurological symptoms may persist for more than a year after the initial infection resolves. The disease may also lead to flaccid paralysis associated with Guillain–Barré syndrome. On postmortem examination, findings include extensive tissue haemorrhage, cardiac damage and brain damage with cerebral oedema and neural degeneration.

Risk factors for the neuroinvasive form of the disease include pre-existing hypertension or diabetes, heart disease or lung disease.

Treatment

There is no specific treatment, with supportive and symptomatic care being the mainstay of therapy. A variety of drug therapies have been tried with varying success, including ribarvin, interferon-alfa, antiepileptics, immunoglobulin and corticosteroids.

Transmission to humans by other means

In September 2005, WNV infection occurred in three of four recipients of organs transplanted from a common donor who was infected with WNV.

Two of the four were found to have the neuroinvasive form of the disease. One was uninfected and the other was asymptomatic. A similar case was reported in 2003.[42]

Transmission has also been recorded via contaminated blood products. Despite a negative test at donation, two clinical cases of WNV occurred in two immunosuppressed patients in Wisconsin in 2006, both of whom received blood from the same donor. WNV transmission through blood transfusion was first reported in 2002, prompting rapid implementation of nationwide screening of blood donations for WNV by 2003. This has been refined since.[43,44]

Transmission may also be possible via breast milk; following a transfusion of possibly contaminated blood, a mother developed symptoms of WNV, and a breast milk sample tested positive for the virus. The infant remained asymptomatic, but antibodies to WNV were demonstrated in a blood sample from the infant 25 days after delivery, when the mother had recovered. The infant had not as far as can be ascertained been exposed to any other source of infection.[45]

Occupational exposure

In 2002, two poultry workers working on a turkey farm in Wisconsin were diagnosed as having contracted WNV. The birds and workers on the farm were found to have a high incidence of antibodies to the virus. After investigation it became apparent that the transmission may not have been mosquito mediated, but through occupational exposure in both birds and humans. The use of insect repellents, masks and gloves for workers at risk is recommended.[46]

Laboratory workers are also at risk and at least two clinical WNV cases have followed accidental inoculation with contaminated material.

Prevention

A vaccine to protect animals, especially horses, against WNV has been developed and is in widespread use in the USA. The vaccination of susceptible feral or domesticated animals could reduce the infective reservoir and, coupled with mosquito control programmes, may drastically reduce transmission rates in endemic areas. It is hoped that a vaccine for human use may soon become available.

The states of the eastern seaboard of the USA have instituted a major programme of detection and monitoring aimed at reducing the impact of any further disease outbreaks. Seventeen states are involved plus New York City and the District of Columbia (Washington State). The programme uses populations of tame birds, which are monitored for the appearance of the virus during the period when the mosquitoes are actively feeding, and transmission is most likely.

All mass 'die-offs' are monitored and viral testing is carried out on recovered corpses as part of epidemic prediction routines. Birds entering the USA as planned imports for the pet trade must be tested for the virus before they are allowed past quarantine.

Attempts are also being made to reduce mosquito populations, using sterilised females, insecticides and other measures. People are encouraged to avoid bites wherever possible, using repellents, nets or screens to reduce the number of insects entering houses or other buildings.

Japanese encephalitis

Japanese encephalitis is also caused by a flavivirus, and is endemic in most rural areas of south-east Asia, especially China, Japan, North and South Korea, and the eastern areas of the former Soviet Union.

Disease in animals

Pigs and some bird species act as the animal reservoir for the disease, usually in rural areas with extensive paddy field cultivation, where the mosquito vectors can breed. The conditions for the disease also exist on the fringes of urban centres, where there is waste land or sites under development. The disease is seasonal, and the infective peak is usually seen between June and September when the mosquitoes are actively feeding, although this will vary from area to area depending upon the prevalent climatic conditions.[47]

Transmission

Transmission to humans follows the bite of a previously infected mosquito.

Disease in humans

Most cases are subclinical and asymptomatic and follow a pre-patent period of between 5 and 15 days; however, in cases where clinical signs are seen there is a high incidence of mortality, with up to a third of patients dying. The clinical course begins with high fever, and neurological symptoms rapidly follow with altered perception, confusion and coma. About 30% of patients who survive demonstrate long-term neural and psychiatric damage associated with neural loss.

In endemic areas, children and elderly people are at the greatest risk. Elderly patients have a high mortality, and children, although surviving the illness, display long-term sequelae. Travellers are unlikely to contract the disease if they are visiting solely urban centres, but there may be a risk of the disease if they are visiting rural areas or are likely to stay in an area for prolonged periods of time.

Treatment and prevention

Treatment is purely symptomatic and supportive. A vaccine is available and those people considered to be at risk while visiting endemic areas should receive a programme of three injections at discrete intervals. A full risk–benefit analysis should be conducted before immunisation takes place because the vaccines are not fully licensed. Vaccine can be obtained through MASTA or Sanofi Pasteur MSD in the UK, and through the CDC in the USA.

While travelling, wherever possible staying in air-conditioned accommodation or using a mosquito net is recommended, coupled with appropriate use of insecticides and repellents.

St Louis encephalitis

St Louis encephalitis is also caused by a flavivirus, widespread in the Americas, and isolated from northern Canada to southern Argentina: 4651 cases were reported across the USA between 1964 and 2005, with most cases being reported in the central and eastern states.[48]

The natural reservoirs are birds and bats, although the pathogen has also been isolated from horses and other mammals. The animals do not display any symptoms. In humans the disease develops after inoculation by infected mosquito bites. The pre-patent period is between 4 days and 3 weeks and, as with many other flavivirus infections, symptoms start with fever. Most cases do not progress to encephalitis, although this is possible, and fatalities have occurred, especially in elderly patients. In Brazil it has also caused haemorrhagic fever in some patients.

There is no treatment, and symptomatic control is the only possible therapeutic intervention.

Other flaviviruses

Powassan virus is another flavivirus found only in North America. The reservoir is believed to be rodents, especially skunks and woodchucks with *Ixodes* tick species acting as vectors for transmission to humans. Few cases have ever been recorded in humans, although approximately 10–15% were fatal. A recent cluster of cases occurred between 1999 and 2001 in Maine and Vermont and were the latest since 1994. Luckily, the ticks that spread the disease between the normal animal reservoir of rodents and their mammalian predators do not preferentially bite humans. Symptoms include gastrointestinal disturbances, decreased kidney function, anaemia, altered mental states, joint stiffness and generalised muscle weakness, with encephalitis. Diagnosis follows isolation of virus from blood or cerebrospinal fluid or positivity for Powassan-specific IgM and neutralising antibody. The CDC recommends that Powassan virus should be included in the differential diagnosis of all encephalitis cases occurring in the northern USA, and particularly in the north east.[49]

As there is no vaccine or specific therapy, prevention of tick bites or removing them as quickly as possible after attachment is the main protection from the disease. Pets should be checked for ticks before they enter the house in at-risk areas.

Kyansur and Omsk haemorrhagic virus are also flaviviruses. Kyansur has been found only in the Kyansur Forest area of Karnatha, India. The natural reservoir may possibly be monkeys, but they may also be victims of the disease, rather than the actual primary host. Transmission follows tick bites. The disease has an abrupt onset, with a biphasic pattern consisting of febrile and haemorrhagic phases followed by CNS involvement, similar to other tick-borne encephalitises. Symptoms include rash, conjunctivitis and pneumonia. Diagnosis is by PCR/ELISA tests.

Omsk haemorrhagic virus is found only in western Siberia, the natural reservoir being rodents, especially muskrats. Transmission is by dermacentor ticks and mosquitoes; it is also possibly capable of being water borne. The diesease that it causes is very similar to cases of Kyansur virus, with an abrupt onset and a biphasic pattern, followed by CNS involvement. The symptoms show the same pattern as Kyansur, including rash, conjunctivitis and pneumonia.

Borna disease

Described more than 200 years ago in the town of Borna, Germany, this is a fatal neurological disease primarily of sheep and horses, caused by an RNA virus of the Mononegavirales order, family *Bornaviridae*. It is interesting that the Monenegavirales order contains the following viral families: flaviviruses (WNV, St Louis encephalitis, Japanese encephalitis), paramyxoviruses (Nipah, Hendra) and rhabdoviruses (rabies, bat lyssa).[50]

Borna disease is unusual in that it appears that the virus itself is not the cause of the symptoms seen – it is the immune response of the victim that causes the underlying damage, which produces the characteristic symptoms.

Disease in animals

The disease occurs in animals in sporadic outbreaks, primarily in central Europe. There is also antibody evidence of infection occurring in Israel, Japan, Iran and the USA in horses. In animals the disease is usually sub-clinical, although more virulent forms may arise and produce fatalities. It is also found in sheep, cattle, rabbits and some exotic species such as llamas and hippopotami. Rodents probably form the wild animal reservoir, especially shrews. It is currently not believed to be present in the UK; however, the Department for Environment, Food and Rural Affairs (DEFRA) is undertaking monitoring of horses and sheep for the presence of this pathogen. The Health Protection Agency is also taking an active interest in monitoring human cases of mental illness where other factors are suspected.[51]

Transmission

The virus is transmitted via nasal secretions, saliva or tears, either directly or by contamination of food or water. There is a pre-patent period of approximately 4 weeks in horses with the disease presenting with non-specific symptoms, usually of fever, loss of appetite, colic and constipation. This can progress to neurological symptoms with loss of coordination, muscle weakness, gait and posture abnormalities, repetitive movements and paralysis as encephalitis develops. The virus invades the CNS by migrating from peripheral initial infection sites down neurons. The illness normally lasts for 1–3 weeks, and those horses displaying the CNS symptoms have up to 100% fatality. Survivors can relapse if stressed.

The disease occurs seasonally in spring and summer and, although this could indicate a possible spread by arthropod vectors, no vector has been identified in Europe, although it has been found in ticks in the Near East.

Disease in humans

There is a possible link with psychiatric illness in humans. The clinical course of infection in humans is not documented, although surveys of patients have demonstrated a correlation between psychiatric disease in humans and the serological evidence of Borna disease virus antibodies showing either active or recent infection. The relationship is most frequent in cases where gait or postural abnormalities are present. Some psychiatric patients who develop fatal meningoencephalitis have also been shown to be Borna disease virus positive.[52]

Treatment

Both ribarvin and amantadine have been used in the treatment of Borna virus. It is unclear if amantadine kills the virus or simply has an antidepressant effect.

Closing comments

Between the first and second editions of this book, the number of zoonotic viruses identified and classified have increased dramatically. The conditions for humans to encounter novel viruses, carried by animals or infected vectors, will continue to occur in the future and, as detection methods change and improve, new pathogens can be identified, and the causatives of previously unidentified or unclassified diseases defined. Just watch this space.

References

1. Randolph SE. Tick borne encephalitis virus, ticks and humans, short and long term dynamics. *Curr Opin Infect Dis* 2008; **21**: 462–7.
2. De Lamballerie X, Boisson V, Reynier J-C *et al*. Chikungunya acute infection and chloroquine treatment. Vector-borne and zoonotic diseases. *J Vector Borne Zoonotic Dis* 2008; **8**: 837–40.
3. CDC. Eastern equine encephalitis – New Hampshire and Massachusetts, August–September 2005. *MMWR* 2006; **55**; 697–700.
4. de Thoisy B, Gardon J, Alba Salas R, Morvan J, Kazanji M. Mayaro virus in wild mammals, French Guiana. *Emerg Infect Dis* 2003; **9**: 1326–9.
5. Charrel RN, de Lamballerie X. Arenaviruses other than Lassa virus. *Antiviral Res* 2003; **57**: 89–100.
6. Salazar-Bravo J, Ruedas LA, Yates TL. Mammalian reservoirs of arenaviruses. *Curr Top Microbiol Immunol* 2002; **262**: 25–63.
7. Weaver SC, Salas RA, de Manzione N *et al*. Guanarito virus (*Arenaviridae*) isolates from endemic and outlying localities in Venezuela: sequence comparisons among and within strains isolated from Venezuelan hemorrhagic fever patients and rodents. *Virology* 2000; **266**: 189–95
8. Ogbu O, Ajuluchukwu E, Uneke CJ. Lassa fever in West African sub-region: an overview. *J Vector Borne Diseases* 2007; **44**(1): 1–11.
9. Lecompte E, Fichet-Calvet E, Daffis S *et al*. *Mastomys natalensis* and Lassa fever, West Africa. *Emerg Infect Dis* 2006; **12**: 1971–4.
10. CDC. Control and Prevention. Update: interim guidance for minimizing risk for human lymphocytic choriomeningitis virus infection associated with pet rodents. *MMWR* 2005; **54**: 799–801.
11. Fischer SA, Graham MB, Kuehnert MJ *et al*. Transmission of lymphocytic choriomeningitis virus via organ transplantation. *N Engl J Med* 2006; **354**: 2235–49.
12. Kilgore PE, Peters CJ, Mills JN *et al*. Prospects for control of Bolivian hemorrhagic fever. *Emerg Infect Dis* 1995; **1**: 97–100.
13. Drosten C, Minnak D, Emmerich P, Schmitz H, Reinicke T. Crimean–Congo haemorrhagic fever in Kosovo. *J Clin Microbiol* 2002; **40**: 1122–3.
14. Ergonul O, Celikbas A, Dokuzoguz B, Eren S, Baykam N, Esener H. Characteristics of patients with Crimean–Congo hemorrhagic fever in a recent outbreak in Turkey and impact of oral ribavirin therapy. *Clin Infect Dis* 2004; **39**: 284–7.

15. Vapalahti O, Mustonen J, Lundkvist A, Hentonnen H, Plyusnin A, Vaheri A. Hantavirus infections in Europe. *Lancet Infect Dis* 2003; **3**: 653–61.

16. Mailles A, Abu Sin M, Ducoffre G, Heyman P, Koch J, Zeller H. Larger than usual increase in cases of hantavirus infections in Belgium, France and Germany, June 2005. *Eurosurveillance* 2005; **10**: E050721.4.

17. Rivers MN, Alexander JL, Rohde RE, Pierce JR Jr. Hantavirus pulmonary syndrome in Texas 1993–2006. *South Med J* 2009; **102**: 36–41.

18. Martinez VP, Bellomo C, San Juan J *et al*. Person-to-person transmission of Andes virus. *Emerg Infect Dis* 2005; **11**: 1848–53.

19. Vincent MJ, Quiroz E, Garcia F *et al*. Hantavirus pulmonary syndrome in Panama: Identification of novel Hantavirus and their likely reservoirs. *Virology* 2000; **277**: 14–19.

20. Padula P, Della Valle MG, Alai MG, Cortada P, Villagra M, Gianella A. Andes virus and first case report of Bermejo virus causing fatal pulmonary syndrome. *Emerg Infect Dis* 2002; **8**: 437–9.

21. Mertz GJ, Miedzinski L, Goade D *et al*. Placebo-controlled, double-blind trial of intravenous ribavirin for the treatment of hantavirus cardiopulmonary syndrome in North America. *Clin Infect Dis* 2004; **39**: 1307–13.

22. Campbell GL, Mataczynski JD, Reisdorf S *et al*. Second human case of Cache Valley virus disease. *Emerg Infect Dis* 2006; **12**: 854–6.

23. Rust RS, Thompson WH, Matthews CG, Beaty BJ, Chun RW. La Crosse and other forms of California encephalitis. *J Child Neurol* 1999; **14**: 1–14.

24. Nunes MRT, Martins LC, Rodrigues SG *et al*. Oropouche virus isolation, Southeast Brazil. *Emerg Infect Dis* 2005; **11**: 1610–13.

25. Madani TA, Al-Mazrou YY, Al-Jeffri MH *et al*. Rift Valley fever epidemic in Saudi Arabia: epidemiological, clinical, and laboratory characteristics. *Clin Infect Dis* 2003; **37**: 1084–92.

26. CDC. Rift Valley fever outbreak – Kenya, November 2006–January 2007. *MMWR* 2007; **56**: 73–6

27. Lin-Fa Wang, Zhengli Shi, Shuyi Zhang *et al*. Review of bats and SARS. *Emerg Infect Dis* 2006; **12**: 1834–40.

28. Guan Y, Zheng BJ, He YQ *et al*. Isolation and characterization of viruses related to the SARS coronavirus from animals in Southern China. *Science* 2003; **302**: 276–9.

29. Towner JS, Pourrut X, Albarino CG *et al*. Marburg virus infection detected in a common African bat. *PLoS ONE* 2007; **2**: e764.

30. Swanepoel R, Smit SB, Rollin PE *et al*. Studies of reservoir hosts for Marburg virus. *Emerg Infect Dis* 2007; **13**: 1847–51.

31. Selvey LA, Wells RM, McCormack JG *et al*. Infection of humans and horses by a newly described morbillivirus. *Med J Aust* 1995; **162**: 642–5.

32. Williamson MM, Hooper PT, Selleck PW *et al*. Transmission studies of Hendra virus (equine morbillivirus) in fruit bats, horses and cats. *Aust Vet J* 1998; **76**: 813–18.

33. Anon. Outbreak of Hendra-like virus – Malaysia and Singapore, 1998–1999. *MMWR* 1999; **48**: 265–9.

34. Goh KJ, Tan CT, Chew NK *et al*. Clinical features of Nipah virus encephalitis among pig farmers in Malaysia. *N Engl J Med* 2000; **342**: 1229–35.

35. Mackenzie JS, Field HE, Guyatt KJ. Managing emerging diseases borne by fruit bats (flying foxes), with particular reference to henipaviruses and Australian bat lyssavirus. *J Appl Microbiol* 2003; **94**(suppl): 59S–69S.

36. Hsu VP, Hossain MJ, Parashar UD *et al*. Nipah virus encephalitis reemergence, Bangladesh. *Emerg Infect Dis* 2004; **10**: 2082–7.

37. Chua KB, Wang LF, Lam SK, *et al*. Tioman virus, a novel paramyxovirus isolated from fruit bats in Malaysia. *Virology* 2001; **283**: 215–29.

38. Reynes JM, Counor D, Ong S, *et al*. Nipah virus in Lyle's flying foxes, Cambodia. *Emerg Infect Dis* 2005; **11**: 1042–7.

39. Wacharapluesadee S, Lumlertdacha B, Boongird K, *et al*. Bat Nipah virus, Thailand. *Emerg Infect Dis* 2005; **11**: 1949–51.

40. Guharoy R, Gilroy SA, Noviasky JA, Ference J. West Nile virus infection. *Am J Health Syst Pharm* 2004; **61**: 1235–41.
41. CDC. West Nile virus update – United States, January 1–November 13, 2007. *MMWR* 2007; **56**: 1191–2.
42. CDC. West Nile virus infections in organ transplant recipients – New York and Pennsylvania, August–September, 2005. *MMWR* 2005; **54**: 1021–3.
43. CDC. West Nile virus transmission through blood transfusion – South Dakota, 2006. *MMWR* 2007; **56**: 76–9.
44. CDC. West Nile virus activity – United States, October 10–16, 2002, and update on West Nile virus infections in recipients of blood transfusions. *MMWR* 2002; **51**: 929–31.
45. CDC. Possible West Nile virus transmission to an infant through breast-feeding – Michigan, 2002. *MMWR* 2002; **51**: 877–8.
46. CDC. West Nile virus infection among turkey breeder farm workers – Wisconsin, 2002. *MMWR* 2003; **52**; 1017–19.
47. Parida M, Dash PK, Tripathi NK *et al*. Japanese encephalitis outbreak, India. *Emerg Infect Dis* 2006; **12**: 1427–30.
48. Spinsanti L, Basquiera AL, Bulacio S *et al*. St. Louis encephalitis in Argentina: the first case reported in the last seventeen years. *Emerg Infect Dis* 2003; **9**: 271–3.
49. CDC. Outbreak of Powassan encephalitis – Maine and Vermont, 1999–2001. *MMWR* 2001; **50**: 761–4.
50. Hornig M, Briese T, Lipkin WI. Borna disease virus. *J Neurovirol* 2003; **9**: 259–73.
51. Hilbe M, Herrsche R, Kolodziejek J, Nowotny N, Zlinszky K, Ehrensperger F. Shrews as reservoir hosts of Borna disease virus. *Emerg Infect Dis* 2006; E-publication.
52. De la Torre JC. Bornavirus and the brain. *J Infect Dis* 2002; **186**: S241–7.

8

Zoonoses of exotic, feral and wild animals

Not all the animals in the world are domesticated. Our domesticated species were once wild and, although in many parts of the world the wild species that were their common ancestor are now extinct, the animals that we now keep as pets or for profit once lived without human intervention. Selective breeding has altered them externally, but genetically they are still very close to their wild cousins, and thus can be susceptible to the same diseases. Domesticated species may also revert to living in the wild, or as close to it as an urban environment allows. These feral species are especially important infective reservoirs, not only for zoonoses, but also for other significant animal diseases.[1]

In the case of feral species the difference between them and domesticated animals, often of exactly the same species, is solely a matter of geography. Some may be escapees, such as racing pigeons that fail to return to their roosts after a race. The large flocks of pigeons encountered in urban centres have been implicated as a reservoir for *Chlamydophila psittaci*, and also cause a significant nuisance with faeces fouling. Cats and dogs can also live a feral existence and are usually reservoirs of the afflictions of their own species, which may not all be zoonoses, such as parvovirus.

The term 'exotics' has been coined to cover species that have been introduced, usually for commercial purposes, into areas or regions where they are not native. Some of these will be kept as pets, ranging from the expected such as caged birds and some rodents (many of which are now bred in country, rather than being imported) to the unusual, such as apes, reptiles, large cats (tigers, etc.) or pygmy hedgehogs. Others will be kept for fur (mink), as curiosities (coypu and edible dormice) or for sport (muntjac deer), or were introduced for other reasons (grey squirrels, catfish, etc.).[2]

Initially confined to farms, estates or other limited and controlled locations, they inevitably escape. With a lack of domestic predators, or with a reproduction rate that far outstrips predation or control strategies, these animals can adapt to the environment, find an ecological niche and establish a wild living population, often to the detriment of native wildlife. Often introduced with less than current standards of quarantine (and therefore capable of carrying unusual bacterial or viral flora), or susceptible to the diseases associated with their closest wild relatives or environmental pathogens, they can form a disease focus.

Some animals have never been domesticated, and can be classed as fully wild or sylvan. Of these some will inhabit only rural or wilderness areas; others will have adapted their mode of survival to living in or around the encroaching urban environment. There are probably now more urban foxes in towns and cities than there are in the countryside.

Wild animals such as foxes, badgers, rats and squirrels have their own associated diseases, some of which are zoonotic. They may also act as amplifying hosts for pathogens, or for the parasites, such as ticks or fleas, that carry zoonotic organisms. Many of these diseases are those of their closest domesticated counterparts, although there are some that are species specific, such as racoon roundworm which given the right conditions may be marginally zoonotic (i.e. rare reported cases in humans).[3]

Currently in the UK, badgers as a reservoir of bovine tuberculosis (*Mycobacterium bovis*) are of particular concern to dairy farmers, although the scientific evidence relating to transmission into cattle is conflicting. As the pathogen has also been found in roe and fallow deer, controlling infected badgers may have no effect, and recently a decision has been made by the British government that, at present, no badger cull will be authorised in endemic areas.

In most urban areas across the UK and the USA, foxes or other wild canids are on the increase and, as they become established in urban areas, they form a potential reservoir for canine zoonoses, especially as they not only hunt but also scavenge, and consumption of other mammalian corpses or food waste is a potential route of spread in certain infections. Rodents as a reservoir for leptospirosis are well recognised, and the emergence of animals resistant to the rodenticides in normal widespread use poses an increasing problem, especially in urban areas. The need to control populations of pest animals and their associated arthropod or intestinal parasites in urban areas is a significant part of the local authorities' focus on maintaining environmental and public health.

Foxes in Europe are known to form a sylvatic focus for *Echinococcus multilocularis*, *Toxocara canis* and *Trichinella* spp.[4] The UK remains at present free of *E. multilocularis*, but it is endemic in Europe and is a significant causative of fatal hydatid disease. The pet passport system (see Chapter 6) is geared to preventing this pathogen among others entering the UK, as is the quarantine regimen in North America.

Other wildlife can also carry some unusual pathogens. In the UK, otters (*Lutra lutra*) and a variety of marine mammals (porpoises and dolphins) have tested positive for atypical *Brucella* spp. Otters have also been found to be carrying liver fluke (*Fasciola* spp.) in southern England. The parasite is potentially zoonotic and believed to have been contracted from imported freshwater fish which have then become naturalised, after escape or release.[5]

Pasteurella multocida has been found in a variety of species including swans, hedgehogs and foxes, and avian botulism has been found in gulls in Scotland.

Other species of wild birds have been found to carry potentially zoonotic pathogens with *Chlamydophila* spp. and trichomoniasis in feral pigeons, and *Clostridium perfringens* having been detected in jackdaws.

There is also a considerable risk that wild animals of similar or related species to domesticated varieties can act as reservoirs of important economic pathogens. Testing by the Veterinary Laboratories Agency (VLA) in the UK has shown that deer can act as reservoirs for such animal diseases as foot-and-mouth disease and bluetongue. A variety of potentially dangerous *Salmonella* spp. have also been found in rodents, wild birds and badgers with *Salmonella dublin* being isolated from fallow deer (*Dama dama*) and foxes (*Vulpes vulpes*). Strains of *Salmonella typhimurium* have been detected in garden birds.[5]

Wildlife are also not static or confined to specific areas as domesticated species are, where the bounds of movement are normally set by agricultural practice. Wild birds migrate, often large distances, carrying with them a variety of pathogens, including importantly viruses such as West Nile or pathogenic influenza such as H5N1.

Transmission pathways

Most feral or wild animals shun human contact, so infections by zoonoses associated with wildlife normally follow changes in circumstance or cultural practice. Natural or man-made disasters such as conflicts may displace people or alter normal life patterns, so that exposure to infected animals or material increases. This pattern is seen in emerging diseases as discussed in Chapter 7. Many of the outbreaks of serious zoonotic disease seen in sub-Saharan Africa have been linked to conflict, e.g. plague and Ebola in The Democratic Republic of Congo (DRC) or Marburg in Angola.

The acronym WIREDs (wildlife-related emerging diseases) has been used for these conditions. It recognises the role of wildlife as a reservoir for pathogens potentially capable of posing a risk to humans or domesticated animals.

Expansion of urbanisation into previously wild environments may lead to unexpected exposures to pathogens, with the emergence of bat-mediated rabies in South America being a particularly unpleasant manifestation of this effect. Alternatively deforestation and agricultural activity on cleared land or other changes in environmental practice can also produce dramatic disease events, as exemplified by the emergence of Nipah virus in Malaysia.

Hunters, ecotourists, animal trappers or handlers, zookeepers, customs officials, quarantine facility or wildlife sanctuary workers can all be exposed as a result of their work or activities. Hunting in the UK is not a mainstream activity, and is normally confined to species bred specifically as game, such as deer or pheasants; however, in Europe it is estimated that there are approximately 10 million people who hunt, generating an annual income of 10 billion euros. In the USA, hunting is both a leisure activity and a way of life, with 700 000 people being employed in hunting-associated enterprises and with an incalculable number of hunters. As discussed elsewhere, hunting can expose hunters to zoonotic infections such as tularaemia, Lyme disease and others that may carry currently unknown risks such as chronic wasting disease (CWD).

Wildlife tourism such as safaris or bush walks are major income generators in many African states such as Kenya or Tanzania, and these can expose participants to a variety of wildlife pathogens.

Bushmeat and the live animal trade

There are also two commercial drivers that appear to increase the risks of wildlife zoonosis spread: the trade in bushmeat and the live animal trade.

Bushmeat is defined as meat derived from wild animals, and in Africa and South America it is a major source of dietary protein. In Africa, in particular, the meat may be derived from a variety of species including apes, rodents and birds, some of which are listed under the Convention on the International Trade in Endangered Species of Wild Fauna and Flora (CITES). Among immigrant populations elsewhere in the world, bushmeat is seen as a delicacy, and returning or visiting nationals or their relatives may bring bushmeat into their new country of residence. Ecologically the trade is also of concern, because, driven by demand from expatriate communities who have the income to pay high prices for bushmeat, it may lead to over-hunting of species, carrying with it risks of extinction.[6]

In the UK approximately 12 000 tonnes of illegally imported meat are seized annually, including bushmeat. To try to estimate the percentage of the seizures that originate from bushmeat sources such as apes or rodents, meat is DNA tested after seizure. In 2007, there were 35 000 seizures, only one of which could be taken to prosecution, with an Egyptian woman being found guilty of the illegal importation of 83 kg of meat and dairy products; she was fined £300. The damage that such imports can cause can be estimated; if the theory that the material that initially caused the devastating foot-and-mouth disease outbreak in the UK during 2001 was illegally imported meat or meat products, it is accepted at £1.2 billion.

In January 2008, the Department for Environment Food and Rural Affairs (DEFRA) in the UK relaunched a campaign to reduce black and minority ethnic (BME) personal food importation under the banner 'Don't break the law, check the rules before travel'. Run by DEFRA in association with Her Majesty's Revenue and Customs (HMRC) and the Food Standards Agency (FSA), the aim is to remind people that it is illegal to bring meat and dairy products from countries outside the EU into the UK. It also aims to explain why the restrictions are in place (prevention of animal and plant diseases), and that many of the products are available legally and safely in the UK. It also highlights the legal penalties that can be applied.

There are concerns that bushmeat seized by customs officials in western Europe or the USA could carry zoonotic or other pathogens such as Ebola; luckily, however, this is probably unrealistic in the case of this virus, because it is likely to have died in meat transported these distances from source. As to other pathogens the picture is less clear and due to the method of preparation, transport method (usually in personal unrefrigerated luggage) and duration of transit, the meat usually carries a large bacterial burden of food-borne pathogens associated with poor butchery techniques or ongoing decomposition.

In fresh bushmeat the risk is higher, with Ebola, simian foamy virus, lymphotrophic viruses and other zoonotic pathogens posing a real risk to consumers. People living in sub-Saharan Africa have been shown to have antibodies to several chimpanzee-borne adenoviruses, probably after infection associated with the butchering or consumption of bushmeat.[7]

This is also true of the legitimate, rather than the illicit, trade in exotic foodstuffs with legally imported meat from reptiles, and other species being identified as capable of infecting consumers, with a variety of pathogens and parasites such as *Toxoplasma* spp., liver fluke, tapeworms and intestinal roundworms.

As a subset of bushmeat, there are also concerns that traditional ethnic medicines, where animal products may be used for therapeutic reasons, could form a source of infection.

The live animal trade in wildlife is now worldwide and is estimated to generate in the region of $US6 billion per annum.[8] It has been implicated in the appearance of zoonoses outside their usual geographical range, such as the outbreak of monkeypox in the USA in 2003 (see below), and also the emergence of diseases such as severe acute respiratory syndrome or SARS (see Chapter 7). The legal trade at least can be regulated, and animals quarantined. No such safeguards are applicable to illicit trading in wild animals; the illegal trade has led to the infection of customs officials with psittacosis and the detection of H5N1 in smuggled birds of prey.[9,10]

Escapees and releases

Animals may be kept for a variety of reasons outside their normal ecosystem, usually for commercial reasons, such as fur or meat farming. These animals do not normally have predators in the external environment outside their area of captivity, and this can be of concern in both animal and zoonotic disease terms, e.g. raccoon dogs, bred in captivity for their fur, escaped from fur farms and now form an important zoonotic reservoir for rabies in eastern Europe. Muntjak deer, once confined to deer parks as an ornamental and game species, are now widespread across the British Isles, and are capable of forming a reservoir for a number of commercially important diseases such as *M. bovis* tuberculosis, foot-and-mouth disease and other diseases.

Paradoxically, animal rights protesters can be responsible for damage to the environment, or altering the zoonotic risk, when they release species into habitats that they do not normally occupy. A release of mink from a fur farm in the West Midlands of the UK led to unquantifiable and continuing predation of mammalian and bird species.

Releases of animals to repopulate areas from which they have withdrawn or become extinct, or for game hunting, has also led to the emergence of animal diseases, some with zoonotic potential, with wild boar forming a reservoir for *Brucella suis* and *Trichinella* spp. which may then be transmitted to outdoor raised commercial pigs.

Zoological parks, circuses and city farms

Zoos, circuses and city farms exist in most countries, often in major cities. Many now have petting areas, where children can interact closely with domestic animals or captive wildlife, either touching or feeding the animals. For many children, and their parents, this will be often the sole contact that they have with animals not kept as pets. Both children and adults may not adhere to good hygiene precautions, and a potential exists for the transmission of zoonoses, including those associated with wildlife or farm animals from this contact.[11]

There have been recurring outbreaks, particularly of *Escherichia coli* O157, across the UK, the USA and many other parts of the world, that have followed visits to petting farms/zoos. An outbreak of *E. coli* infection associated with a petting zoo in Pennsylvania in 2000 led to 55 confirmed cases, with one child requiring a kidney transplantation. *E. coli* is not the only risk; cases of *Salmonella* and *Cryptosporidia* infection have also followed such visits. The incident in 2000 is not the only example; on an annual basis there is at least one report that will reach national media levels of disease outbreaks following such visits. Some further details can be found in Chapter 4.[12]

Many of these outbreaks could be prevented had some simple precautions been taken. Prevention strategies are discussed in Chapter 9, but it is worth reiterating that good hygiene, including hand washing, preventing children from kissing animals, putting objects or fingers in their mouths, especially before washing after contact with animals, will prevent many cases of infection. Proper shoes, appropriate clothing and vigilance by responsible adults are necessary. Guidance can be found for parents, teachers and farmers in the Health and Safety Executive (HSE) Information Sheet AIS 23 (revised).[13]

Exotic pets

Other chapters of this book have already examined some of the more unusual pathogens that exotic pets such as reptiles can carry, including a wide variety of *Salmonella* spp.

As with other aspects of modern life, there are fashions in pet ownership and these can produce some interesting disease risks.

Among the exotic pets currently kept in the USA and Europe are several species of hedgehogs, including Asian, African pygmy and European species. Hedgehogs are known to be reservoirs for foot-and-mouth disease, and therefore in the USA the importation of African species has been banned since 1991.[14]

Hedgehogs have also been identified as hosts for a variety of arboviruses, such as Tahyna, and Bhanja. European hedgehogs (*Erinaceus europaeus*) in Germany have been identified as carriers and amplifying hosts for *Borrelia* spp., the causative organism of Lyme disease, and can be hosts for *Ixodes* ticks, which are capable of spreading the disease to other species including humans.

Among the diseases that they are known to carry are unusual *Salmonellae*, *Mycobacteria*, *Coxiella burnetii*, *Chlamydophila*, *Cryptosporidia* spp., and *Toxoplasma gondii*. Humans exposed to hedgehogs have presented with ringworm.

Prairie dogs are an unusual but popular pet in the USA, although their popularity has declined since the outbreak of monkeypox in 2003; however, they have also been shown to be capable of carrying tularaemia and plague, so, although furry and 'cuddly', they might best be avoided, especially for people in groups at high risk for zoonotic disease.[15]

Examples of diseases associated with wildlife

The following covers some of the better known disease states associated with wildlife. It is not comprehensive but gives a flavour of those pathogens that wildlife can carry.

Raccoon roundworm

An intestinal roundworm found mostly in raccoons, *Baylisascaris procyonis*, causes rare but severe and sometimes fatal encephalitis in a number of other species, including humans.[16]

Transmission follows the ingestion of soil or other material containing raccoon faeces contaminated with worm eggs. Young children are at particular risk.

As human cases are rare, or go undiagnosed, the true prevalence of the disease cannot be estimated, although it is a widespread parasite of raccoons across the USA and Canada. Children presenting with severe encephalitis should be screened for the parasite; however, once clinical symptoms are seen, severe damage or death usually follows.

Treatment with anthelmintics and steroids is usual, and would be decided on a case-by-case basis, although it may not improve clinical outcomes in established infection. Immediate treatment with anthelmintics is recommended in cases of probable infection.

Rat-bite fever (Haverhill fever, Soduku)

Rat bite fever may be caused by two different pathogens: *Streptobacillus moniliformis* or the spirochaete *Spirillium minus*. *S. moniliformis* is seen in North America, whereas *S. minus* is the pathogen responsible for the form seen in Africa and Asia (known as Soduku).

The pathogens are commonly found in the nasal passages of rats and other rodents such as gerbils. Transmission follows ingestion of infected material (specifically known as Haverhill fever when associated with milk or water contaminated with rat urine), handling, or being bitten or scratched by an infected rat, but clinical cases in humans are rare. The organism can also be carried by other animals such as cats, dogs, ferrets and weasels that have been in contact with infected rodents.[17]

After a pre-patent period of 2–10 days (4–28 in *S. minus*), a fever of abrupt onset occurs, associated with rash, joint and muscle pain, headache, diarrhoea and vomiting, often associated with peripheral rash. This can progress to systemic disease with septicaemia, arthritis, anaemia, hypoxia, endocarditis, and liver and kidney failure. If untreated death occurs in 7–10% of cases.[18]

S. minus may also cause an undulant fever, which may recur for months or years if untreated.

It affects children usually more acutely than adults, although there have been fatal adult cases in the USA and Canada, usually in people occupationally exposed to rodents.[19]

Intravenous penicillin is the treatment of choice, and macrolides such as erythromycin have been shown to be effective in penicillin-allergic patients. Tests to identify the causative agent may not be rapid enough to prevent mortality, so presumptive diagnosis and empirical treatment may be necessary in patients with a history of exposure to rodents.

Individuals who handle rodents routinely should adopt safe working practices, including wearing gloves, hand washing after contact, and avoiding accidental inhalation or ingestion of infected material. Wounds inflicted by rodents should be cleaned thoroughly and medical advice promptly sought.

Typhus fever

Cases of typhus fever caused by *Rickettsia prowazekii* have been seen in the USA related to exposure to flying squirrels (*Glaucomys* spp.) or their nests. Classically this is a disease associated with cold mountainous regions of Africa and South America, although historically it has also been seen in Europe, especially after World War II, when there were epidemics associated with increased populations of ectoparasites, especially the human louse (*Pediculus humanus*) in prison camps, or in areas where displaced people were crowded in unsanitary conditions.

Only a few clinical cases have been seen in the USA over the past decades, with approximately 40 being seen in the last quarter of the twentieth century in patients who had no extant human lice, or who could be confirmed as having been in contact with other people who had body lice. They had, however, all had contact with flying squirrels or their nests. It is possible that the infection was transferred by transient contact with squirrel lice or fleas. Infection could also follow contact with infected faeces.[20]

After a prodromal period of 10–15 days, symptoms appear including headache, acute fever, haematuria, joint pain and vomiting.

Treatment is with doxycycline and may have to be prolonged.

Zoonoses of deer

The following two diseases relate to deer. Lyme disease is endemic in certain areas in the UK and the USA. It poses a threat to people exposed to the causative spirochaete *Borrelia burgdorferi*. The second condition, tularaemia, has not been detected in the UK but it is endemic in the rest of western Europe, and the Pet Travel Scheme (PETS) passport regulations insist that animals licensed under the scheme should be treated for ectoparasites to prevent Lyme disease, as well as other tick- and flea-borne diseases.

Lyme disease
Tick-borne borreliosis

Lyme disease is caused by spirochaetes of various *Borrelia* spp. The disease is named after the town of Old Lyme, Connecticut, USA, where a cluster of juvenile arthritis cases in the 1970s were first linked to infection by *B. burgdorferi*. Studies of collected insects and literature surveys on both sides of the Atlantic have identified the organism and the disease was clinically described in the late nineteenth century. Lyme disease is notifiable under public health legislation in Scotland. In England and Wales it is reportable under RIDDOR (Reporting of Injuries, Diseases and Dangerous Occurrences Regulations) 1995 for 'work involving exposure to ticks'.[21]

Transmission

The infection is transmitted by the bite of an ixodes tick, mainly *Ixodes scapularis* or *I. dammini* in North America, which normally preys on deer. In the UK, *I. ricinus* has been identified as the main tick vector and infectious reservoir. Ticks of *Ixodes* spp. are much smaller than common dog or cattle ticks. In their larval and nymphal stages they are no bigger than a pinhead. Adult ticks are slightly larger. Other biting insects, such as mosquitoes and fleas, have also been implicated in transmission, but they are not believed to be an infectious reservoir. They are rather an incidental vector infected by feeding on an infected vertebrate.

Incidence

Reported incidents of Lyme disease have risen in England and Wales in recent years. This probably arises from better recognition of the disease and more thorough reporting. Incidence and prevalence are related to environmental factors. Certain weather conditions, such as drought or high rainfall, can kill the tick before maturation.[22]

During 2006, there were a total of 945 reported cases in the UK, with 768 serologically confirmed cases of Lyme disease in England and Wales and 177 confirmed cases in Scotland. Of the 768 cases in England and Wales, 677 had been acquired in the UK and 91 abroad. The annual figure has increased over the last decade, reflecting greater awareness of the disease, and also greater access by the public to areas where the disease is endemic, both domestically and overseas.

In England and Wales, surveillance by the Health Protection Agency (HPA) has demonstrated that approximately 70% of indigenously acquired infection occurred in the southern counties of England. The main affected areas are the New Forest, Salisbury Plain, Exmoor, the South Downs, parts of Wiltshire and Berkshire, and Thetford Forest. Other endemic areas include the Lake District, the North and West Yorkshire moors, and the Scottish Highlands and Islands.

The HPA has also identified that many of the cases reported in the UK have been acquired abroad, mainly in the USA, Russia, Scandinavia, France, Germany, and other European countries including Poland, the Czech Republic, Slovenia and Slovakia.

Life cycle

The life cycles of the tick and *Borrelia* spp. are closely linked. The female tick lays eggs during the spring of the first year, which hatch into larvae in early summer. The larvae then seek out rodents and birds as hosts. These hosts, being highly mobile, help disseminate the tick over a wider geographical area. The larvae continue to feed over the summer and become dormant

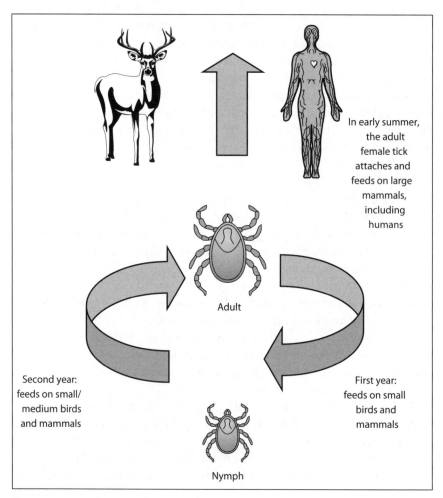

In early summer, the adult female tick attaches and feeds on large mammals, including humans

Adult

Second year: feeds on small/ medium birds and mammals

First year: feeds on small birds and mammals

Nymph

Figure 8.1 Lyme disease: transmission cycle.

in the autumn. The following spring the larvae moult into nymphs which attach themselves to small rodents and other small mammals; in the USA the white-footed mouse plays a significant role as both an interim host for the tick and a reservoir for the disease.[23] In the autumn of the second year they moult again into adults. At this time ticks will attach to a large mammalian host, feeding persistently and mating. The female will then drop off and lay her eggs, starting the cycle again (Figure 8.1).

Borrelia spp. are present in all stages of the tick, acquiring the infection from infected rodents when feeding commences. As the larvae are the most voracious and aggressive of feeders, these actively spread the organism. This correlates with the incidence of infection. Most tick bites that lead to clinical manifestations occur in the period May to July when the larvae and nymphal stages are actively biting. Deer are the preferred host; humans, cats and dogs are incidental hosts, as are cattle and horses. Dogs suffer badly from the arthritic form of the disease.

Disease in humans

In humans, as with other spirochaetal diseases, the course of the disease is undulant, with acute and chronic phases interspersed with long asymptomatic periods. After the initial manifestation there can be a latent period of up to 4 years before further clinical signs are seen.[24]

Initial infection follows a tick bite; it is now believed that the tick must stay attached for a period for transmission to occur. This period can be less than 16 hours: 24–72 hours is believed to give optimal transmission. A localised skin reaction appeared in 60% of English cases. This occurs at the bite site, usually about 9 days after infection due to spirochaetal invasion. This is called *erythema migrans* and it presents as an expanding reddened area. It usually has reinforced borders and can be solid or annular. It may be warm to touch but is rarely itchy or painful.

Later some patients will have flu-like symptoms with fever, malaise and headache. A transient lymphadenopathy may be seen, as may organ involvement with transient hepatitis. Eye problems, including conjunctivitis or optic nerve damage, have been reported.[25] A widespread *erythema migrans* with multiple lesions can occur, often together with other more serious symptoms of neurological damage, cardiac involvement or arthritis. A condition called acrodermatitis chronica atrophicans (ACA) is occasionally seen. This is a serious condition, passing from an initial inflammatory stage to atrophy and pigmentation disturbances of the skin on extensor surfaces of the limbs. Accompanying symptoms include pain, itching and paraesthesia.

Neurological complications may manifest at any time: the incidence in patients aged under 14 years of neurological symptoms is higher than in other age groups. Symptoms range from meningitis, cranial nerve damage and facial palsy to peripheral neuropathies. Subarachnoid haemorrhage and seizures have also been reported. A chronic form of the disease with memory loss, loss of motor skills and dementia is reported, although the linkage to *Borrelia* infection is currently unproven.[25]

Up to 10% of infected individuals in the USA present with associated cardiac problems. These include atrioventricular block, heart failure and myocarditis that resolves on treatment with antimicrobials.

In the USA it is estimated that 14% of sufferers develop arthritis, and in some cases seen in the UK this has been the first symptom resulting in clinical diagnosis. The first symptoms may appear 3–6 weeks after first infection, usually with a single joint involvement, commonly the knee. The jaw, ankles, shoulders, elbows and wrists are also common sites.[26]

The variation in symptoms seen between the USA and the UK seems to be related to a difference in the genus species of the pathogen. In the USA *B. burgdorferi* predominates, whereas in Europe *B. afzelii* and *B. garinii* are more common. Different clinical manifestations are species related, with *B. afzelii* being associated with dermatological symptoms and *B. garinii* with neurological disorders.

Diagnosis

Diagnosis is not easy, because not all patients present with *erythema migrans*, or can remember being bitten by a tick – often the tick will be concealed within clothing when attached and may disengage before detection. Laboratory tests have been notoriously unreliable, due to its genetic ability to vary its outer surface proteins, thus altering its immunological signature. This leads to false-negative test results for enzyme-linked immunosorbent assay (ELISA), polymerase chain reaction (PCR) tests or western blot testing. The Centers for Disease Control and Prevention in the USA (CDC) recommends enzyme immunoassay (EIA) or immunofluorescent assay (IFA) as more accurate.[27]

Treatment

Treatment consists solely of antibiotic therapy. Patients with severe multisystemic involvement, especially where neurological symptoms are present, can be treated with intravenous cephalosporins. Tetracyclines, especially doxycycline, and penicillins, particularly amoxicillin, demonstrate efficacy against most *Borrelia* infections. β-lactams are relatively inefficient and should be used only when other agents are not suitable.[23]

The *British National Formulary* (BNF) recommends that Lyme disease should generally be treated by those experienced in its management. Doxycycline is the antibacterial of choice for early Lyme disease. Amoxicillin (unlicensed indication), cefuroxime axetil and azithromycin (unlicensed indication) are alternatives if doxycycline is contraindicated. Intravenous administration of cefotaxime, ceftriaxone or benzylpenicillin is recommended for Lyme disease associated with moderate-to-severe cardiac or neurological abnormalities, late Lyme disease and Lyme arthritis. The duration of treatment is generally 2–4 weeks; Lyme arthritis requires longer treatment with oral antibacterial drugs.

Prevention

Prevention strategies can be divided into environmental and personal. Many prevention regimens aim to break the ability of the organism to maintain a rodent reservoir, and prevent tick attachment to large mammals or humans. Controlling undergrowth around footpaths, and inspecting and treating livestock for ticks, can reduce the tick population. Controlling access of rodents to commercially farmed deer can reduce infection risks both for animals and for associated human workers.

Personal protection, especially for individuals employed in forestry or other business in endemic areas, consists of wearing long trousers and boots, with the trousers tucked into the socks. Lighter-coloured clothing allows ticks to be spotted before they can establish a potentially infective bite. Prompt removal of any ticks is also important, and examination of the groin, armpits and scalp is particularly important. Outdoor enthusiasts should take similar precautions, especially if camping in areas where ticks are known to be endemic.[28]

Vaccination

Although a vaccine for the prevention of Lyme disease in humans has been developed, it has not been adopted because it is not considered to be cost-effective except for those individuals who live in areas where Lyme disease is endemic and who are frequently exposed to ticks. The associated risks of possible adverse reactions also mitigate against its use, except in exceptional cases where significant benefit can be demonstrated.[29]

Tularaemia
Francis' disease, deer-fly fever, rabbit fever, O'Hara disease

Tularaemia is caused by *Francisella tularensis*, a small Gram-negative coccobacillus. An intracellular pathogen, it can also survive in the environment for extended periods. It has now been found to be able to parasitise life forms as lowly as amoebae and other protozoans. The organism is named after Sir Edward Francis who initially isolated and studied the causative organism at Tulare in California, USA. It occurs in a number of subspecies. *Francisella tularensis* subspecies *tularensis* (type A) also occurs in two distinct subpopulations – A I and A II – with the two subpopulations' distribution being geographically different and linked to the presence of specific vectors and animal hosts (such as different populations of rabbits).

The A I population is mostly seen in central USA and the A II in the western USA.[30]

F. tularensis subsp. *holoarctica* (type C) is distributed across most of the northern hemisphere, with another subspecies, *mediasiatica*, being seen in central Asia and the former Soviet Union; it appears to have less affinity for humans and more for aquatic mammals.

The final subspecies is much rarer and is designated subsp. *novicidia*; so far only a single case has been identified in Australia, outside its normal range of the northern USA.

Francisella spp. appear to produce an endotoxin similar to those produced by other Gram-negative enteric bacilli. An additional twist to the organism is that *F. tularensis* has also been suggested as a possible agent for biological terrorism or warfare. There is some evidence that Israel and Russia have attempted to develop resistant strains for use as weapons.

The organism can also survive in water and penetrate intact skin. As the estimate of inoculum necessary to initiate disease in humans has been set at only 10 organisms, the disease is classified as highly infective. Although not reported in the UK, with the increasing popularity of adventure holidays where trekking or living in wilderness areas forms part of the itinerary, there is a risk of exposure and disease for tourists who might then return home before clinical signs are seen.

There was a recent outbreak in Turkey in 2008, following on from previous ones in the country in 2004 and 2005.[31] A serious outbreak occurred in Kosovo from November 2001 to February 2002, with 715 reported cases. Of those, 170 cases were confirmed as type B tularaemia, and were linked to rodents. Spread to humans was linked to rat-associated ticks, fleas or lice as vectors. There were no cases in peace-keeping or aid workers and no fatalities, as all cases resolved on treatment. An outbreak of long duration occurred in Bulgaria between 1997 and 2005 and affected 285 people.

In the former Soviet Union routine vaccination is carried out, because the disease is considered to be endemic. The disease occurs in sporadic outbreaks across a wide geographical range in western Europe from Scandinavia to Spain. In many of these outbreaks a small and increasing number of cases is seen over a period of time, reaching a peak in incidence and then declining. The same pattern has been seen in the USA where the disease was very prevalent in the 1950s, but has decreased markedly over time, although sporadic outbreaks still occur.

It is not known why the incidence has declined but the use of insecticides, changes in agricultural practice and habitat destruction have all been suggested as factors. Outbreaks such as the Kosovan incident may be associated with boom years for the population of vermin hosts such as rabbits or rats, and thus the blood-sucking parasite population.

The prevalence of the disease shows a marked seasonal bias related, as with Lyme disease, to the life cycle of the ticks that can be the main vector for its spread in certain areas. Most cases reported between May and October are associated with parasite bites. Another peak is seen in the winter relating to hunting, where there is no vector spread but there is direct contact between humans and animals during the skinning and preparation of prey animals. This may explain why most cases are seen in adult males – over 75% of American cases are seen in male hunters.

The reservoir for the disease consists of both wild and domestic animals. It has been found in rabbits, hares, squirrels, deer, snakes, rodents, cats, dogs, cattle, pigs, sheep and goats.[32] The organism has also been isolated from all the life stages of various ticks, and *Dermacentor reticulatus* (dog tick) and *Ixodes ricinus* (castor oil bean tick) are the major European species involved. The organism can persist for many months or years in the tissues of the tick and is carried through moults and can be transferred from mother to offspring. The organism has been isolated from tick saliva and faecal matter, so inoculation of a wound with either substance can provide sufficient inoculum to produce clinical disease. Luckily, not all ticks within a population are infected. Mosquitoes, deer- and horseflies, and fleas have also been found to carry the organism. Whether they are competent vectors of transfer is not proven in all species, although in the USA deer flies are known to be a major vector. It has also been demonstrated that cats are able to transmit the bacterium on their claws, after catching infected prey.[33]

Disease in animals

In animals, the main clinical manifestation of the disease is septicaemia, with high fever, stiffness and loss of appetite. Respiratory involvement may also manifest with symptoms similar to pleurisy. Death follows frequently and rapidly. On postmortem examination, necrotic lesions may be found in the main organs.

Transmission

Humans are susceptible to infection with the organism and it can affect any age or social group.

Infection in humans follows a vector bite, physical contact with an infected animal or an ingested inoculum from water or meat. Human-to-human spread does not occur. As has been previously stated, the organism can also penetrate intact skin and be spread by the inhalation of infected aerosols.

Case history

In February 2004, a 3-year-old boy in Colorado, USA contracted the disease after being bitten by a pet hamster. The boy originally had six hamsters, but they all died shortly after being purchased from a Denver pet store; one of them bit the boy, causing him to become infected. There have been previous cases recorded among hamster hunters in Russia.

Disease in humans

Following infection there is a pre-patent period of 2–10 days before clinical signs are seen. An ulcer appears at the inoculation site and local lymph gland swelling is seen in the lymph nodes nearest to the ulcer as the organism multiplies and proliferates. Initially there may be a high fever, which then subsides and recurs in a cyclical manner. Chills, headache, malaise, anorexia and fatigue are quite common.

Antibody production begins during the second or third week of infection but is usually insufficient to protect against infection.

The disease presents in a variety of forms depending on the route of infection. The CDC classification in the USA recognises six main forms: glandular, ulceroglandular, oculoglandular, oropharyngeal, pneumonic and typhoidal. The classification is useful; however, the clinical symptoms associated with various forms of the disease often present at the same time in the same patient, leading to confusion. The mortality rate for untreated tularaemia is about 8%; early diagnosis and treatment can reduce that rate to below 1%.

The most common type, seen in over 75% of cases, is classified as ulceroglandular following cutaneous inoculation. When the initial ulcers are seen, their location may help to identify the mode of transmission. Ulcers on the upper limbs usually result from exposure to infected animals, whereas ulcers on the lower limbs, back or abdomen usually result from parasitic bites. Glandular swelling follows the appearance of the ulcer, with primary sites again related to mode of transmission. Untreated ulcers can take a long time to heal, with associated persistent lymph node swellings. Most cases will take 3–5 weeks to resolve without treatment; however, symptoms can persist for up to 3 years after the appearance of the disease. Many cases will need a lengthy period of convalescence.[30]

The glandular form presents in a similar manner to the ulceroglandular disease but without skin ulceration, and is responsible for 15–20% of the cases in the USA. Glandular involvement can be acute and severe.

Fortunately, the oculoglandular type of infection is rare. It occurs in no more than 4% of cases in most outbreaks, and less than 1% over a series of outbreaks, although it may appear in single case occurrences where there is only one individual infected. Infected material, e.g. blood, meat, dust or bodily fluids, is splashed into the eye. Following infection the eyelids swell and there is ulceration in the conjunctiva and surface of the eyeball. Localised glandular swelling in the neck may also be present.

Ingestion of contaminated meat or water can lead to the oropharyngeal form. In recent outbreaks, 4–18% of cases have presented with sore throat and pharyngitis. In some individuals, the throat does not appear to be infected on examination. Others show severe inflammation with involvement of the tonsils and swelling to almost total closure. Swelling is seen in the glands of the jaw, throat and neck.

The pneumonic form follows inhalation of infected aerosols; the symptoms and findings in this form vary. As in the other forms, fever and glandular swellings are usually present. Lung involvement may mimic a chest infection or pleurisy.

The last in the list of forms is the typhoidal type. Onset is usually abrupt and follows ingestion of infected material. High fever is seen, with aching joints and muscles, vomiting and diarrhoea. Liver and splenic enlargement is sometimes seen, and usually develops gradually after the acute phase. Skin rashes may also be present.

In all types of infection, some of which will fall into one or more categories, long-term immunity will usually follow infection.

Diagnosis

Confirming a diagnosis is made using clinical samples. The organism is difficult to culture in a laboratory, and also poses a risk to laboratory personnel. Immunofluorescence or PCR methods and serological testing are preferable, and recent advances have been made in producing rapid reliable test methods.

Treatment

The treatment of tularaemia depends on rapid diagnosis and the commencement of antibiotic therapy as soon as possible after clinical signs are seen. Antibiotic use is the only therapy, using single or combination therapy.

Streptomycin with or without the addition of a tetracycline has historically been the mainstay of treatment. Streptomycin is usually given intramuscularly in two divided doses for a duration of 7–14 days. An alternative regimen is 15 mg/kg per day in two divided doses for 3 days followed by a period of 4 or more days at half the previous dose twice daily. Gentamicin has been substituted for streptomycin in a dosage of 3–5 mg/kg per day by intravenous infusion in divided doses for 7–14 days, with the length of the course being linked to patient response. Clinical monitoring of blood chemistry is essential with the use of these aminoglycosides. Chloramphenicol has also been used in the past, but the serious associated side effects have to be weighed against clinical need.[34]

Tetracyclines are effective, but, as they are bacteriostatic rather than bactericidal, the duration of therapy needs to be longer. Doxycycline is given by mouth at a dosage of 100 mg every 12 hours for 10–14 days. Some studies have shown that high-dose erythromycin is suitable for type A infections; however, both type A and B serotypes have demonstrated resistance. Ciprofloxacin has become the treatment of choice in some countries. In an outbreak in Sweden, ciprofloxacin was given by mouth for 10–14 days at a dosage of 15–20 mg/kg daily in two divided doses in children under 10, and at a dosage of 1000–1500 mg daily in two divided doses to adults and children over 10. Norfloxacin 400 mg/day in divided doses for 12 days was used in a single patient in the same outbreak and proved effective. Both ciprofloxacin and doxycycline have the advantage of allowing community treatment because they can be effectively given by mouth, rather than requiring an injection programme, and the use of secondary healthcare resources.[34]

Prevention

A vaccine is available for people considered to be at high risk or where the disease is seen as a public health issue, such as in the former Soviet Union. Vaccination has also been used where the disease is a possible health and safety hazard of employment, e.g. in park rangers and field naturalists in endemic areas. The main human groups at risk of occupational exposure are farmers, shepherds, hunters, veterinary surgeons, meat handlers, cooks and the partners of hunters.

Prevention is the best policy. Avoiding insect bites and implementing hygiene procedures when living or travelling in areas where there is a high prevalence of the disease are essential measures. Use of insecticides and wearing suitable clothing in forested areas – trousers rather than shorts – will prevent many tick bites. Any ticks that succeed in attaching should be removed carefully without crushing them, and whenever possible not with bare hands. Domestic animals suffering from the disease should be treated or culled to prevent spread.

As with leptospirosis, drinking, washing or swimming either by choice or accidentally in infected water should be avoided wherever possible. Hunters and others who handle or butcher wild animals should be advised to wear suitable protective clothing. Wild game should be thoroughly cooked and, as the organism can survive prolonged freezing, suitable precautions should be taken when handling any raw game meat. Antibiotic prophylaxis is not recommended in any risk group.

Viruses associated with primates

The following diseases are included because they pose a risk to humans exposed to them, especially in areas where humans regularly interact with primates, including activities such as hunting, butchering and eating apes.

They also pose a risk for laboratory workers and people who keep this class of animals as pets.

Herpes B virus

Herpes B virus (*Cercopithecine herpesvirus 1*) is found in Asian macaques and other primates, which can be asymptomatic carriers of the pathogen. If transmitted to humans it can cause a fatal encephalitis or severe neurological damage. Cases have occurred in laboratory settings after exposure to infected faeces. In one case death followed infection by material being splashed into the eye of the victim, though the more frequent cause of infection is by inoculation through bites or scratches.[35]

In a survey carried out on free-roaming macaques and workers at a Balinese temple, over 80% of the macaques had antibodies to the virus, and contact between the macaques and workers or tourists was likely to allow transmission to occur (i.e. bites, scratches).[36]

The pre-patent period can be as short as a few days, although it is more normally 2–5 weeks. Neurological symptoms are seen which can progress through paralysis to respiratory collapse and coma. Treatment has to be aggressive using either aciclovir or ganciclovir.[37]

Primate handlers should use eye protection and other protective equipment such as gloves, especially when working with wild-caught primates, and tourists should be encouraged not to come into close contact with monkeys whenever possible.

Monkeypox

First identified in 1958, monkeypox is caused by an *Orthopoxvirus* (designated monkeypox virus [MXPV]), closely related to smallpox and cowpox. It is capable of infecting a range of animals in addition to its normal host of apes and monkeys, especially rodents including squirrels, rats, mice and rabbits. The first confirmed zoonotic case in humans was documented in the 1970s, although it is believed that the virus had previously infected humans, but that the infection was probably mistaken for smallpox.

Most cases are seen in Africa, with The Democratic Republic of Congo and Sudan reporting outbreaks, although the disease probably occurs elsewhere.[38,39] In June 2003, the first and only outbreak so far in the USA began. The primary source of the outbreak was a Texan animal importer, who had purchased from Ghana a mixed group of approximately 800 small mammals in April 2003, composed of a number of species including squirrels, mice, rats, dormice and porcupines; some of these were later identified as being infected with or carrying monkeypox. These animals came into contact with approximately 200 prairie dogs, which were passing through the same facility at the same time. Of the prairie dogs approximately 100 became infected.[40]

The prairie dogs were sold on to an Illinois-based animal distributor, and were subsequently traded on. Following contact with the infected prairie dogs, a number of people who handled or were in contact with these animals became infected with monkeypox. By the time the outbreak was declared over by the CDC in July 2003, 72 cases of suspected monkeypox had been reported with 37 being laboratory-confirmed across 6 states (Illinois, Indiana, Kansas, Missouri, Ohio and Wisconsin). The rapid spread of the disease over a wide geographical area was due to the nature of the animal trade and the holding and distribution mechanisms associated with it.

Prevention of further spread and control of the outbreak was gained by forbidding interstate animal shipments and trade, quarantining premises where infected animals had been found, culling infected or potentially infected animals, and pre- and post-exposure vaccination of at-risk people using smallpox vaccine derived from cowpox (vaccinia).

The main aim was to prevent the establishment of an indigenous focus of infection in wild or captive animals, to prevent a reoccurrence, and this appears to have been successful.

In June 2003, when the outbreak was first recognised, the CDC, on behalf of the Department for Health and Human Services (DHHS) and the Food and Drug Administration (FDA), issued a joint order prohibiting the import of African rodents into the USA.

In November 2003, the joint order became an interim final rule that bans the importation of African rodents and their sale, distribution, transport and release. In addition, the ban applies to rodents with a native habitat in Africa, even if those rodents were captive bred or born outside Africa. Exemption may only be obtained by gaining a permit from the CDC where animals need to be imported for scientific or educational purposes.[41]

The symptoms of monkeypox seen in infected animals vary because some may be asymptomatic, although normally there is conjunctivitis, lymphadenopathy and skin lesions, occasionally followed by splenic and hepatic enlargement, sepsis and respiratory complications, including pneumonia and death.

Transmission to humans follows handling an infected animal, bites or scratches from an infected animal, contact with infected blood or body fluids, handling or eating infected meat or tissues, and fomite spread. Once infected, human-to-human spread can occur by droplet inhalation or contact with infected body fluids or fomites.[42]

In Africa a death rate of 1–10% of clinically infected patients has been seen, although this is reduced by good nutritional status and supportive healthcare. Coinfection with HIV/AIDS may also play a role in mortality levels. In the US outbreak there were no fatalities, although two children required intensive care and one patient had to have a corneal transplantation.

Symptoms in humans are variable; although they normally mimic smallpox, the symptoms are normally milder. After a pre-patent period of approximately 12 days (although this can range from 1 day to 31 days), a high fever of rapid onset occurs with associated myalgia and headache, lymph node swelling and lethargy. Within 1–3 days a vesicular rash occurs, starting normally on the face and spreading, although it may occur on other parts of the body initially. The vesicles burst, turn crusty, scab and then heal normally within 2–4 weeks. In some cases, especially in children, an encephalitis may follow, as may organ failure and death.[43,44]

Treatment is usually non-specific and symptomatic, although vaccination with smallpox vaccine (cowpox derived), or cidofovir, was used to some effect in the US outbreak.[45]

Simian foamy virus

Simian foamy viruses (SFVs) are retroviruses found in primates that are capable of infecting humans.[46] In central Africa and Indonesia, the virus has been found in some humans, especially in hunters, usually after exposure to primates, particularly after bites or scratches inflicted by an infected ape.[47,48] Infection has also been recorded in zoo keepers, laboratory technicians and animal handlers who have been occupationally exposed to primates.[49,50] The virus has been isolated from local people and tourists who have had exposure to monkeys at temples in Bali.[48]

In some areas most apes are infected; however, although the viruses are persistent, they show little or no pathogenicity in the primates, with the animals remaining asymptomatic. The viruses are shed in the saliva, and are also blood and meat borne.

No spread of the virus between humans by sexual contact or other means has been demonstrated, although the virus has been detected in donated blood, and it is likely that transfusion of infected blood could lead to infection.[51]

Although no pathogenicity has been seen in infected humans, in vitro the virus will lyse both human and monkey cells.

Simian immunodeficiency viruses

Human immunodeficiency virus type 1 (HIV-1) and type 2 (HIV-2), which cause acquired immune deficiency syndrome (AIDS) after a prolonged period in humans, were originally zoonotic lentiviruses.[52] Since their initial transfer into humans, they have become capable of relatively easy human-to-human transmission, and have therefore ceased to be considered zoonoses. (HIV infection is not therefore covered further in this volume.)

Apes, monkeys and other primates found across sub-Saharan Africa carry a variety of simian immunodeficiency viruses (SIVs) closely related to extant types of HIV. They are genetically divergent and 'chatter', i.e. produce genetic variations rapidly by swapping or altering their genetic code, so producing diverse pathogenicity and infectivity.

It is possible that new varieties of virus capable of zoonotic transfer to humans and with potential pathogenicity will be transferred from primates to humans in Africa, probably during hunting for, butchery of, or consumption of, bushmeat derived from primates, especially sooty mangabeys or chimpanzees.[53]

A similar situation is observed with lymphotrophic viruses. Human T lymphotrophic virus (HTLV) types 1 and 2 are now widely distributed worldwide and were initially zoonotic.[54] Two new HTLV-designated types 3 and 4 have recently been isolated from humans exposed to monkeys or apes in southern Cameroon.[55] These have probably arisen and crossed the species barrier in a similar manner to the immunodeficiency viruses.

Prevention of spread of wildlife diseases

In agriculture, as a matter of good husbandry practice, feral and wild animal contact should be kept to a minimum wherever possible to reduce disease spread. Good agricultural practice includes reducing mammalian pest species. This has become less routine due to the costs involved and the concerns of the environmental lobby. Control of pests on and around farms is vitally important in the prevention and control of spread of certain zoonoses. It becomes even more significant when the pest and the domesticated species are very closely related; sparrows in a chicken run, or in the feed mill associated with such a unit, would pose a significant risk for avian disease transfer.[56]

Members of the public should be encouraged to be circumspect in their handling of injured wild animals, and children should be educated not to touch corpses of birds or mammals. Normal hygiene routines should be observed, with the use of protective clothing and general hygiene measures. In the event of any injury caused by a wild animal, medical attention should be sought as soon as reasonably practicable. Direct zoonotic transmission is also possible at specialist sanctuaries or rescue units (see Rabies in Chapter 6). Most of these units have standing procedures under which all animals are treated as suspect and as possible biohazards, thus preventing untoward incidents of injury or infective transfer.[57]

Tackling these problems requires a consensus, with healthcare workers, vets and government agencies, at both legislational and practical levels, working in cooperation.[58]

In the USA, an initiative by the American Veterinary Medical Association (AVMA) has led to the establishment of a 'One Medicine Initiative' bringing wildlife, environmental, human and domestic animal health issues together. Supported across professional organisations and government agencies, this coordinated approach aims to prevent and pre-empt disease outbreaks rather than being solely reactive.[59]

Surveillance

In the UK, the VLA has provided surveillance of wildlife diseases since 1998 under the Diseases of Wildlife Scheme (soon to be renamed the Wildlife Health Strategy to be incorporated into the Veterinary Surveillance Strategy, which forms part of the overarching Animal Health and Welfare Strategy launched in 2004). The scheme is government funded and mirrors a scheme run in Scotland and Northern Ireland, with a shared diagnostic database.

The scheme has 16 regional laboratories and investigates and monitors zoonoses, emerging and exotic diseases (such as West Nile virus) and mass mortalities ('die-offs') of birds and animals. It provides DEFRA and other UK government agencies with information and statistics on wildlife diseases.[60]

In Europe, the Office International des Epizooties (OIE) has undertaken surveillance of animal diseases including zoonoses since 1993. The OIE have developed lists of reportable diseases including wildlife diseases, some of which are zoonoses.[61] In general the list contains any disease found in the wild considered to be of an infectious nature that can infect mammals, birds, reptiles or amphibians.

In the USA there are a number of government departments that are involved with the surveillance and response to wildlife diseases. The Wildlife Services unit of the US Department of Agriculture (USDA) Animal and Plant Health Inspection Service (APHIS) aims to support federal and state agencies when a threat to animal or human health is identified that stems from wildlife disease. It has strategic partnerships with many other government departments (such as the Department of Health, CDC, etc.) and also extra-territorial partnerships with geographical neighbours (Canada and Mexico).[62]

Of particular interest is the Wildlife Center of Virginia, and its participation in Project Tripwire. The Wildlife Center of Virginia, a wildlife care centre, had monitored and studied wildlife diseases for some years, and had demonstrated the significance of these conditions for human and domesticated animal health. Project Tripwire began as a cooperative effort to exchange data between wildlife care services to enhance analysis of illness in animals, allowing rapid identification of outbreaks so that appropriate measures can be put in place rapidly. After 11 September 2001, there were concerns over the use of biological weapons, many of which are pathogens that could be carried or infect wildlife. As part of a project to reduce response time to biological incidents a system of epidemic outbreak surveillance (EOS) was developed by the US Air Force Research Laboratory; this was further developed by the Institute of Homeland Security (IHS) which has evaluated and developed Project Tripwire together with the Wildlife Center to produce a system that could monitor patients, diseases and outbreaks.[63]

In Canada, Environment Canada has developed a strategy for wildlife disease. This brings together multiple government and private partners across many disciplines, to produce a coordinated response to the threat of wildlife disease.

Elsewhere in the world there are a variety of schemes that aim to prevent the spread of diseases from wildlife. All these initiatives have one thing in common: they aim to highlight and address the important issues surrounding wildlife as a reservoir of potential pathogens for both humans and domesticated animals, and to prevent or control outbreaks.

References

1. Kruse H, Kirkemo A-M, Handeland K. Wildlife as source of zoonotic infections. *Emerg Infect Dis* 2004; **10**: 2067–72.
2. Chomel BB, Belotto A, Meslin F-X. Wildlife, exotic pets, and emerging zoonoses. *Emerg Infect Dis* 2007; **13**: 6–11.
3. Smith GC, Gangadharan B, Taylor Z *et al*. Prevalence of zoonotic parasites in the red fox (*Vulpes vulpes*) in Great Britain. *Vet Parasitol* 2003; **118**: 133–42.
4. Letková V, Lazar P, Čurlík J *et al*. The red fox (*Vulpes vulpes* L.) as a source of zoonoses. *Veterinarski Arhiv* 2006; **7** (suppl): S73–81,
5. DEFRA and OIE. *Wildlife Diseases in the UK – 2007 Report*. Penrith, UK: VLA, 2008.
6. Fa JE, Peres CA, Meeuwig J. Bushmeat exploitation in tropical forests: an intercontinental comparison. *Conserv Biol* 2002; **16**: 232–7.
7. Wolfe ND, Daszak P, Kilpatrick AM, Burke DS. Bushmeat hunting, deforestation, and prediction of zoonoses emergence. *Emerg Infect Dis* 2005; **11**: 1822–7.
8. Karesh WB, Cook RA, Bennett EL, Newcomb J. Wildlife trade and global disease emergence. *Emerg Infect Dis* 2005; **11**: 1000–2.
9. De Schrijver K. A psittacosis outbreak in customs officers in Antwerp (Belgium). *Bull Inst Marit Trop Med Gdynia* 1998; **49**: 97–9.
10. Van Borm S, Thomas I, Hanquet G *et al*. Highly pathogenic H5N1 influenza virus in smuggled Thai eagles, Belgium. *Emerg Infect Dis* 2005; **11**: 702–5.
11. Bender JB, Shulman SA. Reports of zoonotic disease outbreaks associated with animal exhibits and availability of recommendations for preventing zoonotic disease transmission from animals to people in such settings. *JAVMA* 2004; **224**: 1105–9.
12. Heuvelink E, Van Heerwaarden V, Zwartkruis-Nahuis JTM *et al*. *Escherichia coli* O157 infection associated with a petting zoo. *Epidemiol Infect* 2002; **129**: 295–302.
13. Health and Safety Executive. *Avoiding Ill Health at Open Farms – Advice to farmers* (with teachers' supplement). HSE information sheet. Agriculture Information Sheet (AIS) No. 23 (revised). London: HSE.
14. Riley PY, Chomel BB. Hedgehog zoonoses. *Emerg Infect Dis* 2005; **11**: 1–5.
15. Avashia SB, Petersen JM, Lindley CM *et al*. First reported prairie dog-to-human tularemia transmission, Texas, 2002. *Emerg Infect Dis* 2004; **10**: 483–6.
16. CDC. Raccoon roundworm encephalitis – Chicago, Illinois, and Los Angeles, California, 2000. *MMWR* 2002; **50**: 1153–5

17. Shvartsblat SS, Kochie M, Harber P, Howard J. Fatal rat-bite fever in a pet shop employee. *Am J Ind Med* 2004; **45**: 357–60.
18. Graves MH, Janda MJ. Rat-bite fever (*Streptobacillus moniliformis*): a potential emerging disease. *Int J Infect Dis* 2001; **5**: 151–4.
19. CDC. Fatal rat bite fever – Florida and Washington, 2003. *MMWR* 2005; **53**: 1198–202
20. Reynolds MG, Krebs JW, Comer JA, *et al*. Flying squirrel-associated typhus, United States. *Emerg Infect Dis* 2003; **9**: 1341–3.
21. Stanek G, Strle F. Lyme borreliosis. *Lancet* 2003; **362**: 1639.
22. Smith R, O'Connell S, Palmer S. Lyme disease surveillance in England and Wales 1986–1998. *Emerg Infect Dis* 2000; **6**: 4.
23. CDC. Lyme disease – United States, 2003–2005. *MMWR* 2007; **56**: 573–6.
24. Wormser GP, Dattwyler RJ, Shapiro ED *et al*. The clinical assessment, treatment, and prevention of Lyme disease, human granulocytic anaplasmosis, and babesiosis: clinical practice guidelines by the Infectious Diseases Society of America. *Clin Infect Dis* 2006; **43**: 1089–134.
25. Halperin JJ. Central nervous system Lyme disease. *Curr Infect Dis Rep* 2004; **6**: 298.
26. Steere AC, Sikand VK. The presenting manifestations of Lyme disease and the outcomes of treatment. *N Engl J Med* 2003; **348**: 2472.
27. CDC. Notice to Readers: Caution regarding testing for Lyme disease. *MMWR* 2005; **54**: 125.
28. Hayes EB, Piesman J. How can we prevent Lyme disease? *N Engl J Med* 2003; **348**: 2424–30.
29. Hsia EC, Chung JB, Sanford Schwartz J, Albert DA. Cost-effectiveness analysis of the Lyme disease vaccine. *Arthr Rheum* 2002; **46**: 1651–60.
30. Farlow J, Wagner DM, Dukerich M *et al*. *Francisella tularensis* in the United States. *Emerg Infect Dis* 2005; **11**: 1835–41.
31. Leblebicioglu H, Esen S, Turan D *et al*. Outbreak of tularemia: a case–control study and environmental investigation in Turkey. *Int J Infect Dis* 2008; **12**: 265–9.
32. Meinkoth KR, Morton RJ, Meinkoth JH. Naturally occurring tularemia in a dog. *JAVMA* 2004; **225**: 545–7, 538.
33. Magnarelli L, Levy S, Koski R. Detection of antibodies to *Francisella tularensis* in cats. *Res Vet Sci* 2007; **82**: 22–6.
34. Tärnvik A, Chu MC. New approaches to diagnosis and therapy of tularemia. *Ann N Y Acad Sci* 2007; **1105**: 378–404.
35. Huff JL, Barry PA. B-virus (*Cercopithecine herpesvirus* 1) infection in humans and macaques: potential for zoonotic disease. *Emerg Infect Dis* 2003; **9**: 246–50.
36. Engel GA, Jones-Engel L, Schillaci MA *et al*. Human exposure to herpesvirus B-seropositive macaques, Bali, Indonesia. *Emerg Infect Dis* 2002; **8**: 789–95.
37. Cohen JI, Davenport DS, Stewart JA *et al*. Recommendations for prevention of and therapy for exposure to B virus (*Cercopithecine herpesvirus* 1). *Clin Infect Dis* 2002; **35**: 1191–203.
38. Hutin YJ, Williams RJ, Malfait P *et al*. Outbreak of human monkeypox, Democratic Republic of Congo, 1996 to 1997. *Emerg Infect Dis* 2001; **7**: 434–8.
39. Damon IK, Roth CE, Chowdhary V. Discovery of monkeypox in Sudan. *N Engl J Med* 2006; **355**: 962–3.
40. CDC. Update: multistate outbreak of monkeypox – Illinois, Indiana, Kansas, Missouri, Ohio, and Wisconsin, 2003. *MMWR* 2003; **52**: 642–6.
41. CDC. Control of communicable diseases; restrictions on African rodents, prairie dogs, and certain other animals. Interim final rule. *Fed Regist* 2003; **68**: 62353–69.
42. Fleischauer AT, Kile JC, Davidson M *et al*. Evaluation of human-to-human transmission of monkeypox from infected patients to health care workers. *Clin Infect Dis* 2005; **40**: 689–94.
43. Reynolds MG, Yorita KL, Kuehnert MJ *et al*. Clinical manifestations of human monkeypox influenced by route of infection. *J Infect Dis* 2006; **194**: 773–80.

44. Huhn GD, Bauer AM, Yorita K *et al*. Clinical characteristics of human monkeypox, and risk factors for severe disease. *Clin Infect Dis* 2005; **41**: 1742–51.

45. CDC. Updated interim guidance for use of smallpox vaccine, cidofovir, and vaccinia immunoglobulin (VIG) for prevention and treatment in the setting of an outbreak of monkeypox infections, 2003. Available at www.cdc.gov/ncidod/monkeypox/ treatment guidelines.htm (cited 22 August 2008).

46. Brooks JI, Rud EW, Pilon RG, Smith JM, Switzer WM, Sandstrom PA. Cross-species retroviral transmission from macaques to human beings. *Lancet* 2002; **360**: 387–8.

47. Wolfe ND, Switzer WM, Carr JK *et al*. Naturally acquired simian retrovirus infections in central African hunters. *Lancet* 2004; **363**: 932–7.

48. Engel G, Hungerford LL, Jones-Engel L *et al*. Risk assessment: a model for predicting cross-species transmission of simian foamy virus from macaques (*M. fascicularis*) to humans at a monkey temple in Bali, Indonesia. *Am J Primatol* 2006; **68**: 934–48.

49. Sandstrom PA, Phan KO, Switzer WM *et al*. Simian foamy virus infection among zoo keepers. *Lancet* 2000; **355**: 551–2.

50. Switzer WM, Bhullar V, Shanmugam V *et al*. Frequent simian foamy virus infection in persons occupationally exposed to nonhuman primates. *J Virol* 2004; **78**: 2780–9.

51. Boneva RS, Grindon AJ, Orton SL *et al*. Simian foamy virus infection in a blood donor. *Transfusion* 2002; **42**: 886–91.

52. Hahn BH, Shaw GM, de Cock KM, Sharp PM. AIDS as a zoonosis: scientific and public health implications. *Science* 2000; **287**: 607–14.

53. Kalish ML, Wolfe ND, Ndongmo CB *et al*. Central African hunters exposed to simian immunodeficiency virus. *Emerg Infect Dis* 2005; **11**: 1928–30.

54. Gessain A, Mahieux R. Epidemiology, origin and genetic diversity of HTLV-1 retrovirus and STLV-1 simian affiliated retrovirus. *Bull Soc Pathol Exot* 2000; **93**: 163–71.

55. Wolfe ND, Heneine W, Carr JK, *et al*. Emergence of unique primate T-lymphotropic viruses among central African bushmeat hunters. *Proc Natl Acad Sci USA* 2005; **102**: 7994–9.

56. Anon. *Animal Health and Welfare Strategy for Great Britain*. London: DEFRA, 2004.

57. Advisory Committee on Dangerous Pathogens (ACDP). *Infection at Work: Controlling the risk*. London: HMSO, 2003.

58. Kahn LH. Confronting zoonoses, linking human and veterinary medicine. *Emerg Infect Dis* 2006; **12**: 556–61.

59. Cook RA, Karesh WB, Osofsky SA. Building interdisciplinary bridges to health in a globalized world. Presented at One World One Health Symposium, 29 September 2004, New York.

60. The Report of the Chief Veterinary Officer. *Animal Health 2007*. London: HMSO.

61. OIE. Improving wildlife surveillance for its protection whilst protecting us from the diseases it transmits. Press release 24 July 2008.

62. Reaser JK, Clark EE Jr, Meyers NM. All creatures great and minute. A public policy primer for companion animal zoonoses. *Zoonoses Public Health* 2008; **5**: 385–401.

63. Richardson Z. New network to monitor wildlife for signs of bioterrorism (Wildlife Center of Virginia) Project Tripwire. *Food Chemical News* 29 May 2006.

9

Implications for healthcare

The other chapters in this book have explored the details of zoonotic infection and disease. This chapter explores why these conditions pose a challenge for healthcare professionals and how an understanding of these conditions helps in identifying, treating and offering advice on prevention strategies to patients.

Significance of zoonotic disease

Although some of the zoonotic diseases in this volume are not dramatically significant in daily practice, there are others that cause serious disease, or their prevention complicates the management of severely or chronically ill patients. The estimate from the Health and Safety Executive (HSE) that 300 000 people are potentially exposed to risk of zoonotic disease annually is not insignificant when viewed in terms of economic loss or personal misery.[1]

Zoonoses carry with them a cost, not just in purely monetary terms, and many of them are preventable. It is therefore important that, whenever possible, strategies are implemented to treat appropriately, or prevent these diseases, in order to safeguard scarce resources and thereby benefit patients.

One of the key objectives of this book is to provide a knowledge base to assist assessment of patients seen in pharmacies and other healthcare settings. Information informs and shapes all healthcare practice, and knowledge of these conditions forms a part of the body of skills necessary in primary care. Healthcare practice is changing and there is an increased emphasis on a team approach to dealing with patients. The numbers of patients accessing healthcare services other than through a doctor's surgery is greater than ever before, and the skills and knowledge needed to signpost these patients accurately so that they obtain the best, most appropriate treatment for their conditions are also changing. There is a growing need for practitioners to obtain the widest skills and knowledge base possible to benefit both patients and colleagues.

The majority of zoonoses are untreatable at community pharmacy level, or at other first-contact sites such as walk-in centres or through telephone counselling services. Nor do the healthcare professionals involved at these first-contact sites have comprehensive right of diagnosis and, at present, prescribing rights necessary to treat these conditions effectively. Therefore, after an oral history has been taken or physical symptoms have been noted, all patients who are suspected of being victims of these conditions should be referred to a medical practitioner as soon as possible. It may well be of benefit to write a referral note, especially where there is suspicion of a serious condition, so that the information and observations can be communicated to the medical practitioner. This is especially essential where there may be a period of time between the patient's presentation and the next available appointment at the doctor's surgery, or where it is possible that the symptoms displayed may be transitory, e.g. in the tick bites or tick attachment and *erythema* associated with Lyme disease.

Pharmacists and other healthcare professionals who undertake domiciliary visiting or have regular contact with patients over a prolonged period of time will often have an extensive knowledge not only of the patient but also of his or her domestic situation. This can be a key to understanding either a chronic or an acute exacerbation of a patient's condition, in which a zoonotic disease derived from a companion animal, work or immediate environment may be responsible. There is also an increasing call for health information and activity relating to either health improvement or prevention of illness. For at-risk patients with chronic conditions or who are on continual therapies, a requirement to initiate or enable a risk- or harm-reduction programme is desirable if not yet mandatory.[2]

Disease prevention strategies

There is a body of literature relating to risk–benefit analysis in health issues. Zoonotic disease falls readily into this framework. Many of the risks have already been covered in some detail, so to set the scene for the rest of this chapter it is necessary to consider the benefits associated with animals in a social and domestic context.[3,4]

Benefits of companion animal ownership

Most cat owners, when asked, state that they keep cats for companionship and affection. This group is not alone: other groups of companion animal owners will express similar sentiments, even if their companion animal of choice is a reptile or other creature that is perhaps less cuddly or less demonstrative.

Studies undertaken across the world have shown that bereaved, socially deprived, mentally ill and house-bound individuals all exhibit lower symptom levels, or improvements in their condition, if they have contact with a companion animal. Reductions in blood pressure and improved recovery rates have been demonstrated in male participants in one study. The charity Pets as Therapy (PAT), which takes dogs into residential homes and other long-term care settings, justifiably claims to improve the quality of life of many patients.[5]

Children and adults who have behavioural difficulties or psychiatric conditions have been shown to improve if they have to care for another creature that in return demonstrates affection for them. The evidence appears to be convincing that the benefits are real, and not imagined, with far-reaching implications.[6,7]

These benefits may come at a price, because there may be a risk to a patient from contracting a zoonotic disease. The next part of the process is the risk assessment and, if appropriate, implementation of a harm-reduction strategy.[8]

The assessment process also needs to focus on the already unwell or at-risk patient. It must be remembered that nobody is completely safe, and that individuals who are on their gap year, off to far-flung places to do voluntary service overseas, or outdoor pursuits, may require some health advice, although a full risk assessment and harm-reduction programme are usually inappropriate.

Benefits from domesticated animals

There is another aspect to be considered before passing on to the assessment stage. Domesticated, agricultural and other animals also have a societal role. Traditionally, animals have been kept for their products, be they eggs, meat, milk and milk products, hides for leather, wool, or a wide variety of by-products such as gelatin, glycerin, hair or fats and oils. Although the number has reduced markedly over past decades due to social changes and higher costs, there are also individuals who work with wild or part-domesticated animals, such as pheasant and other game birds or deer, kept solely for hunting.

In social terms, a large number of people derive their employment from involvement in the rearing, husbandry, harvesting and processing of animals and their products. As in many other areas of human endeavour, this carries its own associated risks. Employment in this industry carries with it an enhanced risk from certain pathogens, including some zoonoses. Individuals who have other predisposing factors, which make them more susceptible to contracting disease, may have some difficult choices to make if reducing their risk involves losing the benefit of continued employment.

There are also a number of occupations where exposure to animals is part of the daily routine, but where exposure might be less obvious. Dog wardens, animal rescue workers, roofers, especially when working on roofs where pigeons or other birds have roosted, and zoo and circus employees all stand at greater risk of exposure to zoonotic pathogens than members of the general public.[9]

Risk assessment

In both primary and secondary care settings healthcare workers often gain knowledge relating not only to the medication and/or physical condition of their patients, but also sometimes to their domestic situation, especially when domiciliary visits are undertaken. The presence of a companion animal and a basic knowledge of the likely zoonotic conditions associated with that species might assist in assessing the patient's risk.

A few years ago, a doctor told me that another partner in the practice had been treating an elderly woman for a prolonged period for a recurrent chest infection and persistent dry cough. A home visit had to be made after the woman had become acutely ill and an emergency call had been made. On examination, the woman was found to have a severe pulmonary infection again. It was only as the doctor prepared to leave that the elderly woman said that her cockatoo had been off-colour for a while, and that the vet was now treating it for its wheeze. Serological tests showed the woman to be suffering from psittacosis, and the condition resolved on prolonged antibiotic therapy.

The moral for all healthcare workers that can be drawn from this story is that it is essential, especially when carrying out a risk assessment, to have a comprehensive knowledge of patients and their lifestyle and circumstances. It is necessary to concentrate not just on the disease state, but on the individual as a body with an interesting condition attached.

Accurate observations, asking the right questions and building a picture of the patient's condition are skills that all healthcare workers should develop. There must also be some knowledge of the likely pathogens associated with particular animals and the patient's circumstances.

A risk assessment for other reasons may form part of a patient's discharge procedure from secondary care, and it is essential for the risk of zoonotic disease to be included in an appropriate manner for certain patients. When a patient's history is being taken either formally or informally, any mention of a close association with animals should raise this issue, if only in the mind of the healthcare worker concerned.

To recap, the main identifiable risk groups are children, pregnant women, immunocompromised patients, agricultural and food-industry workers, and elderly or infirm people. The main diseases associated with these groups are summarised in Table 9.1.

Table 9.1 Summary of diseases by risk group	
Risk group	**Main disease threat**
Animal handlers	Leptospirosis *Pasteurella* Rabies *Salmonella* Tetanus
Neonates and children	Cutaneous larva migrans *Escherichia coli* Hookworm *Salmonella* Scabies Tetanus *Toxocara* Toxoplasmosis
Elderly and infirm people	*Escherichia coli* Influenza *Listeria* Psittacosis *Salmonella* Tetanus
Agricultural and food industry workers	Anthrax Brucellosis *Echinococcus* *Escherichia coli* Leptospirosis Orf *Pasteurella* Q fever *Salmonella* Tetanus Tuberculosis (*Mycobacterium bovis*)
Immunosuppressed or immunocompromised individuals	*Campylobacter* Cat scratch disease Cryptococcosis Cryptosporidia *Escherichia coli* *Listeria* *Mycobacterium avium* complex Psittacosis *Salmonella* *Toxocara* Toxoplasmosis Tuberculosis (*M. bovis*)
Pregnant women	Gestational psittacosis *Listeria* *Salmonella* *Toxocara* Toxoplasmosis

Having identified the animals with which the patient comes into regular contact, a review of the possible disease states related to the animal is needed. Detailed information on these diseases can be obtained from the appropriate sections in previous chapters. Listing the diseases can help identify insertion points for control measures to stop transmission or reduce pathogen burdens.

When carrying out an assessment, it is important to remember that it appears that the absolute risk of contracting a zoonotic infection is dependent on additive risk factors. Children on farms, immunocompromised agricultural workers and pregnant food-industry operatives have a greater risk than a similar individual who does not have the additional risk factor. Absolute risk is also dependent upon other factors, such as regular consumption of unpasteurised dairy products; frequent close contact with animals or poor personal hygiene practice adds a further layer of risk.[10]

It should be remembered that patients whose immune system is compromised or inadequate might not be solely those individuals suffering from human immunodeficiency virus/acquired immune deficiency syndrome (HIV/AIDS). This category applies also to patients who are alcoholic, especially if cirrhosis is present, individuals with certain neoplastic diseases where chemotherapy, radiotherapy or high levels of steroids are being used, patients with renal, hepatic or splenic failure, people with diabetes, individuals with certain congenital conditions including cystic fibrosis, those with autoimmune conditions such as systemic lupus erythematosus where immunosuppressant therapy may be used, organ transplant recipients with concomitant immunosuppressant therapy, people who are malnourished and haemodialysis patients.

Patients on high-dose steroids or receiving long-term low-dose steroid therapy also show some loss of immunocompetence. The side effects of such therapy pose a risk to the patient from many pathogens, and from physical damage that may lead to infection. Zoonoses are not the only risk to these patients; however, they should not be ignored.[11]

In essence, an elderly, immunocompromised agricultural worker who keeps pet cats in the kitchen, sleeps with the dogs, does not wash and regularly consumes pints of unpasteurised milk is either lucky or dead.

Harm reduction and prevention

The gold standard for all healthcare has always been preventing a condition from establishing itself, so that therapeutic intervention in clinically advanced symptomatic disease is rendered unnecessary. In zoonotic infection the old adage that 'Ten parts of prevention are better than one part of cure' holds very true. Once contracted there are certain zoonoses that are impossible or extremely difficult to eradicate. Toxocariasis, toxoplasmosis, tuberculosis and psittacosis all pose immense problems in ensuring that a sufferer does not relapse with a further attack after a course of therapy. In some individuals continuous or periodic treatment may be necessary to maintain a cure.[8]

However, prevention, with the implied complete protection that it offers, may be unachievable for a variety of reasons, and often the best that can be attained is a diminution of risk, or a reduction in the harm that an infection may cause. For identified risk groups reducing the risk of contracting zoonotic infections forms an important part of the healthcare professional's role. The usual premise for harm reduction is that an attempt must be made to maintain patients' health, while seeking to alter their overall quality and style of life the least. Realistically, to achieve this end, there is a need for patients to receive as much education and information relating to the risks that they face, and the means of reducing those risks from exposure to zoonotic agents. This can be as simple as promptly cleaning up the cat litter tray, or getting somebody who does not have any predisposing condition to empty the tray. The information provided has to be geared to the patient's comprehension and there may be a corresponding need for counselling or support.

The main plank of any strategy is prevention of exposure or reduction of risk associated with exposure to a pathogen (Figure 9.1). Achieving this in patients who are already ill can be extremely difficult, because there often is a need to change long-standing habits, while trying to hold relationships, employment and private life together. This can be particularly difficult for patients where their condition is unlikely to improve unless they cease to own pets, especially if one of their main sources of emotional comfort is a companion animal, rather than relatives or friends. Harm reduction becomes much less easy in patients who may have an occupational exposure to zoonotic pathogens, where changing employment may be difficult or impossible.

With the current economic and other difficulties that agricultural enterprises face, the last straw may be the loss of a worker, especially in a small operation. The effects for an individual can also be catastrophic, with loss of income leading to far-reaching lifestyle changes.[12]

It is essential that any portion of an overall strategy or measure that can be achieved is seen as a bonus. However resistant the patient may be, and however ill, there is usually something that can be done to reduce risk.

In a chronically ill patient, measures may have to be introduced gradually over long periods. The full spectrum of applicable measures may be attained only as the patient becomes comfortable with the necessary changes. The rate of change has to be driven by the patient, not the health professional, as that could lead to conflict and refusal of the patient to adopt or maintain the necessary measures.

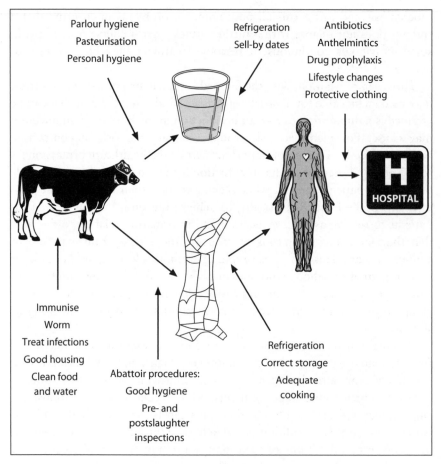

Parlour hygiene
Pasteurisation
Personal hygiene

Refrigeration
Sell-by dates

Antibiotics
Anthelmintics
Drug prophylaxis
Lifestyle changes
Protective clothing

H
HOSPITAL

Immunise
Worm
Treat infections
Good housing
Clean food
and water

Abattoir procedures:
Good hygiene
Pre- and
postslaughter
inspections

Refrigeration
Correct storage
Adequate
cooking

Figure 9.1 Prevention points and strategies for food-borne zoonoses.

It is also essential that this be viewed as a multidisciplinary issue. The traditional core team in community care is expanding. Issues relating to zoonotic infection may cross the boundaries of social work, veterinary care, nursing, pharmacy and medical services. If one practitioner identifies an issue, then communication to other parties is essential. This becomes particularly true when dealing with patients whose condition may be chronic, and who require a large alteration to their lifestyle for risk reduction. The involvement of a veterinary surgeon, employment service advisers or benefit agency personnel – all classes of professionals not traditionally seen as healthcare workers – may be indispensable.[11]

Constituent measures for prevention strategies

Having identified what appear to be the main risk pathogens, the next step is to develop the components for a successful strategy. Table 9.2 provides a

Table 9.2 Summary of prevention measure	
Mode of transmission	**Prevention measures**
Pica/faecal contamination of food, water, clothing or skin	Education and personal hygiene Anthelmintics or antibiotics for animals and humans Prompt removal of faecal matter Disinfection of contaminated areas or items Thorough cleaning and cooking of food Ensuring that water is clean by filtration or chlorination
Aerosol	Use of facemasks (personal protective equipment or PPE)
Saliva	Avoid animal bites and disinfect wounds promptly Vaccinate animals and humans Avoid direct contact with animal's face Muzzle aggressive animals Educate owners not to kiss their pets
Blood	Cover open wounds
Vector mediated	Use repellents Control life cycle at breeding sites Use insecticides/parasiticides Wear suitable clothing
Fomite contact	Clean surroundings thoroughly, and disinfect as appropriate Wear suitable protective clothing while undertaking risk activities
Food	Cook meat and eggs thoroughly Consume pasteurised milk and cheese Wash or clean food thoroughly Refrigerate items correctly. Do not consume past 'best before' or out-of-date items Use common sense and practise personal hygiene

In chronic or extreme cases	Consider drastic changes to lifestyle, including:
	   changing employment
	   avoiding contact with animals
	   permanent removal of animals from domestic environment by rehoming or euthanasia
	   controlling feral or pest animals in vicinity
	   sterilising foodstuffs

summary of the threat posed from method of transmission, mode of infection and the appropriate prevention measures.

The framework shown in Table 9.2 can be used to assemble a list of possible measures, which can in turn be used to reduce transmission and infective risk. It is only a starting point and does not exclude innovation or imagination. Be aware that most of the measures listed are voluntary; there is no legislation that forces companion animal owners to adopt any or all of the recommendations.

This is not true for workers in the agricultural or food industries, or in any other occupation where contact with animals or their products forms part of the normal work routine. People employed in this way have a greater duration and frequency of contact with animals, and therefore an increased likelihood of being exposed to zoonotic pathogens. The protective measures recommended for this group are already enshrined either in statute or in best custom or practice within the associated industry, usually under provisions of established legislation. These are explored at the end of this chapter.[1]

There is also a risk group that falls between the companion animal owner and the commercial extremes. These are people who are employed as animal keepers in zoos and circuses and also the workers in protection societies and animal refuges or rescue centres, who may be volunteers or casual workers. There is a possibility that they can, because of the nature of their work, fall outside the scope of regulatory protection. Best practice would be for these individuals to adopt the measures required in industry; however, this may not be possible. For this group a mix-and-match approach to prevention measures is probably best. Where any doubt exists as to the hazards associated with a particular animal or procedure it is best to err on the side of caution.

Health promotion and education

So far the focus of this chapter has been upon the patient who is already unwell. What of the worried well or the population in general? Healthy pets mean healthy people and vice versa. In general a companion animal that is regularly wormed, properly fed and bedded down will be less likely to harbour infection. The control of ectoparasites, regular veterinary care and domestic hygiene routines with the use of disinfectants, wearing protective gloves when handling faecal matter and preventing the animal biting, licking or scratching any human go a long way to reducing accidental infection rates.[13]

As a prevention measure, the early education of children about the care of animals and good personal hygiene is important in preventing not only immediate disease, but also the establishment of an infective focus (such as toxoplasmosis) which, once contracted, may recur at a later juncture. General advice is usually available from veterinary surgeons, animal charities and other bodies, many of whom provide online advice or information leaflets.

The information relating to prevention measures for patients, their carers, friends and relatives, or healthcare professionals is also not difficult to access. As in many other fields of medicine, there is a great body of information available, particularly on the internet, which is often overwhelming in its quantity, if not its quality. Some of the websites in Appendix 1 provide starting points of proven probity.

As with most medical conditions, many self-help groups are able to provide literature for use in patient education on the risk of zoonotic diseases and the appropriate management of companion animals either to prevent these diseases or to develop harm-reduction strategies.

This is an important field of health promotion where healthcare professionals are well placed to be effective advocates for both patients and their pets. There is a profound need for the void between veterinary care and traditional GP-led community services, where there may be little linkage between the pet and the patient, to be bridged. The problem of health education relating to zoonotic disease is an issue that must be grasped to protect the health of all owners of companion animals.

Healthcare professionals not belonging to the medical profession should consider rapid referral of any patient suspected of having a zoonotic condition to a doctor as soon as is practicable, because most of these conditions will not respond to self-medication.

Treatment

If the disease cannot be prevented, or the risk-reduction strategy fails, the next option is treatment. This is usually with a therapeutic agent, be it an antibiotic, antifungal, anthelmintic or insecticide, although in some conditions (e.g. hydatid disease) surgical intervention may also be necessary.

Resistance, especially in antimicrobial treatment, affects the effectiveness of any drug therapy, and this is becoming an increasing concern. Extensive studies have been undertaken by the Department for Environment, Food and Rural Affairs (DEFRA) and the Department of Health (DH) in the UK, with input from the Health Protection Agency (HPA), to ascertain the extent and significance of the problem. The World Health Organization (WHO) has issued guidelines on prescribing and supplying antibiotics and is also carrying out continuing investigations of its own. The issue is significant when related to zoonoses, because animals are treated with the same antibiotics as humans. Any resistance developing in the animal population can spread into the food chain and thus affect the usefulness of these agents. The display of resistance to certain insecticides and anthelmintics should also be borne in mind when choosing an agent, and monitoring may be necessary to determine the chosen drug's efficacy.[14]

Many cases of zoonotic infection will never reach the stage of symptomatic disease, or be diagnosed, and are resolved by empirical general antibiotic treatment by a patient's GP before full-blown clinical symptoms can manifest. More cases may be seen of certain diseases as blind use of wide-spectrum antibiotics declines.

In many cases of infection where a zoonotic disease is suspected, the rapid use of antibiotics is often imperative. Susceptibility testing may be necessary. Broad-spectrum blind usage, although not desirable, can be the fastest method to prevent progression. Combination therapies or progression to 'reserved' moieties may be necessary, especially if the course of the disease is rapid or morbidity is feared, although this normally requires diagnosis using appropriate tests.

Certain infections may require extended antibiotic therapy with the concomitant problems associated with interactions and choice of a suitable agent for sustained use. In immunocompromised patients there will be a requirement for specialist support in choosing, monitoring and supplying some drugs required for eradication or control of certain organisms, especially resistant strains of tuberculosis and *Cryptosporidia* spp. There may also be a need to keep latent infection suppressed for a patient's lifetime, as in toxoplasmosis, so expert advice is essential.

When choosing anthelmintics for worm infestations, the more unusual parasites may require drugs that are not in routine use and/or available on a named-patient basis only. In these cases support from specialised units can be invaluable. In the UK, IDIS Ltd can provide many of these specialised drugs (see Appendix 2 for details); in the USA the Centers for Disease Control and Prevention (CDC) will provide advice and have a scheme that allows drugs not normally available in continental USA, or not normally used for human treatment, to be supplied. There may also be an issue, where the parasite load is heavy, of the use in a domestic situation of certain products, because rapid death of the parasites can lead to systemic toxicity and allergic reactions.

The use of unlicensed products is a thorny issue, and the initiation of such drugs at primary care level may pose a serious clinical dilemma. It may be necessary to refer a patient to another healthcare provider, if practicable. In cases of more unusual organisms, especially if the condition has been contracted abroad, hospitals specialising in tropical diseases may be the best informed and best placed to undertake treatment. Specimen addresses and contact telephone numbers may be found in Appendix 2.

General supportive therapies may also be needed for symptom control. The use of anti-inflammatory drugs, painkillers, rehydration therapy or antiemetics may be appropriate. In specific conditions, i.e. hydatid disease, surgery may be necessary, requiring unusual drugs or adjuncts depending upon the severity or extent of infection, the organism responsible and the stage in its life cycle. Specialist support can again be invaluable.

The choice of pesticide in arthropod infestations needs to be carefully considered to ensure that no underlying medical conditions are exacerbated. Press coverage of Gulf War syndrome has heightened public fear of pesticide use, but not in a balanced way. This has led to unreasoning fear of all insecticides. On that basis it is necessary to be careful in choosing an agent that will not only eliminate the arthropod concerned, but also not cause or increase the anxiety of patients or their carers.

Hypersensitivity to organophosphates and the emergence of resistant strains of arthropods are matters of concern, and influence the choice of agent. The formulation may also be important; the use of alcohol-based lotions or solutions is contraindicated in people with asthma, and other formulations may be unacceptable to some patients because of odour or consistency.

Wherever possible, detailed information on treatments has been given in the appropriate single-disease sections. However, not all of these therapies are officially approved, so treatment must follow local or national policies or guidelines. The overriding authority is either the national or local formularies when therapeutic choices are to be made, unless the condition is so unusual as to require empirical treatment.

Antimicrobial resistance

The ability of microorganisms to adapt to any conditions and challenges is remarkable. Their ability to develop resistance to currently available antibiotics has become of increasing concern. The emergence of methicillin-resistant *Staphylococcus aureus* (MRSA) and other organisms with multiple resistance to whole classes of antibiotics threatens to return the management strategies for certain diseases to the pre-penicillin era.

Concerns arose over the use of antibiotics related to their use in animals, both in feed as additives either to preserve health or to increase weight gain, and within herd management programmes as routine interventions. In July 1998 a comprehensive review of the issues and data related to antibiotic resistance in the food chain was undertaken by the then Ministry of Agriculture, Food and Fisheries (MAFF; now DEFRA). The House of Lords Select Committee on Science and Technology also reported on resistance to antibiotics and other antimicrobial agents in 2001.[15]

The Advisory Committee on the Microbiological Safety of Food (ACMSF) also reported in 1999, and this led to the establishment by DEFRA of an Antimicrobial Resistance Co-ordination Group (DARC). All of these reports and working groups highlighted the threat to human health, and a report *The Path of Least Resistance* from the Standing Medical Advisory Committee,[16] as well as recommendations made in the UK Antimicrobial Resistance Strategy and Action Plan produced by the NHS Executive in June 2000, led to health authorities being required to develop local prescribing guidelines, and also to the first tranche of animal growth promoters being banned in 1999 (bacitracin, spiramycin, tylosin and virginamycin). The second and final tranche were banned in 2006 (avilamycin, monensin, fluorophospholipol and salinamycin).[17]

A Veterinary Medicine Directorate (VMD) report has also led to the development of guidelines for responsible practice for the use of antibiotics in animals. This is supported by a voluntary scheme endorsed by RUMA – the Responsible Use of Medicines in Agriculture Alliance.

The VLA in cooperation with the Food Standards Agency (FSA) and the HPA continues to survey food-borne pathogens to determine the prevalence, resistance and subtypes of pathogens present in the food chain.

In Europe, in 2001, the European Commission (EC) introduced a 'Community Strategy against Antimicrobial Resistance'. There are 15 actions in 4 key areas: surveillance, prevention, research and product development, and international cooperation. There are also EC recommendations on the prudent use of antimicrobials, and an agreement on the phasing out of growth promoters in animals. The European Union (EU) also has an industry scheme run through the EMEA (European Agency for the Evaluation of Medicinal Products), which seeks to address the need to promote new effective antibiotics.

The European Antimicrobial Resistance Surveillance System (EARSS) consists of 700 laboratories in 28 countries. There are also a variety of schemes under EU or EC auspices; these include Enternet, the European surveillance system for enteric disease which also provides susceptibility testing on salmonella and VTEC (*E. coli*) isolates, EuroTB which undertakes surveillance of tuberculosis (both *Mycobacterium bovis* and *M. tuberculosis*) and developing drug resistance, and the ESAC or European Surveillance of Antimicrobial Consumption, ARPAC (Antibiotic Resistance Prevention and Control) project aimed at the prevention and control of resistance.

The EC also has an outreach programme – Antibiotic Resistance in the Mediterranean (ARMed) – which covers not only European countries in the Mediterranean littoral, but also a wider extended area including Malta, Cyprus, Turkey, Tunisia, Egypt, Morocco and Jordan. The EC and the WHO have a Memorandum of Understanding (MOU) on health including strategies against antibiotic resistance.

From the research available, it would appear that resistance to antibiotics in animal pathogens that may be zoonotic is selected after the introduction of veterinary medicines or growth promoters. This produces bacteria capable of being transmitted to humans by food; these bacteria are resistant to related human antimicrobial moieties, which can then lead to difficulties in successfully treating any disease thus caused. The use of antibiotics in agriculture is of particular concern in zoonotic disease, because the pathogens, by definition, are from animal sources.

The issue is not trivial, as some of the organisms in which resistance has been identified are not resistant to solely one antibiotic class but exhibit resistance across a range of antimicrobial groups. Multi-antibiotic-resistant pathogens of particular concern are those resistant to fluorinated quinolones

(*Salmonella* and *Campylobacter* spp.), macrolides (*Campylobacter* spp.), virginamycin (enterococci) and avoparcin (enterococci).

There is also evidence that resistance has increased. Recent reports from UK government agencies show that *E. coli* resistance to ciprofloxacin has increased up to 23% in 2006, up from 1% in 1993; resistance in the same organism to third-generation cephalosporins has risen to 11% in 2006, up from 2% in 2001. Resistance to cephalosporin is also up from 2.2% in 2001–3 to 12% in 2006, and resistance to ampicillin/amoxicillin has gone from 52% in 1993 to 60% in 2006. Resistance to gentamicin, which was 1% of isolates in 1993, has reached 8.5% in 2006. Most of Europe demonstrates the same or in some cases higher levels.

In 2006 *Campylobacter jejuni* was 30% resistant to ciprofloxacin and *C. coli* was 37% resistant. Erythromycin resistance is low in *C. jejuni* and runs at 38% in *C. coli.*

The other food-borne zoonotic pathogens considered to be of significance are the *Salmonella* spp., still deemed to be responsible for most serious food-poisoning cases. *Salmonella typhimurium* DT104 and other strains of *S. typhimurium* and *S. virchow* have been isolated that are fluoroquinolone resistant. In addition, 58% of *Salmonella* DT104 isolates are resistant to ampicillin, chloramphenicol, streptomycin, sulphonamides and tetracyclines. The R serotype of this pathogen is additionally resistant to trimethoprim and quinolones, posing a real problem in treatment terms. In non-typhoidal salmonellae the most worrying is the resistance to nalidixic acid coupled with decreased susceptibility to ciprofloxacin.[18]

The fear is that resistance may be transferable from animal to human enterococci, which continue to pose problems in immunocompromised patients. Plasmid-transferred resistance has been demonstrated in two strains isolated in Madagascar of *Yersinia pestis*, the zoonotic causative pathogen of plague, and of considerable concern and significance in terms of world health, especially in the developing world. One strain is streptomycin resistant – previously the main drug of choice for treating plague – and the other is resistant to chloramphenicol, tetracyclines and sulphonamides – the second-line alternatives.

The WHO believes that there is evidence for arguing that, wherever possible, antibiotics should not be extensively used in agriculture, especially where the use is purely to accelerate animal growth to market weight, rather than to treat clinical disease. The emergence of vancomycin-resistant bacteria shows links to the use of the related compound avoparcin, and the introduction of pristinamycin into human therapy has been compromised by the past use of virginamycin in animal feed.

The WHO has set out a document containing global principles for the containment of antimicrobial resistance in animals intended for food. This suggests that all antimicrobials used for growth promotion should be phased out as soon as possible. Governments are exhorted to refuse or revoke licences for these products. There is also a recommendation that antibiotic use in animals should not be seen as a replacement for good husbandry.[14]

Direct impact of antibiotic resistance on healthcare

This issue is of considerable concern in a secondary care setting where seriously ill patients are treated regularly, and where health policy, especially on prescribing practice, is pioneered. The emergence of MRSA and *Clostridium difficile*, in particular, along with other resistant pathogens in hospital premises, has provoked a measured response with the introduction of antibiotic policies in these establishments. With the move to primary care trusts (PCTs) and the introduction of regional or area formularies, consideration has been given to issues of seamless care and antibiotic hierarchies. Coordinated policies for primary and secondary care on antibiotic prescribing may slow the emergence of resistant pathogens.[19]

The situation in the USA is similar, with the CDC driving the prudent use of antibiotics, and a cross-governmental consensus across a wide range of national, and state, bodies working towards rational and agreed strategies to prevent resistance in both human and veterinary spheres.

Antimicrobial resistance in therapy for immunocompromised patients has also become an issue. Regimens for the treatment and continued prophylaxis of the main zoonotic pathogens seen as a threat to these patients must be decided through specialist units, with the support of microbiological laboratories and consultants to ensure that moieties can continue to be effective and available.

In conclusion, there is a need for coordination between not only secondary and primary care, but also animal and human health specialists and governmental bodies to ensure that, in the future, the therapeutic gains derived from antibiotic use are not lost.

UK legislation

A brief mention has previously been made of the HSE/COSHH (Health and Safety Executive/Control of Substances Hazardous to Health) regulations. As in any other realm of healthcare, practice goes hand in hand with the law. It is almost inevitable that some of these rules and regulations cover aspects of zoonotic diseases. Wherever possible these regulations have been indicated in the sections or chapters relating to the condition caused by the responsible pathogen. The following section assembles some of the more significant measures.

The Health and Safety at Work etc. Act 1974

This act and the statutory instruments and regulations made under it confer a duty of care on employers to ensure that they do not expose their employees to risks in the work place. It requires all employers to draw up a health and safety policy statement, and to provide protective clothing or equipment as required by health and safety law. Likewise, all employees must ensure, as far as possible, their own safety when working.[1]

There is also a requirement to report injuries and certain diseases (including zoonoses) to the HSE. This is covered by the Reporting of Injuries, Diseases and Dangerous Occurrences Regulations (RIDDOR) 1995. These replaced the previous regulations, and came into force in England, Scotland and Wales on 1 April 1996. Under these rules there is a responsibility for an employer or self-employed person to report a case of any disease listed in Schedule 3 of the regulations, once it has been diagnosed in writing by a doctor, and when the person concerned is currently employed in an associated work activity.

The following zoonotic diseases are included in the Schedule:

- Anthrax
- Avian and ovine chlamydiosis
- Brucellosis
- Leptospirosis
- Lyme disease
- Q fever
- Rabies
- *Streptococcus suis*
- Tuberculosis.

In addition there is a catch-all clause, where any disease that may have stemmed from work activities has to be reported, including those possibly contracted from handling dead bodies or tissues of animals or humans. The section on work-induced lung disease also covers such pathogens as *Chlamydophila psittaci*, *Mycobacterium avium* complex and *Cryptococcus neoformans*.

Management of Health and Safety at Work Regulations 1992

These regulations are made under the Health and Safety at Work etc. (HASAW) Act 1974, and require employers to carry out an assessment of the risks in their work place, implement suitable risk control measures and carry out health surveillance on employees. They must also inform employees of any risks in the work place (including zoonoses) and give suitable and adequate training to educate their workers in good practice and prevention measures.

Control of Substances Hazardous to Health Regulations 1999

The COSHH regulations are also made under the HASAW Act 1974. They classify the pathogens that cause zoonoses as hazardous substances. Under these rules employers and self-employed people are required to assess the risks to health from work activities that involve hazardous substances and prevent or, where this is not reasonably practicable, adequately control exposure to the hazardous substances.

Employers must promote good occupational hygiene, with the emphasis on safe working practices, personal protective equipment (PPE) and personal hygiene. Safe working practices include avoiding injury from tools or equipment, correct disposal of contaminated sharps, and avoiding other high-risk activities such as handling placental matter or dead animals with the bare hands. PPE should be used whenever necessary, and must be adequate and appropriate for avoiding infection. The use of gloves, respirators, waterproof aprons, face shields, special overalls or other clothing and footwear, when carrying out tasks such as examining animals or assisting at birth, is recommended. All PPE should be CE marked and to the appropriate British Standard (BS).

Personal hygiene should be promoted with adequate washing facilities, provision of hot water and soap, and a means of drying the hands.

The regulations also lay emphasis on the need for common-sense precautions regarding wound care, first aid, disinfection of animal bedding and housing, mucking out regularly and other precautions that prevent disease transmission. Good husbandry practice of regular worming, prompt vaccination and high standards of care and cleanliness are suggested as appropriate measures to assist disease prevention.

Leaflets, advice and information on the HASAW Act and the other legislation made under it can be obtained from http://www.hse.gov.uk.

Notifiable disease legislation

There are measures separately enacted that require disease notification for animals or humans. As zoonoses affect both categories, the main legislation for both is discussed below.

Statutory notifications of infectious diseases (human)

The requirement to notify cases of certain infectious diseases first came into force in the late nineteenth century. It is tackled by two strands. The first, health and clinically based aims to undertake disease surveillance, works through the HPA; the second is based around a network of public health 'proper officers' (who may not be health based) appointed by local authorities who collect and collate information which is passed to the Office for National Statistics.

The health-based system is geared to providing rapid detection of epidemics or mass outbreaks of potentially serious disease. The system is currently administered by the HPA Centre for Infections, and other regional surveillance centres, and is known as Notification of Infectious Disease System (NOIDS). Based on clinically based activity through diagnostic laboratory reporting, and clinical reports of disease through the Local and Regional Service (LARS) of the HPA, it is fed by the responsibility for notification which rests upon 'the attending medical practitioner', who may range from any doctor in any care setting to the proper officer of the local authority. To gain the speed necessary to prevent epidemics, notification does not rely on clinically proven diagnosis; a presumptive diagnosis is enough, with later confirmation or cancellation.

Under this legislation food poisoning should also be notified. This was defined in respect of the regulations using a DH definition, which states that food poisoning is 'any disease of an infectious or toxic nature caused by or thought to be caused by the consumption of food or water'.

Although this is a wide definition, it does cover all cases; however, it does not permit differentiation between causative organisms, but the resulting notification allows some statistical work to take place.

In the public health arena, there is a formal reporting system covering a number of diseases under the Public Health (Infectious Diseases) Regulations 1988. In Scotland the Public Health (Notification of Infectious Diseases) (Scotland) Regulations 1988 require similar notification but also include Lyme disease and toxoplasmosis. In Northern Ireland the equivalent legislation is the Public Health Notifiable Diseases Order (Northern Ireland) 1989.

Diseases notifiable under the Public Health (Infectious Diseases) Regulations 1988, which are considered to be zoonoses, are (in alphabetical order):

- Acute encephalitis
- Anthrax
- Food poisoning
- Leptospirosis
- Meningitis caused by *Haemophilus influenzae*, or other viruses either specified or unspecified
- Plague
- Rabies

- Relapsing fever
- Tetanus
- Tuberculosis (*M. bovis* and *M. tuberculosis*)
- Typhus fever
- Viral haemorrhagic fever (i.e. Ebola)
- Viral hepatitis.

Note: because of advances in diagnosis and symptom classification, some of the categories framed at the time of the regulations now include under their general headings conditions that might be caused by zoonotic agents. In those cases the heading has been left open.

Notifiable disease in animals

A variety of measures is in place that requires notification of cases of certain infectious diseases in animals. As in human cases, the notification is based on presumption, not necessarily clinical proof, and the diagnosis may be confirmed or cancelled after examination of suitable samples by the Veterinary Laboratory Service.

Cases of notifiable diseases must be reported on suspicion to the divisional veterinary manager of DEFRA. Once confirmed, action will be taken in accordance with animal health or other legislation.

Many of the measures relating to notifiable diseases in animals overlap, and relate to previously endemic conditions that have now been eradicated or controlled. Others relate to organisms that are classified as emerging, or are seen as posing a significant threat were they to arrive in the UK. Examples are Hendra virus and *Echinococcus multilocularis*. The latter condition is specifically mentioned in the legislation and procedures underpinning the Pet Travel Scheme (PETS), which defines specific measures to prevent the introduction of this pathogen into the UK (see p. 201).

It should be noted that, in addition to the statutory reporting legislation, there are a number of industry or trade association schemes for voluntary reporting of diseases that may not be covered by legislation, but which could cause economic loss to the agricultural industry.

Concerns that zoonotic pathogens could emerge or re-emerge also underpin the following legislation:

- The Specific Animal Pathogens Order (1998) and the Specified Animal Pathogens Order (Northern Ireland) 1999 cover three zoonotic pathogens that are not currently seen in the UK, but that could cause considerable damage were they to be introduced, namely *Trichinella spiralis*, equine morbillivirus and *Echinococcus multilocularis*.

- The Zoonoses Order 1989 and the Zoonoses Order 1991 (Northern Ireland) are specifically framed to cover the monitoring of *Salmonella* and *Brucella* spp. from food-producing animals, their products, environment or feeding stuffs.
- The Zoonoses (Monitoring) (England) Regulations 2007 came into force on 1 October 2007, and are aimed at controlling zoonotic outbreaks (and specifically highly pathogenic or HP H5N1). They allow designated inspectors to enter any premises at all reasonable hours to determine if an outbreak has occurred. In addition it has a provision relating to wild animals, allowing samples to be taken that might otherwise be in contravention of legislation protecting wildlife species from any sampling or disturbance.

Notifiable diseases in the USA

In the USA, the CDC have responsibility for the National Notifiable Diseases Surveillance System. Surveillance of infectious disease started in the USA in the late 1800s, and by the early twentieth century an annual summary of serious notifiable diseases was being produced. In 1961, the CDC was given the mandate to collect and publish data relating to notifiable diseases; however, state reporting to the CDC still remains voluntary, although reporting to state authorities is mandatory at state and county level.

The list of diseases that are considered notifiable varies slightly by state; however, every state reports the internationally quarantinable diseases in compliance with the WHO regulations. The CDC publishes statistics and data relating to notifiable infectious diseases in the *Morbidity and Mortality Weekly Report* (MMWR). Of the diseases included in the list, which alters periodically, many are zoonotic, but not all.

Nationally Notifiable Infectious Diseases List, United States 2008 (Zoonoses only)

- Anthrax
- Arboviral neuroinvasive and non-neuroinvasive diseases
- Eastern equine encephalitis virus disease
- Powassan virus disease
- St Louis encephalitis virus disease
- West Nile virus disease
- Western equine encephalitis virus disease
- Botulism
- Botulism, food borne
- Botulism, infant

- Botulism, other (wound and unspecified)
- Brucellosis
- Cryptosporidiosis
- Giardiasis
- Hantavirus pulmonary syndrome
- Haemolytic–uraemic syndrome, post-diarrhoeal
- Listeriosis
- Lyme disease
- Novel influenza A virus infections
- Plague
- Psittacosis
- Q fever
- Rabies
- Rabies, animal
- Rabies, human
- Rocky Mountain spotted fever
- Salmonellosis
- Severe acute respiratory syndrome-associated coronavirus (SARS-CoV) disease
- Tetanus
- Trichinellosis (trichinosis)
- Tuberculosis
- Tularaemia.

Other US legislation

Non-Americans looking at the plethora of rules and regulations made at a variety of levels within the US system (i.e. national, state, county, etc.) soon become very confused because the system varies from state to state, and some standards are voluntary whereas others are mandatory. National governmental organisations such as USDA (US Department of Agriculture), the FDA (Food and Drug Administration) and the health departments set rules where possible, and enforce them nationally; however, because of the complexity and size of the physical area of the USA, and the strength of state legislatures, there may be other standards and regulations in addition to national law. Readers are advised to check both national and local statutes to ascertain what rules and legislation apply locally, and which diseases are notifiable in both animals and humans, along with quarantine rules, etc.

Points to ponder

To round off this chapter and the book, there are a few random topics relating to medical aspects of zoonoses that need some consideration.

Choice of companion animal

When individuals choose a pet, they do not routinely consult either a vet or a doctor. In most cases, the decision may not have any significant consequences for the health of the pet owner or family; however, where there is a seriously ill or potentially at-risk individual in the equation, either as a sole owner or within a family group, the decision process may be more crucial. The more exotic the pet, the more unusual the range of bacteria and other pathogens that it can carry.

As discussed elsewhere in this book, reptiles and other exotic pets are recognised as carrying unusual strains of *Salmonella* spp., stray kittens can carry a variety of very interesting pathogens and a bird from a pet shop could be the last straw for an already distressed respiratory patient. The other aspect is that a young animal may be tractable and adorable, but the adult may be less appealing and a lot more difficult.[11]

Guidance as to the suitability of a pet is readily available, usually from veterinary surgeons or groups such as the Pet Health Council. When knowledge is gained that a patient or family is contemplating obtaining a new companion animal, it is essential that they be encouraged to seek the available advice before they take on a creature that could pose a health risk.

Xenotransplantation and transgenic animals

One of the dreams of the late twentieth century was the availability of an inexhaustible supply of organs, especially hearts and kidneys, for transplantation from genetically engineered animals. Although still a matter of science future rather than pure science fiction, the realisation of this dream is still probably some years away. The ability of a company to produce Dolly the Sheep and Percy the Pig was certainly impressive.

The scientific application of cloning technology, with the possibility of manipulating the genetic material of animals to achieve therapeutic breakthroughs, has become more accepted. The existence of transgenic sheep capable of producing human insulin or growth hormone gives hope for many patients and opportunities for profit for drug companies. The use of hearts from transgenic pigs has been suggested as a solution for the chronic shortage of these organs from human donors.[20]

In any of these future initiatives it is necessary to exclude all zoonotic pathogens from the material or organs used. The risks are greater than accidental exposure to the pathogen, because there will be a deliberate introduction of a quantity of animal tissue or material by surgery, or possibly injection. In natural transplantation with human organs, the same risks apply, demonstrated graphically by the development of rabies in patients who received infected organs. After the emergence of variant Creutzfeldt–Jakob disease (vCJD), it has been demonstrated that under laboratory conditions prions have been transferred to unrelated species by tissue transplants.

In the USA, transplants from non-human primates have been banned, not only to preserve primate numbers, but also to prevent the spread of zoonotic pathogens, especially viruses, because of these concerns. These organisms may be benign in the normal host but could be pathogenic in humans. Of concern is that any pathogen once across the species barrier could modify to pass from person to person if there is a process such as viral recombination, a process that probably occurred in the emergence of HIV.[21]

The other closest animal source to humans of organs are those derived from pigs; these are also capable of carrying porcine endogenous retroviruses, which are not known to be pathogenic in humans, but might become so.

This has led to a number of bodies passing policies and making recommendations including the EU and the WHO to reduce or prevent xenotransplantation. Thus, sadly, it appears that turning science fiction into science fact still remains a distant, if not unrealistic, dream in this field of endeavour, until safety concerns can be addressed.

References

1. Anonymous. *Farmwise*. London: Health & Safety Executive, 2005.
2. Zinsstag J, Schelling E, Wyss K, Bechir M. Potential of cooperation between human and animal health to strengthen health systems. *Lancet* 2005; **366**: 2142–5.
3. En Health. *Environmental Health Risk Assessment – Guidelines for assessing human health risks from environmental hazards*. Department of Health and Ageing and enHealth Council, Canberra, 2002.
4. European Academies Science Advisory Council (EASAC). *Combating the Threat of Zoonotic Infections*. London: Royal Society, 2008.
5. Wells DL. Domestic dogs and human health: An overview. *Br J Psychol* 2007; **12**: 145–56.
6. Schoen AM. The healing power of pets. In: Gorrel C (ed.), *Kindred Spirits*. New York: Broadway Books, 2001.
7. Siegel JM, Angulo FJ, Detels R, Wesch J, Mullen A. AIDS diagnosis and depression in the Multicenter AIDS Cohort Study: the ameliorating impact of pet ownership. *AIDS Care* 1999; **11**: 157–70.
8. Guay DR. Pet-assisted therapy in the nursing home setting: potential for zoonosis. *Am J Infect Control* 2001; **29**: 178–86.
9. Bender JB, Shulman SA. Reports of zoonotic disease outbreaks associated with animal exhibits and availability of recommendations for preventing zoonotic disease transmission from animals to people in such settings. *JAVMA* 2004; **224**: 1105–9.
10. CDC. Compendium of measures to prevent disease associated with animals in public settings, 2005: National Association of State Public Health Veterinarians, Inc. (NASPHV). *MMWR* 2005; **54**(RR-4): 1–13.
11. Kahn LH. Confronting zoonoses, linking human and veterinary medicine. *Emerg Infect Dis* 2006; **12**: 556–61
12. Department for the Environment, Food and Rural Affairs (DEFRA). *Zoonoses Report UK*. London: Defra, 2006.
13. Wong S, Gorczyca K, Forrow L, Angulo F. The healthy pets, healthy people project: A collaborative effort between medical and social communities for persons with AIDS and HIV. International Conference on AIDS, 9–14 July 2000. 13: abstract WePeD4495.

14. World Health Organization. *Overcoming Antimicrobial Resistance – World Health Report on Infectious Diseases*. Geneva: WHO, 2000.
15. Report of the House of Lords Select Committee on Science and Technology. *Resistance to Antibiotics*, 3rd report. London: House of Lords, March 2001.
16. SMAC (Standing Medical Advisory Committee), Department of Health. *The Path of Least Resistance*. London: HMSO, 1998.
17. Advisory Committee on the Microbiological Safety of Food. Report from the Defra Antimicrobial Resistance Co-ordination Group (DARC) on the Government's Actions to address the Recommendations of the ACMSF report on Microbial Antibiotic Resistance in Relation to Food Safety – ACM/730 March 2005.
18. Collignon P, Angulo FJ. Fluoroquinolone-resistant *Escherichia coli*: food for thought. *J Infect Dis* 2006; **194**: 8–10.
19. Powers JH. Antimicrobial drug development – the past, the present, and the future. *Clin Microbiol Infect* 2004; **10**(suppl 4): 23–31.
20. World Health Organization. Animal to human transplantation – future potential, present risk. Press release. Geneva: WHO, 2 May 2005
21. Muir DA, Griffin GE. *Infection Risks in Xenotransplantation*. London: Department of Health, 2001. Available at: http://www.doh.gov.uk/pub/docs/doh/76035_doh_infection_risks.pdf.

Appendix 1

Web resources

Without access to the literature resources available through the internet, it is unlikely that this book would ever have been written. The world-wide web offers the resources of a comprehensive library, with access to a wide range of peer-reviewed scientific papers, at the touch of a keyboard or the click of a mouse.

It is not just technical texts that are available. Many government departments, both at home and abroad, have their own websites, where information on legislation, statistics and breaking news can be found.

The uniform resource locators (URLs) listed below represent a brief selection of those sites that were used in the research for this publication. The addresses offer the opportunity for students to locate additional information or research topics in depth.

Some of the sites listed require visitors to register before they are able to use all of the facilities. At the time of writing none requires any fee for access. An attempt has been made to arrange the sites in a semblance of order; however, the list is not exclusive or necessarily comprehensive, as new sites appear daily. These sites offer a jumping-off point for further investigation.

European

Council of Europe	http://www.coe.int
European Centre for Disease Control and Prevention	http://www.ecdc.europa.eu
European Food Safety Authority (EFSA)	http://www.efsa.europa.eu
Institut Pasteur	http://www.pasteur.fr
MedVetNet	http://www.medvetnet

International

Arabian Horse Association   http://arabianhorses.org
Emedicine   http://www.emedicine.com
Food and Agriculture Organization   http://www.fao.org
(FAO) of the United Nations
International Association for   http://www.paratuberculosis.org
Paratuberculosis
Merck Manual   http://www.merckvetmanual.com
Office International des Epizooties   http://www.oie.int
(OIE)
ProMED reports   http://www.promedmail.org
Eurosurveillance   http://www.eurosurveillance.org
World Arabian Horse Association   http://www.waho.org
World Health Organization (WHO)   http://www.who.int

The UK

Animal Health Distribution   http://www.ahda.org.uk
Association (AHDA)
Animal Medicines Training   http://www.amtra.org.uk
Regulatory Association (AMTRA)
Association of British Pharmaceutical http://www.abpi.org.uk
Industry (ABPI)
British Association for Pure Bred   http://bapsh.co.uk
Spanish Horses
British Broadcasting Corporation   http://news.bbc.co.uk
(BBC) news
British Equine Veterinary   http://www.beva.org.uk
Association (BEVA)
British Horse Society   htttp://bhs.org.uk
British Medical Association (BMA)   http://www.bma.org.uk
British Medical Journal (BMJ)   http://www.bmj.com
British Small Animal Veterinary   http://www.bsava.com
Association (BSAVA)
British Veterinary Association (BVA) http://www.bva.co.uk
British Veterinary Poultry   http://www.bvpa.freeserve.co.uk
Association (BVPA)
Central Scientific Laboratory (CSL)   http://www.csl.gov.uk
Chartered Institute for   http://www.cieh.org.uk
Environmental Health (CIEH)
CJD Surveillance Unit   http://www.cjd.ed.ac.uk

Department of Agriculture and Rural Development (Northern Ireland) (DARDNI)	http://www.dardni.gov.uk
Department for Environment, Food and Rural Affairs (DEFRA – formerly MAFF)	http://defra.gov.uk
Department of Health (DH)	http://www.doh.gov.uk
Department of Health, Social Services and Public Safety (Northern Ireland)	http://www.dhsspsni.gov.uk
Department for Transport (DfT)	http://www.dft.gov.uk
Department of Trade and Industry (DTI)	http://www.dti.gov.uk
Farmers' Weekly	http://www.fwi.co.uk
Food and Drink Federation	http://www.fdf.org.uk
Food Standards Agency (FSA)	http://www.food.gov.uk
Foreign and Commonwealth Office (FCO)	http://www.fco.gov.uk
Health Protection Agency (HPA)	http://www.hpa.org.uk
Health Protection Agency Communicable Disease Surveillance Centre (Northern Ireland)	http://www.cdscni.org.uk
Health Protection Scotland (HPS)	http://www.hps.scot.nhs.uk
Health and Safety Executive (HSE)	http://www.hse.gov.uk
Institute for Animal Health (IAH)	http://www.iah.bbrsc.ac.uk
Institute of Food Science and Technology (IFST)	http://www.ifst.org
The Lancet	http://www.thelancet.com
Meat and Livestock Commission (MLC)	http://www.mlc.org.uk
Medicines and Healthcare products Regulatory Agency (MHRA)	http://www.mhra.gov.uk
Milk Development Council	http://www.mdc.org.uk
National Farmers' Union (NFU)	http://nfuonline.com
National Institute for Health and Clinical Excellence (NICE)	http://www.nice.org.uk
National Office of Animal Health (NOAH)	http://www.noah.co.uk
National Pig Association (NPA)	http://www.npa-uk.net
National Public Health Service for Wales	http://www.nphs.wales.nhs.uk
National Sheep Association (NSA)	http://www.nationalsheep.org.uk

North West Zoonoses Group	http://www.northwest-zoonoses.info
The People's Dispensary for Sick Animals (PDSA)	http://www.pdsa.org.uk
Pet Food Manufacturers' Association (PFMA)	http://www.pfma.org.uk
Pet Health Council (PHC)	http://www.pethealthcouncil.co.uk
Royal College of Physicians	http://www.rcplondon.ac.uk
Royal College of Veterinary Surgeons (RCVS)	http://www.rcvs.org.uk
Royal Pharmaceutical Society of Great Britain (RPSGB)	http://www.rpsgb.org.uk
Royal Society for the Prevention of Cruelty to Animals (RSPCA)	http://www.rspca.org.uk
Scottish Executive Rural Directorate	http://www.scotland.gov.uk
Scottish Environment Protection Agency (SEPA)	http://www.sepa.org.uk
Scottish Farmers' Weekly	http://www.nfus.org.uk
Society for Companion Animal Studies	http://www.scas.org.uk
Society of Practising Veterinary Surgeons (SPVS)	http://www.spvs.org.uk
Veterinary Laboratory Agency (VLA)	http://www.defra.gov.uk/corporate/vla
Veterinary Medicine Directorate (VMD)	http://www.vmd.gov.uk
Veterinary Products Committee	http://www.vpc.gov.uk
Welsh Assembly Government	http://www.wales.gov.uk

The USA

American Veterinary Medical Association (AVMA)	http://avma.org
American Association of Wildlife Veterinarians	http://www.aawv.net
American Horse Council Foundation (AHCF)	http://www.horsecouncil.org
American Quarter Horse Association	http://www.aqha.com
Animal and Plant Health Inspection Service	http:/www.aphis.usda.gov
Centers for Disease Control and Prevention (CDC); includes National Institute for Occupational Safety and	http://www.cdc.gov

Health (NIOSH), *Emerging Infectious Diseases* (EID) and *Morbidity and Mortality Weekly Report* (MMWR)

Center for Food Safety and Applied Nutrition (CFSAN)	http://vm.cfsan.fda.gov
Department of Agriculture (USDA)	http://www.usda.gov
Department of Health and Human Services	http://www.hhs.gov
Food and Drugs Administration (FDA)	http://www.fda.gov
Food Safety and Inspection Service (FSIS) – part of USDA	http://www.fsis.usda.gov
Medscape	http://www.medscape.com
Nature	http://www.nature.com
New England Journal of Medicine	http://www.nejm.com
Pan American Health Organisation	http://www.paho.org
Pets as Therapy (PAT)	http://www.petastherapy.org
Pets are Wonderful Support (PAWS)	http://www.pawssf.org
Pubmed (National Library of Medicine and National Institutes of Health)	http://www.pubmed.gov
Science	http://www.sciencemag.org
Scientific American	http://www.sciam.com
Therapet	http://www.therapet.com
Wildlife Disease Association	http://www.wildlifedisease.org

Canada

Canadian Association of Zoo and Wildlife Veterinarians Health Canada	http://www.cazwv.org

Appendix 2
Useful addresses

BCM Specials Manufacturing
D10 First 114, Nottingham NG20 2PR, UK
Tel: +44 (0)800 952 1010

Bio Products Laboratory (BPL)
Dagger Lane, Elstree, Herts WD6 3BX, UK
Tel: +44 (0)20 8905 1818

Centers for Disease Control and Prevention
1600 Clifton Road, Atlanta, Georgia 30333, USA
Tel: +1 (0)888 232 6348
Website: http://www.cdc.gov

The Hospital for Tropical Diseases
Mortimer Market, London WC1E 6AU, UK
Tel: +44 (0)845 155 5000 or +44 (0)207 7387 4411
Website: http://www.thehtd.org

IDIS Ltd
IDIS House, Churchfield Road, Weybridge, Surrey KT13 8DB, UK
Tel: +44 (0)1932 824 100
Website: http://www.idispharma.com
US contact tel: +1 (0)651 503 7327

Scottish National Blood Transfusion Service (SNBTS)
Protein Fractionation Centre, Ellen's Glen Road, Edinburgh EH17 7QT, UK
Tel: +44 (0)131 536 5700

Tommy's, the baby charity
Nicholas House, 3 Laurence Pountney Hill, London EC4R 0BB, UK
Tel: +44 (0)870 777 30 60
Email: info@tommys.org

Creutzfeldt–Jakob disease and variant Creutzfeldt–Jakob disease

The National CJD Surveillance Unit
Western General Hospital, Crewe Road, Edinburgh EH4 2XU, UK
Tel: +44 (0)131 537 3073
Fax: +44 (0)131 343 1404

CJD Resource Centre
National Institute for Biological Standards and Control, Blanche Lane, South Mimms, Potters Bar, Hertfordshire EN6 3QG, UK
Tel: +44 (0)1707 641 000
Fax: +44 (0)1707 641 050

CJD Support Network
PO Box 346, Market, Drayton, Salop TF9 4WN, UK
Tel: +44 (0)1630 673993
Helpline: +44 (0)1630 673973

National Prion Disease Pathology Surveillance Center (NPDPSC)
Institute of Pathology, Case Western Reserve University, 2085 Adelbert Road, Room 418, Cleveland, Ohio 44106, USA
Tel: +1 (0)216 368 0587

Index